Where Children Live: Solutions for Serving Young Children and Their Families

Advances in Applied Developmental Psychology
Irving E. Sigel, Series Editor

Vol. 1 Advances in Applied Developmental Psychology
edited by Irving E. Sigel, 1985

Vol. 2 Continuity and Discontinuity of Experience in Child Care
edited by Donald Peters and Susan Kontos, 1987

Vol. 3 Parent Education as Early Childhood Intervention: Emerging Directions in Theory, Research and Practice
edited by Douglas R. Powell, 1988

Vol. 4 Ethics in Applied Developmental Psychology: Emerging Issues in an Emerging Field
edited by Celia B. Fisher and Warren W. Tryon, 1990

Vol. 5 Parent–Child Socialization in Diverse Cultures
edited by Jaipaul L. Roopnarine and D. Bruce Carter, 1992

Vol. 6 The Psychological Development of Low Birthweight Children
edited by Sarah L. Friedman and Marian D. Sigman, 1992

Vol. 7 Coming Home to Preschool: The Sociocultural Context of Early Education
edited by Richard N. Roberts, 1993

Vol. 8 Child Abuse, Child Development, and Social Policy
edited by Dante Cicchetti and Sheree L. Toth, 1993

Vol. 9 Two-Generation Programs for Families in Poverty: A New Intervention Strategy
edited by Sheila Smith, 1995

Vol. 10 Sibling Relationships: Their Causes and Consequences
edited by Gene H. Brody, 1996

Vol. 11 Interacting with Video
edited by Patricia Greenfield and Rodney R. Cocking, 1996

Vol 12 Mastery Motivation: Origins, Conceptualizations, and Applications
edited by Robert H. MacTurk and George A. Morgan, 1995

Vol. 13 Applied Developmental Science: Graduate Training for Diverse Disciplines and Educational Settings
edited by Celia B. Fisher, John P. Murray, and Irving E. Sigel, 1996

Vol. 14 Caribbean Families: Diversity Among Ethnic Groups
edited by Jaipaul R. Roopnarine and Janet Brown, 1997

Vol. 15 Verbal Interaction and Development in Families with Adolescents
edited by Manfred Hofer, James Youniss, and Peter Noack, 1998

Vol. 16 Children of the Dispossessed: Far-West Preschoolers 30 Years On, Second Edition
by Barry Nurcombe, Philip DeLacey, and Susan-Lee Walker, 1999

Vol. 17 Where Children Live: Solutions for Serving Young Children and Their Families
edited by Richard N. Roberts and Phyllis R. Magrab, 1999

Vol. 18 Partnerships in Research, Clinical, and Educational Settings
edited by Roger Bibace, James J. Dillon, and Barbara Noel Dowds, forthcoming

Where Children Live: Solutions for Serving Young Children and Their Families

edited by

Richard N. Roberts
Early Intervention Research Institute

and

Phyllis R. Magrab
Georgetown University Child Development Center

Ablex Publishing Corporation
Stamford, Connecticut

Printed in the United States of America

Library of Congress Cataloging-in-Publication Data

Where children live : solutions for serving young children and their families/edited by Richard N. Roberts and Phyllis R. Magrab
p. cm. — (Advances in applied developmental psychology ; v. 17)
Includes bibliographical material and index.
ISBN 1-56750-440-X (cloth) — ISBN 1-5670-441-8 (paper)
1. Handicapped children—Services for—United States.
2. Parents of handicapped children—Services for—United States.
I. Roberts, Richard N. II. Magrab, Phyllis R. III. Series: Advances in applied developmental psychology ; v. 17
HV888.5.W44 1999
362.4′083—dc21 98-5578
CIP

Ablex Publishing Corporation
100 Prospect Street
Stamford, CT 06901-1640

Contents

List of Contributors

Adrienne L. Akers, Early Intervention Research Institute, 6580 Old Main Hill, Utah State University, Logan, UT 84322-6580

Susan D. Mackey Andrews, Solutions Disability Program, Policy, Financing and Technology Consulting Services, 21 Grove St., Dover-Foxcroft, ME 04426-1254

Diane D. Behl, Early Intervention Research Institute, 6580 Old Main Hill, Utah State University, Logan, UT 84322-6580

Glenna C. Boyce, Early Intervention Research Institute, 6580 Old Main Hill, Utah State University, Logan, UT 84322-6580

Suzanne M. Bronheim, Georgetown University Child Development Center, 3307 M St., NW, Suite 401, Washington, DC 20007

Sharon Carnahan, Rollins College, 1000 Holt Avenue, Winter Park, FL 32789-4499

Gary J. De Carolis, Department of Health and Human Services, Center for Mental Health Policy, Child Adolescent and Family Branch, 5600 Fishers Lane, RM 18-49, Rockville, MD 20857

Peter Evans, Organization for Economic Cooperation and Development, Centre for Educational Research and Innovation, 2 rue du Conseiller Colignon, 75016 Paris CEDEX, France

Linda D. Goetze, Early Intervention Research Institute, 6580 Old Main Hill, Utah State University, Logan, UT 84322-6580

Thomas R. Gordon, University of South Florida BEH339, 4200 E. Fowler Ave., Tampa, FL 33620-9200

Maureen Greer, Indiana Family and Social Services Administration, Division of Family and Children Bureau of Child Development, 402 W. Washington St. W 386, Indianapolis, IN 46204-2739

Mark S. Innocenti, Early Intervention Research Institute, 6580 Old Main Hill, Utah State University, Logan, UT 84322-6580

Therese R. Johnson, Office of the Director, Department of Human Services, 120 North 200 West, Salt Lake City, UT 84103

Carnot E. Nelson, University of South Florida BEH339, 4200 E. Fowler Ave., Tampa, FL 33620-9200

Phyllis R. Magrab, Georgetown University Child Development Center, 3307 M Street, NW - Suite 401, Washington, DC 20007-3935

Richard N. Roberts, Early Intervention Research Institute, 6580 Old Main Hill, Utah State University, Logan, UT 84322-6580

Roxane Kaufman, Georgetown University Child Development Center, 3307 M Street, NM, Suite 401, Washington, DC 20007-3935

Nancy Strifler, Georgetown University Child Development Center, 3307 M St., NW, Suite 401, Washington, DC 20007

Amy Locke Wischmann, Georgetown University Child Development Center, 3307 M Street, NM, Suite 401, Washington, DC 20007-3935

Foreword

Irving E. Sigel

The volume of essays brought together by R. N. Roberts and P. R. Magrab is an important collection of papers relevant at the turn of the 20th century. The message of this volume is that effective delivery of child and family services, a comprehensive theoretical model, is needed so that efficient delivery can take place, as well as an evaluation of the quality of those services. This becomes particularly important these days because of the changing nature of communities, not only in the United States, but globally. Since humans first lived in organized communities, there has been service to the sick, the needy, the abused, and the aged. Over the millennium, these services have been provided by religious and secular agencies. The advent of the Industrial Age and the concomitant urbanization in many western European countries resulted in community services brought under the auspices of government agencies. This shift in responsibility for the welfare of the citizenry, from voluntary charitable organizations to government agencies, was more characteristic of European countries such as Germany, France, and the Scandinavian countries. In the United States, voluntary philanthropies have provided the major support for community service to children and families. Many of these charitable foundations are still functioning, for example, the YMCA. However, in the middle of the 20th century, when the catastrophic Great Depression hit the United States, a major shift in the role of government took place, led by President Franklin D. Roosevelt's New Deal. The federal government initiated various community services, such as childcare services, employment opportunities for unemployed family members, and health services for children and mothers. These community efforts were continued during World War II. Childcare was still needed because women were entering the industrial workforce. The post-war period was one of considerable social change with the changing geographical demography. Population shifts with the growth of suburbs and exurbs led to changes in community organization. The population shift from the cities to the suburbs resulted in different compositions of communities. The populations that remained in the cities were often marginal and consisted of members of minority groups. As a result of changes in the international political scene and worldwide conflicts, further population shifts occurred with the arrival of poor immigrants from Asia, South and Central America, Eastern Europe, and Africa. Most of these newly arriving members of society gravitated toward the cities and required help in getting settled and becoming economically self-sufficient.

During the 1950s and 1960s, various forms of community organizations developed. One of the big changes was the development of overarching community organizations such as the United Way. These organizations brought together diverse private agencies working in collaborative and cooperative ways to collect funds and distribute them equitably on the basis of combined need. Such organizations not only provided help as needed, but also had the secondary effect of winnowing out fraud and inefficiency among the services. This collection of private nonprofit community service organizations works in conjunction with various local, state, and federal agencies. Ideally, such cooperation could blanket the community with what is needed. Coverage for the various community needs, such as foster care, preschool education, family health services, and the like, is not always met. The complexities that arise may be a function of cultural differences between recent immigrant groups, where the difficulties that these families face in getting settled may be due to differences in cultural values. Attitudes toward child rearing and family relations may not necessarily fit into the categories or values that agencies define (for example, differences among some immigrant groups in family values compared to mainstream U.S. families). Attitudes toward poverty and level of employment may also differ. Such cultural differences complicate service delivery, since most agencies deliver service in the conventional American style.

It is the case that such issues have been prevalent since the beginning of the 20th century, when large groups of immigrants entered the United States from Europe. In those early days the model of community service was conceptualized differently than in the latter half of the 20th century. In those early days, the "melting pot" thesis prevailed in contrast to the cultural pluralism that is prevalent today. The change may be due to the legacy of the New Deal, which ushered in new programs of service heretofore unknown in the United States (for example, social security and unemployment insurance). It may well be that the attitude toward government or public support for helping various constituents in the community, instead of relying primarily on voluntary private agencies, has been increasingly accepted, so that government interventions addressing a number of social problems facing the communities are acceptable.

In this volume, the authors show the increase in social legislation that is directed toward community service for children and families. The changing composition of communities and the awareness that the needs of children and families are of different orders of complexity has forced the public sector to shift its perspective from families being self-sufficient and denying their cultural heritage to working with their cultural values with the help of community agencies—essentially a more accepting attitude toward diversity.

Another legacy that still exists is the proliferation of narrowly focused special interest volunteer agencies. For example, there are organizations that limit their services to children with cerebral palsy, cystic fibrosis, and diabetes. Aside from these medical issues, there are services for children who need foster care, some of whom need adoption, while others need a combination of these services.

Financial support for each of these groups comes from different types of sources: volunteer, public funds, and different levels of government—federal, state, and local agencies. Not only are there overlapping jurisdictions and funding programs, but often their functions are not well defined, so there may be redundancy, and, consequently, a waste of time, energy, and funds, as well as human tragedies, where the child or family does not fit any single category. In addition to these sources of conflict, there are value issues among the various community leaders in just what is the legitimate role of government or service. These are issues that are addressed in the theoretical sections of this volume.

Such reports have been particularly evident in larger urban centers where the caseloads are high, the personnel are not well trained, and the bureaucracy is great. It is usually in these large urban areas that new immigrants collect, because of kindred spirits and the availability of economic opportunities.

It is from this set of circumstances that Roberts and Magrab have fashioned a volume that defines and conceptualizes the organizational issues facing communities in their efforts to organize the diverse elements in a community to provide effective services. The authors' construction of a theoretical framework by which to analyze existing community services and develop a coherent functional and practical approach for the community is equally important. To support their argument and methodology, they present some case histories of communities that have become effective service providers.

What is unique about this volume is the way in which the authors have integrated the service questions at each government level. Hence, services funded by the federal government are discussed within that context, and similarly for states and local communities. What is a particular treat in this compilation of chapters is the attention paid to the community-based services on a global level. For any of these programs to work, there has to be an interdisciplinary approach that appears like a new discipline for the study of community service organizations.

The chapters are organized with a seamless integration of social and economic fields. A number of chapters complete the volume by describing exemplar programs that provide services for child abuse, mental health, or what is termed "high-risk families." In effect, they demonstrate how their approach can work—a welcome success story in these days of many community service program failures.

In sum, the development of the major thesis in this volume is that given a theoretical model, it becomes possible to devise strategies for developing programs and criteria for evaluating them, and, in the long run, helping them to become effective. Thus, *Where Children Live* is an apt title, generating an approach for creating model community service programs to provide the necessities for various needy constituents. By advocating a national coalition of service programs, as well as an international perspective, Roberts and Magrab and their co-authors have brought together a comprehensive systematic approach to communities serving their citizens in need.

Where Children Live is a natural extension of the Advances in Applied Developmental Psychology series because it extends our coverage and concerns for children and families in their natural habitats.

section I

Introduction to the Concept of Community

This volume provides a context for, and examples of, an emerging paradigm shift in the field of human services toward one in which the services and supports for families with young children are provided where and how they can be most helpful—that is, where children live. This first section begins by defining *community* and by providing a set of principles that will be reflected in the examples that follow in subsequent chapters. The concept of community as the place where children live will be described as both a psychological and physical place. The activity settings that make up the daily routines of children and families are the reflection of both of these aspects of community. A common theme emerges in these first chapters, which explicates the need to provide formal and informal supports to families within these everyday activity settings, rather than outside of the context of the family's life. Community support efforts both incorporate and transcend traditional views of primary, secondary, and tertiary prevention through models of service and support, which are: 1) universal as opposed to targeted; 2) built on individual family strengths, rather than on needs or deficits; 3) routinely involve both formal and informal systems of support; and 4) do so in partnership with those who live within and make up the community.

chapter 1

The Meaning of Community

Phyllis R. Magrab
Georgetown University Child Development Center

INTRODUCTION

In an increasingly technological and mobile world, maintaining social networks and supports to respond to the needs of families and children and to combat families' ever-growing sense of isolation is a paramount challenge for our society today. As we expand to global markets and international frontiers for organizing our economies, we cannot lose sight of the day-to-day demands on families and children. Over the decades, the shared interests of people living close to one another has formed the basis for a major tier of support and resources. Much debate has occurred in recent years over the erosion of such supports, commonly thought of as community.

This book focuses on families of young children and how community networks, both formal and informal, strengthen their roles as caretakers, nurturers, and teachers. Communities that respect the values, self-determination, and priorities of families and translate their needs and desires into appropriate resources, supports, and services are effective communities. Often, families can chose where they live in concert with their values, work, and need for services. In some instances, for a variety of reasons, families are unable to exercise choice and must adapt to their environs. Ideally communities should meet the needs of all their inhabitants; yet, in an age of scarce and unequally distributed resources, this can be difficult to achieve. It is the intent of this book to consider the broad range of life circumstance of families of young children and how all communities can provide effective supports.

You may ask, why focus on communities? The answers are several. First of all, it has been said that "Control of nuclear arms will be in the marketplace," a metaphor for the power of the community. At the level of community, issues can be addressed by *all* and creative solutions can emerge that embrace the views and needs of *all*. Through respectful and trusting relationships that emerge in communities from members having to create shared solutions for multiple types of problems and issues, even the most complex problems can be addressed.

Second, this is a time in history in the United States where great value is being placed on the devolution of government. Increasingly more responsibility is being given to localities to be responsive to families and to develop and support needed services. Accompanying this phenomenon are major reforms in the health, education, and welfare systems. As these reforms occur, significant attention has been given to two extremes: program development and broad policy. How these come together in the immediate environment where families actually live is a critical matter. Communities become the entity that can ensure that solutions are family-driven and linked to natural networks of support as well as to more formal services (Farrow, 1996).

Third, as infrastructures are put in place for families who have young children with special needs, service systems must be established that allow families to receive services close to home in a coordinated way. Families who have children that require complex services must be recognized as an integral part of their community. A universal value of "communities for all" should prevail; communities should be encouraged to sustain support for all of their members. An inclusive society implies inclusive communities where families and children of all diversity can benefit from the networks and resources within.

Last, communities are a very significant force for change. Within communities rests a capacity important for organizing movements to improve the conditions that affect families and children. The future of our society lies within the strength and talents of our children. Alongside families, communities and the resources they represent are the harbingers of our future.

If one examines the contemporary directions of political intellectual thought in America, community plays a major role, regardless of political orientation (Fowler, 1991). The altruistic, affective view of the 1960s, community as participatory democracy—the place where we find our origins and roots—implies the community's psychological strength of freedom and empowerment. In the republican view of the 1980s and 1990s, citizenship, politics, and rational interactions are the basis for vigorous communities. Would that there be a convergence of the two extremes of political perspectives on community. Nonetheless, the eclipse of the community has been a concern across the continuum of political thought. The reemphasis on its value has been tied to survival—survival of the globe, humanity, nature, and even the earth itself.

DEFINING COMMUNITY

Community is an elusive concept. It means different things to different people and is defined differently in the literature for different purposes. In part, it is the significance of the concept that dictates the plethora of definitions; in social sciences there appears to be an inverse relationship between the importance of a concept and the precision with which it is defined (Lyon, 1987). In this instance, the concept of community is important to a large number of social scientists representing diverse approaches and areas of interest.

Generally speaking, the term community implies something both geographic and psychological (Warren, 1978). Community can be thought of as a framework for living rather than as a political jurisdiction—a complex network of people, institutions, shared interests, locality, and a sense of psychological belonging (Warren, 1978). Political boundaries of a village or a city do not necessarily coincide with the shared life, shared institutions, and behavior that constitute local community (Warren, 1978). In America, it has long been recognized that communities do not consist of discrete and separate entities but that communities exist within communities. People's lives are intertwined with the institutions that serve them locally; this becomes an essential element for families of young children. A sense of solidarity and significance is also a core concept in the definition of community. The assumption of a geographic basis for defining community, thus, can be challenged and the term can apply to persons united as a community of interests. For the purposes of this book, the importance of geography will prevail because of the intent to consider the notion of community as it ultimately relates to local supports and services to families of young children.

Historic Overview of the Definition of Community

In the western world, the concept of community, as we know it today, is primarily linked to two major revolutions: the French Revolution and the Industrial Revolution. In medieval Europe, a rural agrarian economy prevailed. As a result, the family and church dominated most individuals. Apart from those who lived as royalty or within the castle confines, the population worked in the fields and produced for themselves, with family members working side by side. The two revolutions resulted in great change. In France, the revolt against royalty and feudalism diminished the role of the church and a thrust towards individualism began to emerge. With the Industrial Revolution, employment shifted to the cities, families became divided, and money and labor became the primary means of exchange. By the mid-19th century urban large-scale societies became the norm.

It is within this context that theories of social change and the community developed. In 1887, Ferdinand Tonnies in the book *Gemeinschaft und Gessellschaft* (now published as *Community and Society*, Loomis, 1963) characterized community types as a mechanism for studying social change. He contrasted two basic types of groups: *gemeinschaft*—where the relationship of sympathy among members is a primary feature and the group has value in and of itself such as kinship and neighborhood groups and *gessellschaft*—where the focus is on the group's purpose or task, a more rational, goal-oriented, formalized group such as the city or state. Tonnies's conception of social groups has had a lasting influence on the study of community through characterizing the rational versus irrational actions, the functional specificity and diffuseness, and the integration of roles within and without the systems of the community.

The earliest attention to defining and studying communities in the United States began at the University of Chicago in the early 1930s. Parks (1936) established community as a central concept in the study of social change and identified three core characteristics: (a) a population territorially organized, (b) a population more or less completely rooted in the soil it occupies, and (c) a population whose individual units live in a relationship of mutual interdependence. Almost 20 years later, Hillery (1955) conducted the most comprehensive analysis of the concept. Analyzing 94 various definitions of sociologists and anthropologists, he concluded community can be defined as the social interaction of people living in a given geographic area who have common ties. The most common characteristics he identified included a feeling of self-sufficiency; a common life; a consciousness of homogeneity; a possession of shared ends, norms, or means; a collection of institutions; an emphasis on features of localism; and a feeling of group uniqueness. Updating Hillery's work, Sutton and Munson (1976) examined community definitions published between 1954 and 1973 and found that 70 percent emphasized structural entities such as specific population, place, or location and 12 percent included social interaction as part of the definition.

Theories of Community

Stonewall (1983) argues the importance of going beyond merely defining "community" to evolving specific theories of communities. Theories, she points out, make sense of definitions. Addressing, in this case, the essential elements of people, time, and space, she identifies five theoretical frameworks to study community: human ecology, structural functionalism, conflict theory, social-psychological approaches, and network exchange analysis. For each theory she delineates its main features and limitations.

1. *Human ecology* compares human communities to plant and animal communities using Darwinian thinking to characterize how groups survive with limited resources. The emphasis is on the process of cooperation and competition.
2. *Structural functionalism* emphasizes the community as a system of institutions held together by shared values. The anthropologic study of culture—norms, values, morals, and folkways that govern collective life—underpin this theoretical perspective.
3. *Conflict theory* relies on studying what divides communities, how class segments are pitted against each other, conflicting over property, status, and power. Communities become battle grounds of antagonistic forces.
4. *Social psychological* approaches and *network exchange analysis* are more recent theories and are still evolving. Social psychological approaches examine social life within community—the processes of communication, negotiation, and consensus building.
5. *Network exchange* analysis portrays the community as a complex pattern of ties among people through which resources, feelings, and demands are exchanged. Exchange works through established patterns of reciprocity or distributive justice.

These theoretical frameworks are useful for understanding communities. Each provides a unique lens with its own strengths and weaknesses. Each offers different aspects of dimensions such as people, history, process, and boundaries.

A Functional Model of Community

When people live together in groups in close proximity, there is a significant affect on their daily activities. Warren (1978) asserts that by community, one means the organization of social activities to provide people with local access to those broad areas of activity that are necessary to day-to-day living. Community is defined through the functions it performs. While this is a narrowing definition of community, it provides a very useful model to examine the supports and services families of young children need and receive.

Warren organizes these activities around five major functions that have local relevance, although they may not necessarily be exclusively the responsibility of the community: production-distribution-consumption, socialization, social control, social participation, and mutual support.

1. *Production-distribution-consumption* implies that the community participates in this process for goods and services in a manner that is desirable for its inhabitants. In our broadening economies, often all these elements are not contained within the community boundaries.
2. *Socialization* is the process through which knowledge, social values, and behavioral patterns are transmitted to individual members of the society. This is principally the responsibility of families and schools.
3. *Social control* is how a community encourages the behavior of its members to conform to its norms. Multiple entities contribute to this function, such as government, police, courts, schools, churches, and social agencies.
4. *Social participation* represents the way in which all community members are included in the social life of the community and how the community provides access to work settings, religious groups, and other social organizations.
5. *Mutual support* is the connection and interdependence of community inhabitants. In times of need, the exchange of labor or helping families in distress is typically the role of the family, neighborhood groups, friendship groups, and local agencies.

To understand community differences with respect to these functions, the structure of the community can be addressed on four dimensions: local autonomy, the coincidence of service areas of local units, the psychological identification with the locality, and the horizontal pattern of relationships of various local units.

1. *Autonomy* is the extent to which the community is independent of or dependent upon extracommunity resources and services to perform its major functions.
2. *Coincidence* is the extent to which the responsibility of local units such as schools, health systems, and churches coincide. At times communities lack a geographic center with major units having very different boundaries.

3. *The psychological identification with a common locality* represents the importance of the community as a reference for its inhabitants and is characterized by the sense of relationship felt among the inhabitants.
4. *Horizontal pattern* is the structural and functional relationship among local units and the extent of their interconnection and interdependence. These patterns represent the opportunity for collaboration and change of systems within a community.

Application of Definition and Theory

One of the most frequently asked questions when one embarks on either the study of a community or the development of community programs is "What is the community?" While the discussion thus far suggests that community is not necessarily a formally defined geographic area, some group must determine the boundaries of the geographic area in question, keeping in mind some of the defining characteristics discussed thus far. Where does the community begin and where does it end? What are the boundary edges that separate it from other geographic areas and why have those boundaries been chosen? A city block, a county, an informally defined geographic area—all could demonstrate the key characteristics of a community. Often it is difficult to determine where the boundaries are. For example, boundaries can be drawn that seem to be natural ones but leave the surrounding rural areas unlinked, or the designated community can be imbedded in a larger community with unclear relationships.

Geographic communities are an open system. As the boundary or edges separate a community from the rest of the world, the community survives through its own internal activities and through exchanges with the environment across the boundary. It is always difficult to establish where the real boundary is and even the residents may disagree. The following check list (see Figure 1.1) summarizes some of the major characteristics of the concept of community and can be useful in analyzing whether a designated area demonstrates a significant number of these characteristics such as people, space, shared institutions and values, interaction, distribution of power, and social system.

Once having identified a geographic area as the community, in order to address issues and actions, a community can profile itself along dimensions related to history, composition, attitudes, economic life styles, networks, population, needs, resources, and connections outside the boundaries to develop a common sense of who the community is. Effective communities typically have a good understanding of their assets and resources. The Community Profile in Appendix A represents

- ❑ Geographic boundaries
- ❑ Complex network of people
- ❑ Emphasis on features of localism
- ❑ Common life
- ❑ Shared goals and interests
- ❑ Feeling of group uniqueness
- ❑ System of institutions held together with shared values
- ❑ Social structure
- ❑ Feeling of self-sufficiency
- ❑ Mutual support among inhabitants
- ❑ Sense of psychological belonging
- ❑ Sense of solidarity

FIGURE 1.1. Determining the Community Checklist.

a useful outline for such an endeavor, particularly related to supporting families of young children.

EFFECTIVE COMMUNITIES

Once a geographic context is agreed upon, understanding how communities can be effective in serving and supporting families of young children is of particular importance. There are some common characteristics that either promote or mitigate against the effectiveness of a community to support the needs and desires of its inhabitants. These include:

1. vision,
2. history,
3. organizational design,
4. leadership,
5. decision-making processes, and
6. capacity-building strategies.

Vision

The importance of a shared vision to drive the purposes and functions of a community is paramount. Sharing a view of the future represents the most important context for community effectiveness. Vision encompasses the values, promise, and hope that energizes and amalgamates persons of diverse views and backgrounds to a common end. Developing a vision is an opportunity to have all voices in a community included and all creativity engaged. Families of young children need to be assured that their hopes and dreams are part of the community's vision. Caring communities will create opportunities to involve these families as they look towards their future and plan for the present. Without a vision, there is no unifying ideal for the community to strive towards.

History

Community is a place of change, not a fixed structure. That change over time creates a history that has considerable meaning for understanding both the present and the future effectiveness of any community. There is the history of a community's vision and purpose, of its successes and failures, and of its growth and decline.

The literature suggests that geographic communities have a describable life cycle. Identifying the stage of development of a given community in that cycle provides insight into its capacities and its future. The following five differentiated stages have been delineated:

1. The *early phase* of development typically involves immigration into an area to form a small town or village.
2. The *developing phase* represents a time of growth production and immigration structuring.

3. The *mature phase* implies a readjustment of the community with peripheral growth such as suburbs.
4. The *declining center phase* is usually characterized by inner city decay and satellite growth.
5. The *assimilation phase* involves reconstruction with new resource distribution and functional allocation.

The ability of a community to respond to these phases of growth and decline forms an important historical perspective. How has a given community evolved over the past 10-20 years and how is it likely to evolve? For example, growth pressures often result in expanded social services, the need for rapid transportation, escalating budget costs, and suburban sprawl. The decline of local areas often involves the migration of business out of the community reducing the tax base and marking the need for redevelopment of affected areas. Growing conflict historically emerges among social groups as there is competition for scarce revenue for special-interests.

There is a history of relationships in the community as well that impinges on the community's effectiveness in meeting the needs of its inhabitants. That history is often critical to understand in order to evolve creative plans for the future. In considering the recent history of a specific community, knowing to what extent there have been continuity and stability of participation and leadership as well as sustainable resources is useful to a planning process. The historic relationships between and among agencies, organizations, businesses, and citizen groups can play a facilitating role or become barriers to effective problem solving in the community. Effective communities understand where they are in a cycle of change, recognize the historic relationships that have existed in the community, and use this sense of their past to inform and guide the planning for their future.

Organizational Design of the Community

Reminding ourselves that communities identify themselves in ways that are not necessarily consistent with formal governmental structures, the effectiveness of a self-defined community is contingent upon the infrastructure it establishes. The relationship of the infrastructure to formal local governance, of course, is one of the defining features. Local governance is a formal mechanism for linking communication, information sharing, planning, and implementation. With respect to young children and their families, local governance has a significant role in finding ways of delivering services that are effective in meeting family needs.

The differences in formal organizational structure among communities whose boundaries may be a city block, a neighborhood, a town, a county, or a cluster of rural inhabitants is striking; yet, the features of their organizational design that make them effective typically have considerable similarity. Those features can be placed on a continuum with two extremes:

1. *Participation*: inclusive membership open to all individuals and groups *or* exclusive membership marginalizing some citizens;
2. *Communication*: open, respectful, and supportive *or* hierarchical and closed;
3. *Information sharing*: well-established, broad based lines *or* poor flow with few established mechanisms;
4. *Utilization of resources*: creative and nurtured with attention to skills and strengths of the community *or* untapped strength and skills of community members;
5. *Resolving conflict*: interest-based negotiation strategies with opportunities for facilitation and mediation of differences *or* nonexistent mechanisms with little attention on how to resolve conflict among individuals and competing factions;
6. *Vitality and motivation*: dynamic energy in the community *or* static and apathetic atmosphere;
7. *Commitment to the community*: a cohesive sense of the importance of the community as composed of individuals and groups with differing needs and wishes *or* an unwillingness of individuals and groups to assume responsibility; and
8. *External relationships*: fluid linkages to outside groups *or* few connections outside the community.

The collaborative strategies that frame the organizational design for a community usually represent the key source of success in accomplishing the community's agenda. Either through a governing entity or through developed mechanisms, there must be a way for a wide range of local agencies, organizations, businesses, and citizens to come together to develop and implement creative, collaborative, and cost effective solutions to community problems such as those of families with young children. To achieve a successful organizational design in a local community that addresses the needs of families of young children as well as other community problems, the community must have collaborative strategies for the following:

1. involving a broad range of participants;
2. agenda setting around community problems including defining problems, establishing goals, setting priorities, and planning for action;

3. developing new service capacities and making better use of overlapping resources;
4. coordinating fiscal strategies—including maximizing federal entitlements and better use of existing dollars; and
5. maintaining accountability for outcomes, both child/family outcomes and process outcomes (Building a Community Agenda, 1991).

Currently there are innovative organizational concepts that embody the collaborative features of effective organizational design and have shown promising trends such as neighborhood networks. Neighborhood networks are deliberate, ongoing, and structured arrangements among public and private sector organizations and informal and formal supports for the explicit purpose of responding more immediately and flexibly to family needs and to promote the well-being of children (Farrow, 1996). They focus on neighborhood inhabitants' strong commitment to "place." Accountability and governance structures are redefined based on geography and have considerable neighborhood ownership. They involve the community's own organizations and incorporate natural helping networks.

Neighborhood networks are effective because the services are brought close to home, are more accessible and welcoming, and are more likely to be used. Usually they imply new flexible funding arrangements, professional development, and organization for the network. Typically the public sector operates in more creative and productive ways. Neighborhood networks involve a new set of interactions among workers referred to as "radical teaming." These interactions go beyond joining staffs; workers see themselves as team members doing whatever it takes. Recent economic programs like the Enterprise and Empowerment Zones, designated urban or rural areas that provide economic incentives to the community for creative community arrangements and employment opportunities, promote this capacity. Neighborhood networks do not all look alike; their structures are different but they all have the characteristics noted above. These networks serve as a bridge between public sector involvement and neighborhood advocacy.

The importance of building effective partnerships to achieve collaboration has been underscored in the last decade (Melaville, Blank, & Asayesh, 1993). Building partnerships between different service delivery systems, different levels of government, formal agencies and informal organizations, professionals and parents, and community residents and outsiders is key to effective organizational design in communities. The term "collaboratives" has emerged to define these partnerships. In the chapters that follow, a more in-depth look at the role of organizational design and systems' building for families of young children will be presented to include systems of services, fiscal strategies, evaluation of outcomes, and specific community examples.

Leadership

Building a community agenda and acting on that agenda is a highly political process that requires skilled leadership to shepherd its success. Such skilled leadership has a marked affect on the accomplishments of a community. Leaders are important to establishing direction and a vision of the future; to aligning people with the agenda and communicating the goals; to motivating, inspiring commitment, and energizing the group to overcome barriers; and to affecting and producing change. Providing vision in the context of reality with ethics and courage, the leadership diamond model of Koestenbaum (1991) is a useful framework for thinking about community leaders.

Leaders have been viewed through history in differing roles. When one thinks of a leader, often, the first qualities that come to mind relate to the leader's personality and character. In 1947, Weber (1947) coined the concept of a charismatic leader, a person who is set apart from ordinary men and women and has exceptional power or qualities not accessible to ordinary people from which is derived a social authority over others. Popular interpretations link this to a leader's personality but a single charismatic personality type has not been borne out in the literature. Such leaders are likely to appear in political and religious movements and certainly play a role in community agendas.

Newer conceptions of leaders and their roles place less importance on such extraordinary personal characteristics and more on the range of roles a leader must assume. The contemporary notion of transformational leadership (Bass, 1991), where leaders broaden and elevate the interests of all the group and look beyond themselves for the good of the group, represents a leadership for change. It is a facilitative conception of leadership that implies community collaboration and collective accountability. Communities are inspired and persuaded to new ways by such leadership.

The connective leadership model of Lipman-Blumen (1996) is very appealing for understanding effective leadership in communities. Recognizing that in this decade there are new challenges for leaders—shorter time frames, fewer second chances, need for innovative solutions, goals that must reach beyond the initial problems, thinking for the long term despite short term pressures—leaders must draw on a broad range of behaviors. Leadership has to emphasize mutuality and common interests as well as inclusiveness through addressing the issues of diversity. Lipman-Blumen asserts that *connective leaders* join their

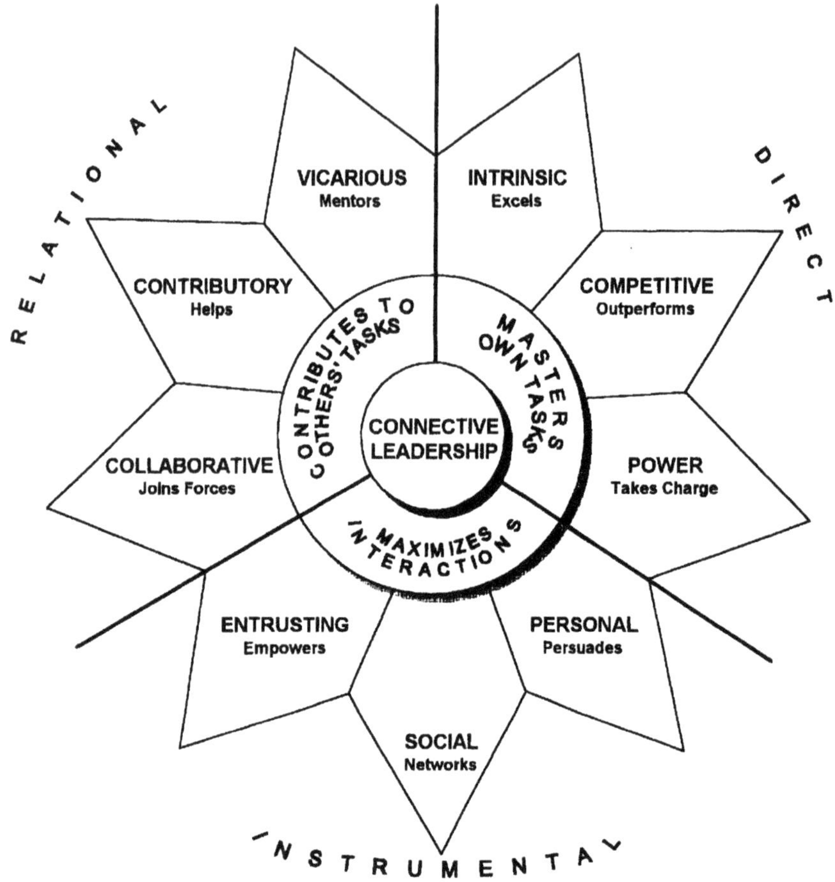

Source: Lipman-Blumen (1996).

FIGURE 1.2. The connective leadership model.

dreams to the dreams of others, strive to overcome common problems, create a sense of community, encourage active constituents, join with other leaders, nurture potential leaders, and demonstrate authenticity through dedication. They prefer the "politics of commonality" and take the widest view of what is needed.

The connective leadership model (see Figure 1.2) consists of three major sets of behavioral styles: direct, relational, and instrumental. The *direct style* is to confront tasks individually using mastery, competition, and power. It typically is an expression of individualism. The *relational style* represents a preference to work in groups to attain a goal. It speaks to interdependence through joining forces, helping, and mentoring. The *instrumental style* implies using oneself and others as instruments toward community goals through networking, empowering, and persuasion.

Leaders have access to all these behaviors. Through their instrumental style they act as brokers and matchmakers. They use relationships in multiple ways to carryout their task, but they can also lead the charge. The connective leadership model gives leaders diverse ways to take action and to identify the leadership strategy they might apply to a given situation. Connective leaders recognize that leadership embraces all varieties of behavior and they combine many strategies to achieve their goals. They use themselves as versatile leadership instruments. Critical to the model is the issue of timing, choosing the appropriate behavior for the specific moment. Importantly, leadership studies demonstrate that leadership is not merely a set of inborn traits; it can be learned.

As the leadership paradigm has shifted from independence to interdependence and from competition to collaboration, it is obvious why leadership models focus less on the individual and more on the group. The issues of shared leadership and leadership teams permeate the recent literature. When one examines the variety of functions a leader performs, it is easy to understand why, in a community, it is effective when the leadership roles are shared. Some of these leadership functions include:

1. shaping vision and purpose;
2. focusing on key priorities;
3. creating a learning environment and incentives;
4. insuring that the tasks necessary to plan and carry out the group's goals are accomplished;
5. guiding the planning process;
6. facilitating productivity and creative interaction of the group;
7. clarifying responsibilities and assignments;
8. sustaining commitment;
9. supporting actions and change as needed; and
10. assuring accountability.

There are a variety of factors that affect the pattern of leadership in community groups. Importantly, leader and member behaviors affect each other. Contributing to the patterns of leadership in the community are factors related to the leader, forces in the community, and the specific issue or situation being addressed. With respect to the leader, his or her values, confidence in the group, own needs, and skills will influence his or her role. Forces in the group that interact include the group's interest and commitment to the problem, readiness to assume responsibility, skills and expectations of members, and roles of members in formulating goals and plans. The external situation such as the pressures of time, the organizational barriers of members, and the consequences of the groups actions further affect leadership patterns.

To understand barriers to effective leadership, community groups should ask themselves question such as:

1. Is the leadership overpowering?
2. Is there an unwillingness to assume leadership roles?
3. Is the group able to confront the leader or resolve the issue of absence of leadership to maintain their effectiveness?

Decision-Making Processes

Cottrell (1977) describes "competent communities" as those that collaborate effectively, have consensus on goals and priorities, agree on how to implement goals, and work together on actions. This implies a well developed and effective decision making-process in the community.

Making satisfactory decisions can be difficult for a community group. To move forward successfully, a trust, openness, respect, and mutual reliance must evolve within the community. The interaction of the group and the process for making decisions that develops is key to establishing group confidence and success. There are two basic elements in a decision-making process: the shared human experience of the members and the task at hand. An effective process addresses both.

With respect to the shared human experience, all members must feel as if they contribute something that is essential to the decision-making process to sustain their commitment. They must be able to participate in giving or seeking suggestions, information, and opinions. To establish a positive atmosphere, group members need to assure that all voices are heard, encourage other members as needed, address the interests of all, have ways of relieving tension, and mediate conflict situations. The most effective groups are those where members can fill a diversity of roles.

Understanding who the decision makers are and their respective styles is helpful in embarking on a collaborative decision-making process. The following characterizes decision makers and how they make decisions along a continuum:

1. Top-down decision makers...Consensus building decision makers
2. Little community knowledge...Knowledge of community vision, assets, and strengths
3. Rigid in approach...Flexible/adaptable
4. Crisis oriented...Driven by long term goals and objectives
5. Personality oriented...Issue oriented

6. Elitist...Democratic
7. Disconnected from community members...Accessible to community members

In reaching and implementing decisions, clarifying the roles, capabilities, and responsibilities of the participants is important. All members have other masters, such as a home agency or organization, and must balance the needs of the community with responsibilities to others. There may be fiscal and other ramifications that may inhibit their participation. At times participants may have similar capacities and expertise. Clarifying boundaries and overlapping territories is an important negotiation among such group members.

Specific human factors play a major role in the decision-making process. Varying degrees of fear and suspicion of individuals entering into the decision-making process influence the effectiveness of the process. Problems of apathy, impotence, and competitiveness can fragment and diffuse the energy of the group. When there is competent leadership within the group and an inclusive process established, these problems can be resolved.

Putting in place a problem-solving process that supports inclusive decision making in the community is essential for success. Characteristics of an effective collaborative decision-making process include:

1. Identifying and addressing the interests of all members,
2. Focusing on the communication process with an emphasis on active listening and well-framed statements,
3. Creating opportunities for generating options, and
4. Establishing clear mechanisms for evaluating options.

Beginning with an interest-based orientation is important to success. Usually in decision making, each participant focuses on an outcome he or she has previously thought up and much of the discussion centers on justifying those outcomes. This represents a position oriented process which limits the opportunities for success. A position is *what* someone wants as compared to an interest that is *why* someone wants what he or she wants. For example, your position may be that you will only support funding a particular school; whereas, your interests may be that there is an opportunity for children in the community to have an education that is culturally respectful, close to home, accommodating to family schedules, and so forth. Those interests open up the possibility for multiple creative solutions—not just the one solution—funding a particular school. When all participants explain their interests, why they want what they want, many more common options and alternatives become possible. Interest-based decision-making allows everyone to work together to collectively solve problems in a way that everyone is satisfied and no one feels as if he or she has compromised. Decisions tend to be durable and effective.

Where there is clear purpose, informality, open communication, active participation, respectful disagreement, consensus decisions, and shared leadership there is a greater likelihood of success and sustainable decisions and actions in the community. Groups are more likely to establish a good process when goals are attainable, and there is a stability of participation. When members are competent and accountable to make decisions, exercising personal competence is valued, and harmony is fostered in the group. It is a process where everybody wins. The following checklist (Figure 1.3) is a way to assess the decision-making process of a community group.

	YES	NO
1. Most members are committed to the mission of our community group.	❑	❑
2. Our community group has formulated clear goals.	❑	❑
3. The atmosphere in our group makes it easy to make a useful contribution.	❑	❑
4. Our group encourages all members to participate.	❑	❑
5. All members interests are addressed by the group.	❑	❑
6. Our community group is productive in meeting its goals.	❑	❑
7. Most members participate in important decisions.	❑	❑
8. Our meetings are run effectively.	❑	❑
9. Members are clear about their responsibilities to the group.	❑	❑
10. Members trust and respect the other members of the group as we work toward our goals.	❑	❑
11. Our group is able to act on our decisions.	❑	❑
12. Most members feel good about being a part of this collaborative effort.	❑	❑
13. There is recognition for a job well done.	❑	❑
14. Most members feel good about the outcomes of our work.	❑	❑

FIGURE 1.3. Assessment of decision-making process.

Red-flag questions whose answers suggest an ineffective decision-making process include:

1. Is there widespread apathy in the group?
2. Is there conflict within the group that continuously prevents the team from resolving issues or focusing on the task?
3. Is the group continuously unable to reach effective decisions?
4. Does the group spend a lot of time on problems or issues without taking any action?

Often it is the soul and conscience of the community to further change and maintain success. The blend of people who can exhibit humor, tolerance, and patience, marks the community's ability to work towards collaborative agreement. Recognizing the need for a decision-making process that is inclusive, collaborative, and respectful—and implementing it—is key to the effective functioning of a community.

Capacity-Building Strategies

Local solutions that evolve through a collaborative decision-making process must be translated to action. Capacity building involves identifying strengths and assets, acknowledging existing resources, creatively enhancing these assets, and developing new capacities.

There are a number of very good concrete examples of community programs that emphasize capacity-building strategies that can serve as examples for communities addressing issues of families with young children. The private-sector/voluntary organization, United Way, has recently dedicated its resources to this end. United Way facilitates community wide strategic planning, provides support for organizing community leaders, and provides training for neighborhood and community leaders in capacity-building approaches. Their goal is to revitalize all types of neighborhoods through increasing the capacity of local citizens to care for themselves and each other addressing the issues of affordable housing, creating jobs and economic opportunity, nurturing grass-roots leaders, and catalyzing a powerful community vision building process.

Another useful example of a community capacity-building effort is Healthy Communities, Healthy Youth, which unites communities to build assets through a community wide commitment to asset building. Relationships are key to their process. They begin with a positive vision to which everyone contributes; they engage people throughout the community, they build on quality information, and they resist the temptation to create new programs. A hallmark of their efforts is taking time to motivate and educate and to celebrate commitment and successes. Their efforts embrace innovations from the community and they encourage networking among communities. Specifically, a community is mobilized through talking with leaders, friends, neighbors, and other citizens about the potential for asset building. Community-wide events are sponsored to discuss asset building and to gather information about what is currently happening in the community. A cross-section of leaders and other citizens are involved to develop plans for increasing the capacity of the community to meet its vision.

Effective communities identify their existing resources and build on them using internal planning, cooperative arrangements, and commitment to the process. They do not give up but constantly broaden their net to accomplish their goals.

COMMUNITIES SUPPORTING YOUNG CHILDREN AND THEIR FAMILIES

All communities are unique and therefore have different concerns, needs, and resources; yet, it is commonly agreed that the core of effective communities includes public safety, a strong economy, health care, educational opportunities, a clean and healthy natural environment, and an ability to meet the needs of the diverse inhabitants (Lyon, 1987). The effective community maximizes the quality of life for all.

For young children and their families, communities represent an essential source of support and resources. Responsive communities for families of young children establish systems of services that are comprehensive and coordinated, utilize informal as well as formal networks, and maximize state and federal programs. As communities respond to the voices of families of young children, the national effort to establish in all communities a "Community Vision for Young Children and Their Families" should be addressed: how we know when the supports and services that families of young children need are in place in the community and that the communities themselves are assisted with this work.

The rest of this book speaks to the specifics of supporting a community vision for families of young children: systems building, collaboration strategies among partners, resource development, accountability to the mission and goals, and specific examples of effective communities. Communities are the heart of our country and in them lies the potential for nurturing the future of our society.

APPENDIX A
COMMUNITY PROFILE

As you prepare this community profile the following observations may be useful:

- Rural communities have existing communication and power structures which are often informal.
- Community members often prefer to be in charge of their own destiny and wish to be the planners who will create services for their area.
- Communities usually have developed mechanisms for dealing with outsiders and have established some type of linkages with them depending upon need. Linkages may range from formal arrangements with state officials to sporadic phone contacts with tertiary providers.
- Services to children with special needs are closely linked to community attitudes. Key power sources (whether the judge, the school board chairman, or the wealthy farmer) have considerable influence on resources for families.
- Community planning must relate strategies to the immediate "felt" needs of the people residing in the community.

Mark box with a **check** for a mild problem
and a **star** for a major problem.

Community History/Composition/Attitudes

❑ 1. What sense of community is shared by members of the community?

____

____

____

❑ 2. What is the degree to which education and health care are valued within the community?

____

____

____

❑ 3. Are there strong family ties within the community?

____

____

____

❑ 4. Does the community take care of its own? What is the level of volunteerism occurring within the community? How much church activity takes place within the community?

____
____
____

❑ 5. What is the community attitude towards outsiders?

____
____
____

❑ 6. How willing are community representatives to work with problems?

____
____
____

❑ 7. What is the community's history with creative problem-solving? with conflict?

____
____
____

❑ 8. How does the community pull together when resources are threatened?

____
____
____

❑ 9. What is the average age of residents? How does this influence the concern for services?

____
____
____

❑ 10. What is the level of community involvement in planning new services?

____
____
____

- ❑ 11. Are minority groups represented in the community leadership?

- ❑ 12. What is the political climate for change within the community?

- ❑ 13. How old is the community? Were community structures completed prior to accessibility requirements? What community revitalization efforts are taking place?

- ❑ 14. Are individuals with disabilities participants in the day-to-day mainstream of the life of the community? Do they feel segregated?

Economic Lifestyles

- ❑ 1. What is the major economy of the community?

- ❑ 2. Has an economic boom or bust occurred in the last 10 years?

- ❑ 3. What is the tax base within the community? What is the ratio of taxpayers to nonincome citizens?

- ☐ 4. Do residents trade within the community?

- ☐ 5. What is the rate of homelessness?

- ☐ 6. What community economic activities affect treatment programs, i.e., times of harvest or seasonal festivals in resort communities?

Networks

- ☐ 1. What mechanisms are utilized to communicate information within the community?

- ☐ 2. What meeting places are utilized daily by residents?

- ☐ 3. What is the availability of computers or FAX machines?

- ☐ 4. What formal and informal community power structures exist?

- ☐ 5. What are the community linkages with academic institutions?

- ❑ 6. What are the community linkages with tertiary institutions?

____
____
____

Population

- ❑ 1. How large is the population? Percent of children? Percent of adults?

____
____
____

- ❑ 2. How clustered is the population?

____
____
____

- ❑ 3. How mobile is the population? What means of transportation are typically used?

____
____
____

Geographic Barriers and Climatic Barriers

- ❑ 1. What is the terrain of the community?

____
____
____

- ❑ 2. What geographic inhibitors to transportation are there? Are airplanes or boats required for access? Is there regular delivery of commodities to the community?

____
____
____

- ❑ 3. What is the climate of the community? seasonal changes?

____
____
____

- ❑ 4. Does the community experience hazardous weather necessitating special precautions? (e.g., What is the condition of roads and how are they affected by weather?)

____
____
____

- ❑ 5. How many miles must people drive to obtain primary medical care services? other services?

____
____
____

- ❑ 6. What percent of children must receive services in another community?

____
____
____

Connections with Regional and State Systems

- ❑ 1. To what extent are community wishes known to regional and state planning groups? Is the local community group part of the planning process?

____
____
____

- ❑ 2. Is there county support of local efforts?

____
____
____

- ❑ 3. Who represents local citizens in state and regional issues? Are they informed of local needs?

____
____
____

- ❑ 4. What regional planning and service mechanisms exist?

____
____
____

☐ 5. What is the degree of support received from state agencies?

____

____

____

Adapted from: Nancy Fire, *Planning Services for Rural Children with Special Health Care Needs*, Georgetown University Child Development Center (1991).

REFERENCES

Bass, B. M. (1991). From transactional to transformational leadership: Learning to share the vision. *Organizational Dynamics, 18*, 19-31.

Building a Community Agenda (1991). *Building a community agenda: Developing local government entities*. Unpublished manuscript, Center for the Study of Social Policy, Washington, DC.

Cottrell, L. S. (1977). The competent community. In R. Warren (Ed.), *New perspectives on the American community* (pp. 535-545). Chicago: Rand McNally.

Farrow, F. (1996). *Creating better futures for children, youth, and families. System Change at the neighborhood level*. Center for the Study of Social Policy for the National Leadership Symposium on Community Strategies for Children and Families: Promoting Positive Outcomes.

Fire, N. (1991). *Planning services for rural children with special health care needs*. Washington, DC: Georgetown University Child Development Center.

Fowler, R.B. (1991). *The dance with community: The contemporary debate in American political thought*. Lawrence, KS: University of Kansas Press.

Hillery, G. A., Jr. (1955). Definitions of community: Areas of agreement. *Rural Sociology, 20*, 779-791.

Koestenbaum, P. (1991). *Leadership: The inner side of greatness*. San Francisco: Jossey-Bass.

Lipman-Blumen, J. (1996). *The connective edge: Leading in an independent world*. San Francisco: Jossey-Bass.

Lyon, L. (1987). *The community in urban society*. Philadelphia, PA: Temple University Press.

Melaville, A., Blank, M. J., & Asayesh, G. (1993). *Together we can: A guide for crafting a profamily system of education and human services*. Washington, DC: U.S. Department of Education and U.S. Department of Health and Human Services.

Parks, R. E. (1936). Human ecology. *American Journal of Sociology, 17*(1), 1-15.

Stonewall, L. (1983). *Country life, city life*. New York: Praeger.

Sutton, W., & Munston, T. (1976, August). *Definitions of community, 1954-1973*. Paper presented at the Annual Meeting of the American Sociological Association, New York.

Tonnies, F. (1963). *Community and society*. (C. P. Loomis Trans., Ed.). New York: Harper Torch Books. (Original work published 1887)

Warren, R. L. (1978). *The community in America* (3rd ed.). Chicago: Rand McNally.

Weber, M. (1947). *The theory of social and economic organization*. (A. M. Henderson & T. Parsons, Ed. & Trans.). New York: Oxford University Press.

chapter 2

Supporting Families Where Children Live: Community Principles in Action

Richard N. Roberts
Utah State University

The title of this book, *Where Children Live,* directs us both to a physical and a psychological place in our efforts to help families create the range of supports that young children need for optimal developmental outcomes. The fullness of children's lives goes beyond their apartment, house, trailer, day care center, playground or family car as they travel from place to place. Each of these physical places has meaning and is filled with other people and activities that teach the full breadth of everyday knowledge and human interaction as young children participate in the scripts of their daily lives. Tharp and Gallimore (1988) said it well by suggesting that "In every culture natural teaching transmits skills of immense variety and power—a 'curriculum' of far greater complexity than anything created in school. Such interactions awaken and arouse mind, communication, and expression and assist the instantiation of culture and society" (p. 20).

As human service providers and applied developmental psychologists work with families to affect this natural curriculum in ways that support young children, it is important to remember that educational, health, childcare, and social service systems must interweave their services and supports to children and families in places that are part of the fabric of where children live. Where children live is not in a social service, educational, or health system. They live in families that are wonderfully diverse in communities across the country that also express this same diversity. These communities are made up of families that support each other in work, play, religious life, recreation, governing structures, education, health care, birth, life, and death. The title also reminds us that the resources used to support children where they live are not equitably distributed across the country and an increasing number of children are being forced to live in ecological disaster zones as graphically described by such authors as Garbarino, in his work, *Raising Children in Toxic Environments*; Kozol, in *Amazing Grace* and Kotlowitz in *There are no Children Here*.

This chapter will articulate a set of principles that help define the manner in which services and supports need to be provided at the community level. Later chapters will explore specific issues in children's lives in families with particular health, educational, or ecological challenges. In each case, a common theme that ties all of these special populations together is that families are better able to achieve optimal outcomes when they live in communities where there is a system of supports available to its members that is at the same time:

1. Responsive to family challenges, priorities and strengths,
2. Developed in partnership with constituents,
3. Reflective and respectful of the cultural norms and practices of the families participating,
4. Accessible to everyone,
5. Affordable to those who need assistance, and
6. Organized and coordinated through collaboration so that resources are equitably distributed in an efficient and effective manner.

These themes mentioned above are those that form the basis of the goals of projects discussed in some detail in later chapters.

A second theme in this chapter, and indeed within this book, is that communities are but a logical entry point into a support system that extends through all the places children live throughout their busy week. Though some children may spend their days in a community with relatively little movement outside of it, others are in continuous movement from one community to the next. For example, some children may live in families where their mothers and fathers live in different homes in different communities. These children may commute back and forth from one family to the other over time. Other children may live in one community with their family and yet their parents work in another community. Their daycare center may be closer to their parents' work than their home. Other children may be involved in a more mobile lifestyle such as those within migrant farming communities. For migrant families, the community may be those people who move together from one work site to the next while the physical and geographic communities in which they live change throughout the seasons. The support structures involving policy, service, training, and financing at the county, state, and federal levels must reflect, adapt, and embrace this diversity to make it possible for families to use the supports they need in their local situations. These bureaucratic structures must also begin to value the community as a source of strength and solutions facing families. In doing so, the role of higher bureaucratic structures emphasizes the need to ensure equitableness, assists in providing resources, and strengthens local efforts to achieve common goals.

COMMUNITIES AS THE LOGICAL SYSTEMS ENTRY POINT

Families live in a complex web of social interactions that include work, daycare, schools, religious groups, shopping malls, grocery stores, medical care facilities, playgrounds, recreational opportunities, law enforcement centers, human resource centers, and a host of other activities that fill everyday lives. While these interactions may involve one or many communities, the supports that foster a family's ability to use them come from many different ecological contexts. Figure 2.1 suggests the relationships of the bureaucratic levels of support that surround the community and hence, a family. It would be possible to enter into an analysis of a system of supports at any level depicted in this figure and productively examine the policies and practices that either support or hinder the ability of families to provide for their members and children.

From our perspective, it is most logical to begin that investigation at the community level because it is most proximal to the family itself and it is often the first place where support for families with young children can be found. Ideally, at the community level, private and public agencies and family representatives within a geographical area work together to develop noncompeting collaborative partnerships to make services and supports more accessible and acceptable to families. In some areas, there may be a county or city geopolitical structure serving to unite communities, while in others no such structure may exist. At the state systems level, these same private and public agencies support, assist, and coordinate local efforts and systems development. At the federal agency and legislative levels, functions related to broad national initiatives, funding models, and coordination among federal and nonprofit agencies should be occurring (Roberts, Akers, & Behl, 1996; Roberts, Rule, & Innocenti, 1998).

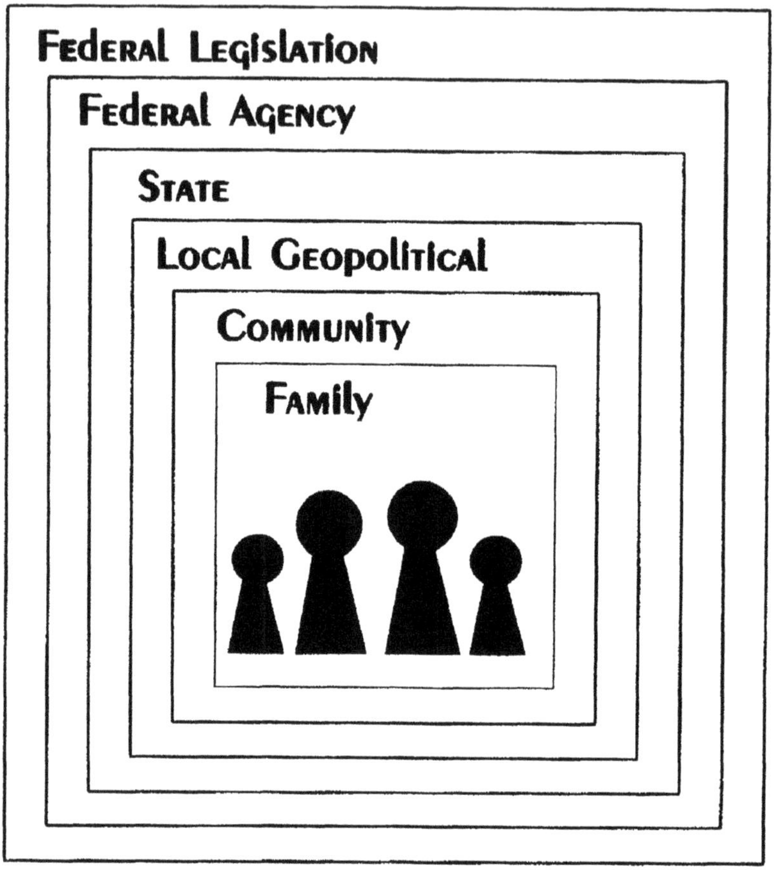

FIGURE 2.1. Ecological context. Reprinted by permission from Roberts, Rule, and Innocenti (1998).

MODELS OF COMMUNITY INFLUENCE ON CHILD DEVELOPMENT

A number of psychological/sociological models have been developed to trace neighborhood-environmental influences on children's development. Jencks and Mayer (1990), for example, suggested four broad mechanisms through which neighborhoods could mediate children's experience in their families. These included:

1. Epidemic models in which norms are transmitted through peers like a social contagion;

2. Collective socialization in which the community exerts influences on adults toward common perspectives that in turn influence children;
3. Presence of institutional resources within a community that can promote certain opportunities and prevent other problem behaviors from occurring; and,
4. The proximity of well-off neighbors can have a perverse influence on development by reducing motivation in less advantaged children as they perceive themselves to be disadvantaged.

Other models suggest an intergenerational social reproduction of disadvantage (Wilson, 1987). Children raised in areas of concentrated poverty may be isolated from conventional values and networks that would support their development of mainstream conventions. Coleman (1988) describes the impact of social capital on development as the capacity to be able to draw on social relationships to implement goals. Thus, the amount of support that one has in reserve can be drawn upon in times of need to get things done. As Furstenberg and Hughes (1997) have described, if parents have limited resources they may not choose to invest in community building, which continues to exacerbate already difficult conditions. It is within this context that formal and informal systems of support at the community level may make the difference as they work in partnership to enhance the social capital within families or to decrease social isolation in support of child and family well-being.

Child and Family Well-Being as the Community Goal

Families and their young children are most likely to be able to profit from the use of supports when they are *meaningful* to the situations families face with their children, *sustainable* over time given the variety of competing demands placed on families and *congruent* with families' cultural and religious beliefs (Bernheimer, Gallimore, & Weisner, 1990). Assistance that meets these criteria is most likely to fit into the ecological lives of families. A broader question may be asked, however, "To what end are these services and supports provided?" One way to approach this question is from the context of child and family well-being as the most appropriate basic outcome for a community-based system of services. The concept of child and family well-being draws heavily on the work of such authors as Brofenbrenner (1979), Maslow (1954), Weisner and Gallimore (1994), and White, Kaban, and Attanucci (1979). The mutual interdependence of goals for child and family well-being are tied to those levels of support and constraints emanating from county, state, and federal measures of well-being. By defining and promoting supports needed by families to effectively draw on the resources that are within their communities, the connection between human services and our efforts to foster effective, educated, productive citizens becomes more clear. The ecological models outlined over 20 years ago by Brofenbrenner (1979) continue to serve as an appropriate beginning framework for communities to define their roles in this process as the place where children live.

In addressing child and family well-being, the distinctions made by our diagnostic and categorical systems of care become somewhat artificial. Broad indicators for the quality of life of a child who has been enrolled in a program for the prevention of child abuse and neglect are no different from those for a child who is enrolled in a program for special health care needs or for a child who is enrolled in a program for daycare because his or her parents work. Basic principles of child and family well-being are understood best as a universal construct that can be applied to all families independent of their particular circumstances. As suggested by Tolstoy (1960) in the opening sentence of *Anna Karenina,* "Happy families are all alike; every unhappy family is unhappy in its own way" (p. 1). "Happy families," as described by Tolstoy, are ones that have developed a way to achieve a sense of well-being for their members. This concept is incorporated into Maslow's (1954) assertion that a good society is one that fosters the fullest development of human potential and the fullest degree of humanness so that needs are met in such a way that independence rather than dependence is encouraged. Independence is equated with a sense of competence and mastery that allows the individual to reach his or her own potential.

The services and supports that foster independence, competence, mastery, development, and humanness are ones that are responsive to families, created in partnership with families, and are respectful of families' cultural and ecological constraints. The very nature of the individual circumstances and adaptations that families have made in seeking assistance outside their own resources suggest the truth in the second half of the above Tolstoy quote. Each individual family is "unhappy in its own way" and individualized, family-centered plans that address both the ecology and the culture are most effective in addressing those factors leading to "unhappiness" or a lack of well-being. When these constructs are operationalized into actual practice, plans, and activities in which families are involved are more likely to be sustainable, congruent, and meaningful within individual and family lives.

The basic needs described by Maslow's (1954) hierarchy are ones that must be addressed for well-being to be achieved. Without going into great detail, these can be broken down into: (a) physiological needs that form the basic biological functions of food, shelter, sleep, sex, comfort, wellness, and health; (b) safety needs; (c) love and belonging; (d) self-esteem; and (e) self-actualization. For families with young children, each family member must first be assured that the more basic physiological, safety, and love and belonging needs are met, and then continue to build on these experiences that contribute to their self-esteem and to their full potential.

A valuable lesson with respect to establishing priorities in addressing needs in practice was learned by this author from a group of teenage pregnant and parenting women. As we began a project with community organizations providing services to pregnant and parenting teens, we conducted a needs assessment survey that separately asked teenagers who were involved in social service programs within this community, and the service providers who provided those services, to rank order a number of needs that could potentially be met by these agencies. There was a surprisingly high negative correlation between the rankings of the teenagers and the service providers. That is, those services that the teenage mothers ranked very high on their list of needs were ranked as lower priorities by the service providers. Those services that were ranked high by service providers as being needed by parents were ranked low by those same teenage parents. For example, teenage mothers ranked as their highest priorities services associated with (a) finding a stable place to live; (b) having assistance in obtaining food stamps and other means of feeding their children, such as the WIC program; and (c) finding stable daycare for their children so that they were able to attend school. In contrast, service providers listed as primary importance, (a) information on child development and health; (b) counseling on birth control; and (c) counseling on family and partner relationships. Neither the agencies nor the teenagers were wrong in their list of needs. Rather, the ordering of priorities vastly differed between the two groups. The teenagers identified items much more basic on Maslow's needs hierarchy that needed to be met first before the higher needs seen as priority by the service providers could be addressed. The resulting discussion between the two groups helped each clarify for the other the rationale for their ordering and a method to come to agreement on how to proceed in jointly developing a service system that addressed concerns in turn (Roberts & Calkin, 1989).

The concept of family well-being as being an appropriate outcome for community-based services has reached a growing acceptance among both policy makers and service providers over time. Bailey and Simeonsson (1988), for example, indicated that family quality of life was a useful indicator of outcomes and policy initiatives and the Accreditation Council on Persons with Disabilities (The Council, 1998) has listed a number of appropriate ways of being able to measure an individual's quality of life and that of his/her family. Indeed, improved quality of life may be the only acceptable outcome of policies, the resulting programs and services.

FAMILY ACCOMMODATIONS AS ADAPTIVE RESPONSES TO CHANGES

As families seek a sense of well-being for themselves and their children, tradeoffs or accommodations must be made between the various needs of each of its members and the resources available to them. The best fit in this dynamic interaction of accommodation and resource allocation is the one that will provide for the maximum sense of family well-being for the family as a whole. The accommodation domains as developed by Gallimore and colleagues (1993) suggest both a model for examining how families' circumstances are altered by the course of events in their lives and a way of measuring the impact of those changes on the family's ability to meet the needs addressed by Maslow. Table 2.1 describes 10 accommodation variables suggested by Gallimore, Weisner, Bernheimer, Guthrie, & Nihira (1993) and gives examples of each as well. These categories suggest domains by which negotiations must take place each time the family structure changes. Thus, the birth of a child, a divorce, the loss of a job are all occasions for redistribution of the family's resources in time, money, and talent. The fit that emerges should give family members their best sense of managing, coping, and well-being. For example, even though the child's birth may well be a joyful event within the family, it creates a number of stressors that must be addressed in order for the family to return to a more homeostatic state. A family's own resources in time, money, and talent are rarely sufficient by themselves to make all the accommodations necessary to meet all of its needs. Even the more basic needs on Maslow's hierarchy may require additional assistance and support for an adequate level of health and safety to be reached and maintained.

For families with young children, for example, both parents may be working or a single mother may be holding a full-time job. The issue of childcare becomes an important concern on which the remaining resources for the family may depend. Without adequate childcare, a parent may not be able to work either temporarily or maintain employment over the long term. He or she must provide for the well-being of the young chid. The needed childcare may be provided by a grandmother/father living near by or another family member. Alternately, there may be family daycare available at a neighbor's home or a daycare center on the way to work. Each of these options requires different accommodations with respect to their costs in time, money, or personal relation-

TABLE 2.1.
Ten Accommodation Variables and Examples of Each

Variable	Example
1. Family subsistence and financial base	a. Mother stayed home because child "needed" her; later went back to work to afford speech therapy; b. Father turned down contract for third year working abroad in part to get child services in Los Angeles.
2. Accessibility of health and educational services	a. Mother drove child to intervention program, waited at grandmother's house; b. Parents each took time from work to make trips to doctor; it took split-second timing to transfer child.
3. Home and neighborhood safety and convenience	a. Family planned move to a larger house to accommodate wheelchair; father built special chairs and table; b. Home was child-proofed; nothing breakable in child's room.
4. Domestic task and chore workload for family	a. Mother put less priority on house and housework and higher priority on helping child; b. Mother got up at 4 a.m. to do laundry, housework, had no paid help.
5. Child care tasks	a. Child's older sisters voluntarily assisted—mother did not mobilize help outside family circle; b. Complex job assignments for child care were given to father, mother, grandmother, etc.
6. Child play groups and peers	a. Child was allowed to play only inside with sibling's friend, not outside with neighbor children; b. Mother started play group for child in neighborhood.
7. Marital role relationships	a. Father left family partially because he could not accept child who had delays; b. Joint parent decisions (e.g., parents slept separately for 6 months due to child's sleeping problems).
8. Social support	a. Extensive support networks: relatives, parents, church, boy scouts; b. Mother lived rent-free with grandparents; grandfather helped teach child.
9. Father's role	a. Father took over on weekends, as he commuted long distance and had long working hours during week; b. Father gave up drinking, went to church, was helping rather than adding to mother's workload.
10. Sources of parental information and goals	a. Father's former girlfriend was speech therapist; she led family to transfer child to that clinic; b. Mother received advice from grandmother (RN) grandfather (special education teacher), and her own former special education teacher.

Source: Gallimore et al. (1993).

ships. If a family member provides day care, the costs to the family are different than if a center-based program is used though each requires its own set of accommodations. The decision with respect to which option is used depends both upon the availability of any given option and its perceived cost versus its perceived benefits to family well-being.

As in the above example, any solution to a situation that inhibits child and family well-being over the long term will emerge when the accommodations are found in services and supports within communities that are meaningful, sustainable, and congruent with the family's life style over time. To the degree that this occurs, families are more likely to be able to, in Maslow's words (as cited in Tribe, 1982), "...foster the fullest development of human potential and the fullest degree of humanness within each of its members" (p. 40). The less likely those services can be provided within the community context, the higher the stress to the family. As stress increases, the more "unhappy" the family becomes and the less likely that short-term solutions will work because they are not meaningful, sustainable, or congruent within that family's life.

For example, a child with a disability may spend most of his or her day time in center-based daycare because the parents work and the daycare setting is the best fit overall for this family. Early intervention services for this child and family may be provided in several settings. The best option would be to involve the family, the daycare center, and the early intervention program in the Individualized Family Service Plan (IFSP) so that it includes activities in each of the child's most significant settings. Daycare providers, family members, and early interventionists would be involved, understand the issues, and provide meaningful input into the planning process. If the daycare provider is left out of the loop, and the therapist works exclusively with the child in a setting that involves neither the parents nor the daycare provider, then the effects of such a program will neither be meaningful, sustainable, nor congruent with the ongoing activities of this child's life. The chances of services being most helpful are enhanced when all of the partners involved throughout the child's day are included in the planning and implementation process of the IFSP.

ACTIVITY SETTINGS AS THE UNIT OF ANALYSIS FOR COMMUNITY SERVICES AND SUPPORTS

This chapter began with the assertion that children live in places that are, at the same time, both physical and psychological. For this reason, the context and activities that make up the day for a young child are important units of analyses in service and support planning with families. Activity settings are a convenient and effective way to analyze the contexts in which children spend their days learning and interacting with other people. The activity setting is the place in which everyday interactions are played out (Gallimore, Goldenberg, & Weisner, 1993; O'Donnell, Tharp, & Wilson, 1993; Roberts, 1993b, Roberts, Rule & Innocenti, 1998; Tharp & Gallimore, 1988; Wertsch, 1985). An activity setting is a dynamic combination of both an ecological description of the physical place in which human interaction occurs and a description of the cultural attributes that influence that activity over time. Activity settings are the expression of the daily routine of a family as it goes about its everyday tasks. These daily routines are the building blocks and the evidence that assist us in understanding the mix of the personal and cultural values, and the environmental constraints, pressures, and resources on how a family meets its daily needs at each level of Maslow's hierarchy. As described by Bernheimer and Keogh (1995), "the daily routine, 'is composed of the common stuff' of family life. The things that are done and the things that are not done.... They reflect the mix of personal and cultural values as well as the constraints, pressures, and resources in the environment" (p. 420). Activity settings are composed of both the psychological and the physical components of each of the interactions that a family is involved in over the course of a day. Gallimore, Goldenberg, and Weisner (1993), have suggested a model for analyzing activity settings that has been very useful in our work. Activity settings are composed of: (a) the people involved, (b) their values and tasks, (c) the operations and task demands before them, (d) their scripts for conduct, and (e) the purposes and motivations of the participants.

This type of analysis becomes important at the point in which service providers begin to think about the kinds of interventions that may be developed with and for a family at the community level. Everyday activities for families involve mundane tasks such as getting breakfast or dinner ready, getting children ready for daycare, as well as the interactions families may have with human services providers such as a family service worker, home visitor, an early intervention program's staff member or the physician providing well-baby care. Any of the above interactions can be usefully examined with respect to whom, why, what, and to what end each interaction occurred. It is a window into helping the service provider to understand the family and his or her own contribution to whether services were provided in ways that truly supported the family's needs and beliefs.

Take, as an example, two young children with a physical disability receiving physical therapy. In one case, the parent takes the child to the local recreation center in the community for the parent-tot swim class.

The physical therapist meets the mom and the instructor as the class begins and helps the mother adapt the activities to the physical capabilities of her young daughter. The instructor works with this mother and her child along with the other six mother-child pairs in the class.

In the second case, the physical therapist meets the parent and child at the early intervention program, engages both mother and child in exercises and discussion helping the mother with important lessons in positioning during feeding and other important activities. The therapist also spends time alone with the child working specifically on muscle strengthening exercises while the mother joins a support group of parents with children with disabilities. Table 2.2 describes each of the activity setting components for these two scenarios.

In the example in Figure 2.2, two different ways of supporting families in the community are presented. Each model has its strengths. The purpose of the exercise is to demonstrate how the physical activity of a parent-toddler swimming class or an early intervention program therapy session can be understood as the activity setting that shapes both the physical activity and the psychological mind set of all of its participants.

Both parents want to be able to play and teach their children useful skills while building on their strengths. Both receive support from the other parents and their community in doing so. The mother in the swimming class receives support from other parents in the swim class, but also finds it helpful to involve herself in a parent-to-parent support program in her community so that she can have time with parents of other children with special needs. The parent who is involved in the early intervention program receives support from the physical therapist and other parents of children with disabilities, but must look elsewhere for opportunities to integrate her child in activities with other children her age from the community.

The physical therapist must make different arrangements in each setting and approach the time spent with the parents in different ways with different purposes. In the swimming lesson example, the therapist comes as the support facilitator to help figure out how to adapt the activity that any parent and child should be able to enjoy together. For this particular family, the physical therapist becomes a consultant who fades his or her involvement over time as the parents feel comfortable and competent in the new situation with her child. The center-based early intervention program may take on many of these same roles, but in a setting where other typically developing children and their parents are not present and that is not part of the normal everyday activities of the community.

As a consequence of these different activity settings with their different purposes, motives, and people involved, the nature of the partnerships

TABLE 2.2.
Family–Professional Activity Setting Analysis

Persons involved	Values	Operations and task demands	Scripts	Purposes
mother child physical therapist swimming instructor for other parents/children	1. Mother: Being included in everyday activities with other moms and babies is important to me and my child. 2. Physical Therapist: I help parents see their child's strengths and build on them in their everyday routines whenever the parents want that to happen 3. Swimming Instructor: Its important that all of my classes are open to the entire community.	1. Mother and physical therapist meet with swim teacher before classes begin to talk through how the three of them can work together. 2. Physical therapist fades out her attendance over time; keeps contact with mom.	Mother: 1. Finds community-based activities for daughter. 2. Participates in activities with daughter. 3. Meets regularly with parents of other children with disabilities in Parent-to-Parent meetings	1. Parents participate actively and fully in activities of our own choosing in our community with support as needed from Parent-to-Parent group and others. 2. Physical therapist helps mother and swimming instructor feel comfortable in the swimming class together
mother child physical therapist other parents/children at the early intervention center	1. Mother: The Early Intervention Center is a place where I gather support and my child learns new skills 2. Physical therapist: I help parents see their child's strengths and help them learn exercises they can incorporate into the child's daily routine.	1. Meet weekly together at early intervention program. 2. Learn new exercises each week. 3. Practice exercises as part of daily activities at home. 4. Talk to other parents of children with disabilities. 5. Share their experiences.	1. Mother: I have to learn what my child's strengths are and work on incorporating new skills into our every day lives 2. Therapist: I have to teach the mother how to be her child's therapist. I have to help build skills in this child's repertoire.	1. Learn the skills I need to help my daughter learn the skills she needs.

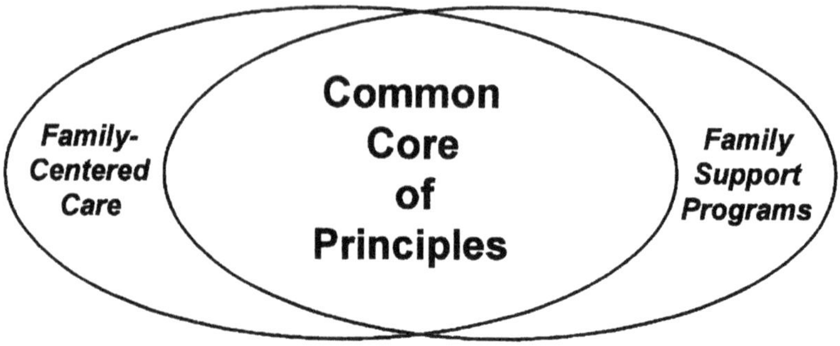

FIGURE 2.2. Relationship between family support programs and family-centered care. Reprinted by permission from Roberts, Rule, and Innocenti (1998).

between the parent, the human service provider, and the community is altered in important ways. A partnership that is equal between these three elements is one that shares common characteristics as described in more detail in Roberts, Rule and Innocenti (1998). In Table 2.3, the characteristic of successful family professional partnerships are briefly presented. The roles taken on by family and informal support systems within a community hopefully mirror these constructs that represent equal partnerships in child rearing, problem solving, and community building.

PRINCIPLES OF CARE

The six principles of care mentioned earlier in this chapter are reflected throughout this book as the primary categories by which we understand programs that are most likely to increase the sense of well-being of families with young children. Though this discussion will artificially separate the principles into distinct categories, together they reflect an approach that squarely identifies the well-being of a family and its children as the primary focus of community supports and interventions. More attention will be paid to the principles involving partnerships with family members at the individual family level, systems development level, and as partnerships related to cultural competency. Many of the remaining principles are covered more fully in other chapters. For example, accessibility and coordination issues are themes in chapters by Boyce and colleagues, Akers and Behl, Kaufman and Wischmann, and Bronheim and Striffler. Issues of affordability (Principle Five) are addressed specifically in Chapter 4 by Goetze and Mackey Andrews.

TABLE 2.3.
Common Characteristics of Family-Professional Partnerships

Author	Characteristics
Vosler-Hunter (1988)	1. Mutual respect for knowledge and skills 2. Honesty and clear communication 3. Understanding and empathy 4. Mutually agreed-on goals 5. Shared planning and decision making 6. Open and two-way sharing of information 7. Accessibility and responsiveness 8. Joint evaluation of progress 9. Absence of labeling and blame
Dechillo et al. (1994)	1. Caring, nonblaming attitude toward the family 2. Shared information 3. Recognition of the family as a key resource 4. Recognition of the limits and of the existence of other responsibilities 5. Shared responsibility and power in the relationship, including joint decision making and problem solving
Dunst and Paget (1991)	1. Mutual contributions and agreed-on roles 2. Desire to work together to meet those mutually agreed-on goals 3. Shared responsibility for taking actions to achieve 4. Loyalty, trust, and honesty in all dealings in the partnership 5. Full disclosure of all information between partners 6. Parental locus of decision making in exercising their rightful role to decide what is in the best interest of their family and its members

Note: Reprinted with permission from Roberts, Rule, and Innocenti (1998).

As the principles are applied to a community's capacity to provide for the well-being of families, it is important to understand that the activity settings in which these principles will be enacted. The individuals who construct the activity setting out of the physical place embody these principles in their interaction with one another.

The manner in which activity settings are constructed says much about the purposes and motives and the values and beliefs of those individuals who are constructing them. For example, early intervention programs that serve children with disabilities in segregated settings can be contrasted with early intervention programs that serve children within the context of the everyday routines of those children outside of a particular program that is set up only for children with disabilities. In a segregated program, this activity setting has been constructed to assist service providers to be able to provide grouped activities for young children and to efficiently provide therapies as needed. Therapy sessions provided in the context of situations in which all children are involved such as those described in the swimming lesson earlier have a different set of beliefs and attitudes with respect to how services should be provided. This activity setting is one in which an underlying belief asserts that services and supports should be available to all children, with adaptations made as necessary, in order that all children independent of their disability or special circumstances are able to profit from these experiences.

Principle One: Responsiveness to Family Challenges, Priorities, and Strengths

Families experience a wide range of care in their interactions with service providers ranging from that which is family-centered to that which is agency-centered. As an example, Mr. and Mrs. Johns were the parents of a young child, Tom, who exhibited serious behavioral and medical problems. As Tom moved through the early intervention programs, special education preschools, and special education in the elementary and middle schools, his parents were amazed at the different approaches that service providers used in working with their family. In some cases, they were welcomed in meetings and their advice was solicited with respect to the decisions being made. Meetings were held at a time and a place that made it possible for them to attend. In some instances, the meetings were arranged and held in the family's home or at the local church down the street when it was known that childcare and transportation were chronic problems for them. In working with other agencies, sometimes the Johns found out about a meeting after it occurred and no one helped them understand the implications of the decisions being made. In one extreme situation, the family found out about an educational placement decision after their son had been placed in another classroom without their knowledge or consent.

Within other community programs, this same range of family-centered to agency-centered experiences were seen. For example, the Johns made it a point to take their son, Tom, to all of their older son's basketball games. Efforts were made by the local high school staff to ensure that there was room set aside for Tom's wheelchair and that seats were saved for his parents to be able to sit next to him throughout the game. Likewise, when the social worker was helping Mrs. Johns find appropriate after school care for her son, she asked the mother what assistance she would need or like to have in finding such a placement. The parents discussed the options among themselves, then with the social worker, and laid out their preferences with respect to the types of opportunities that they would like to see for him. The social worker, working closely with the family, helped them find placements that met their list of needs that included an inclusive setting for Tom with the appropriate adaptive equipment that would make it possible for him to interact with other children while he was there. In this example, not only is an equal partnership developed between the family and the social worker, but the family's preferences and concerns are taken into account and serve as the driving force for the policies as they are developed.

The central feature of a family-centered program is that it recognizes that the family is the major constant in a child's life and that many of the supports needed in parenting are found within informal structures organized around the family. Issues such as discipline, daily routines, childcare, religious education, and planned health practices are resolved and carried out within this informal structure. Although not all of these activities are carried out by the parents or even the family members, basic decisions are made at the family level by the family that set the stage for their occurrence. Roberts, Rule, and Innocenti (1998) defined family-centered care as the following: "family-centered care...occurs when a service provider assists a family in decision-making that honors and respects family preferences. This form of assistance helps families use the informal structures that are already available and helps to make decisions about more formal systems with which they choose to interact" (p. 56). The ongoing decision-making process in which families engage as they continue to strive toward meeting their family's needs and achieving a sense of well-being is a complex one. Such issues as identification of family concerns, assistance in setting goals and choice of one strategy over another, and even a decision about whom and how someone should be working with a family, are all part of the decision-making process known as family-centered services. The degree to which families are the ultimate decision-makers in this process is one measure of family-centered care.

Families are constantly making decisions about their own well-being and are constrained in this decision-making process by a number of beliefs that are part of both of their ecological and their cultural worlds. In order for agencies to work most effectively with families, they must be responsive to and understand the different perspectives and constraints that families bring to them as they seek services of one kind or another. It is only through understanding the ecocultural context in which families make decisions and the activity settings that result from them that service providers can enter into a family's world.

Families will rarely, if ever, describe their particular cultural beliefs or their particular ecological constraints clearly to a service provider or a human service agency. For the helper to effectively discover with each family the accommodations that have been or must be made, information from several sources must be understood: (a) the *family information* with respect to how the family spends their time with their children, what they believe they are doing, how they do it, and what they expect as outcomes are all important; (b) *program information* on the range of possible intervention services to families within the constraints of the agencies; and (c) the *family working with the program information* in making decision with respect to which solutions will work best for them. When all of these information sources are taken into account, services are more likely to be sustainable, meaningful, and congruent with the family's life. As Gallimore, Goldenberg and Weisner (1993) stated, "...interventions can build upon commonalities between families and interventions, rather than always assuming chasms that must be bridged" (p. 548).

It is important to distinguish between family-centered care as we have been discussing it and family support programs as they have been developed. The family-centered care and family support programs share a common set of principles. There are some unique differences between the two.

Dunst, Johansen, Trivette and Hamby (1991) suggested a continuum of family involvement in family-centered care from ones that are completely professionally dominated to ones that are family centered. Professionally dominated ones are ones in which the decisions are made almost completely by service providers and families are seen as incompetent in their ability to make decisions for themselves. As Dunst and colleagues (1991) describe the family-centered model, "Professionals are seen as agents and instruments of the family, and intervene in ways that maximally promote the family decision-making autonomy and competency "(p. 118).

Family support on the other hand, is a movement that recognizes that all families need support in one form or another and that none are islands unto themselves. In this context, public and private policies and programs should be ones that support families in their ability to achieve well-being as they go about their daily activities. Such programs as the Family Resource Coalition (Weisbourd, 1994), work described by Weiss and Halpern (1990), and Weiss and Jacobs (1988) suggest the wide range of state- and community-level initiatives that seek to create a more secure safety net for all families within communities. Several of the chapters within this book also directly address family support activities at the community level as part of their programs. Dunst and colleagues (1991) identified six principles that exemplify contemporary family-centered practice as the intersection between family-centered care and family support programs:

1. Enhancing of sense of community;
2. Mobilizing resources and supports;
3. Sharing responsibility and collaborating;
4. Protecting family integrity;
5. Strengthening family functioning; and
6. Engaging in proactive human services practice.

As Roberts, Rule and Innocenti (1998) noted, the distinction between the two is perhaps best understood by viewing family-centered care as the philosophical base of service systems that insures that families are treated as equal partners in decision making with formal, public, and private human service agencies. Family support, on the other hand, is more broadly conceived and recognizes that each family requires some type of support and that communities and society at large have a responsibility to actively participate in helping to provide such support. Both family-centered care and family support services are important components of community options for increasing child and family well-being.

Principle Two: Development of Systems in Partnership with Constituents

As human service providers, educators, and community planners move from expert models of service delivery to ones that are more participatory, this principle of developing programs and systems of care in partnership with those constituents who will be using them has become more and more of a central feature in community development activities. As evident in our analysis of activity settings, the very process of who is participating in decision-making affects the nature of the activity setting. Part of the post modernist perspective of research involves an understanding that reality is more firmly based on the subjective experiences of those people who are involved in it, and that those experiences are irrevocably tied to places that constitute our understanding of the activity setting (Denzin & Lincoln, 1994).

The view that programs can only be developed and evaluated meaningfully in partnership with constituents is evident in several different levels of the human services field. First, at the individual family level, it is becoming more commonplace that Individualized Family Service Plans (IFSP) must be developed working collaboratively. Service providers and family members should work together to develop the plan that will lead to the goals that the families have set. At the next level, partnership with constituents is equally as important, in the sense that program development and implementation must occur in full partnership with those people who will be using those services. The only avenue through which family concerns can be fully represented in program development is to have those concerns represented by families. By having family members involved at the IFSP level and at the program development and policy level, services move from doing *for* families to doing *with* families. This paradigm shift is a critical development in a program's life.

An example of this paradigm shift occurred recently within one of the projects under the Opening Doors project (Roberts, Behl, & Akers, 1998). In this project, communities throughout the country work within a participatory action research model with researchers and evaluators in helping to create programs that are more accessible, more appropriate, and goal oriented. In one community, the planning group had been working to develop mental health services for very young children. Though the planning group was making progress, it was made up entirely of service providers. Over time, as the program continued to work with the Opening Door's staff, the issue of having meaningful parent input and involvement in the program continued to emerge. The concerns raised by the service providers involved their belief that they needed to have everything perfect before families should be able to enter into the process. That is, they did not want families to observe them struggling with significant issues, but would have preferred to have the system in place and then have families come in and approve it.

Over several months, as we talked with the planning group, resistance to the idea of asking families to participate in a meaningful way in the program was gently erased to the point that the planning group decided to invite a large representation of families to the next meeting and began to include them as ongoing members of the committee. The decision was reached during a meeting in which the group was setting goals for itself over the course of the year. One of the goals involved inclusion of family members as participants in the process. As the discussion within the group developed, it was apparent that this needed to be the first priority for the group. When the group facilitator asked to rate some of the other priorities, one of the group members said, "Well, that would be dumb. We have to wait until we have the parents here in order to make those decisions as a group with parents." A true paradigm shift and a new activity setting were formed as a function of including parents in the process.

Remember back to the elements of an activity setting that included five descriptors. Prior to having parents involved in the planning meetings, the planning group was completely comprised of service providers. After the inclusion of parents, the makeup of the planning group included service providers, parents of young children with mental health issues, and adolescents who had received mental health services.

TABLE 2.4.
Values' Shift by Including Families in Activity Settings

Persons involved	Values
Service providers prior to family involvement	• We are the experts • We know what is best for families • Families must not see our weaker side and know our decision-making process • It is important to have all our ducks in a row before we approach families so that we will not upset them
Families seeking family involvement in decision making	• Our experiences with the service system are valuable • We have a role to play in making plans for ourselves and other families • We will ensure that service providers hear our voices in the development of service models
Service providers and families as they work together as a coordinated team	• We are part of a team • We each know some of the answers, but we do not know all the answers ourselves • It is important to understand the perspective of parents and people who are receiving services from programs in order for all of us together to make them better

Table 2.4 suggests the shifts in values as parents become involved in the process. The values expressed by the service providers both implicitly and explicitly prior to involving parents included comments such as the following: "We are the experts. We know what is best for families. Families must not see our weaker side and know our decision-making process. It is important for us to have all our ducks in a row before we approach families so that we will not upset them." After having parents involved, the implicit and explicit values expressed by the service providers reflected views such as: "We are part of a team. We know some of the answers, but we do not know all of the answers ourselves. It is important to understand the perspective of parents and people who are receiving services from our programs in order for us together to make them better." Values implicitly and explicitly expressed by the parents included such ideas as: "Our experiences with the systems are valuable. We have a role to play in making plans for ourselves and other families. We will ensure that service providers hear our voices and that the development of service models will address these values and concerns."

This example exemplifies why constituent involvement is so important. Not only do families feel more comfortable knowing that their voices are heard, but service systems cannot do their jobs correctly without such input. It has been the voices of such family-driven groups as *Federation for Children with Special Needs, Family Voices, Family Resource Centers*, and so forth, who have thoughtfully, but assertively changed the rules in decision making with respect to children with special needs. Other examples of this paradigm in action have been the evolution of meaningful parent involvement within local Head Start programs.

Prior to having parents involved, the operations and task demands for service providers included attending meetings, giving input as a team member, and making decisions as well as implementing those decisions. After parents were involved, the parents and the service providers together shared roles of attending the meetings, providing input acting as a team member, making decisions, and implementing those decisions. Service providers, prior to having families involved, included bringing information from their program to the meetings, conveying information from the meetings back to their program, and implementing policy changes as they felt necessary within their own programs as a function of the discussions at the planning meetings. They were to inform families of decisions as they were made without accepting or requesting feedback.

Scripts for conduct for families at the point were to be compliant—to do what they were advised so that their child would get better by following the instructions of the professionals within their individual programs. After parents were involved, the scripts for conduct for both changed dramatically. The scripts for conduct for the professional included respecting the family as an equal partner, ensuring that the family's points of view were heard, particularly in the meetings, and to act as a facilitator for families as they came to the meetings to help them feel comfortable in their new roles. The families, at the same time, provided input into the decision-making process, helped set the goals, and expressed their family preferences with respect to how services should be provided.

Prior to family involvement, the purpose of professionals attending the planning meeting was to create a system of mental health services for families with children. After having families involved, the purpose of the group was to create a system of mental health services with families that were maximally useful to families and most efficient for service providers in the community.

As can be seen in this example, constituent involvement in program development is an important component of community development. It builds capacity within both the service system and families to interact with one another in a different way and makes the services that have been provided the most meaningful to families over time. Though in this example, parent involvement has worked to the betterment of the operation of the committee, the transition from service provider dominated to equal partnerships within the policy level of systems development is not always this smooth. Families who have been excluded from having their voices heard in the policy arena frequently take an adversarial role toward the system in order to begin the process.

Principle Three: Respect for Cultural Norms and Practices

An ecocultural model, by its nature, incorporates cultural values of families and the community as a principle in a system of care. Families come to interact with the service system with a set of cultural beliefs and attitudes that affect the way that they understand the problem, expect to be treated, interact with service providers and other staff, and the types of outcomes they anticipate as possible. Many times, these belief systems and attitudes are quite different from those represented by the service providers themselves. This duality in the service system, that contrasts parents and family expectations and beliefs to those of the service system providers, have been discussed in a number of contexts (e.g., Cross, Bazron, Dennis, and Issacs, 1989; Roberts, Rule and Innocenti, 1998). For families to effectively participate in programs at both the individual family level and at the systems level within a community, services have to be offered in a way that makes sense within the context of their cultural and ecocultural characteristics.

This issue has become more visible within the last two decades as the changing demographics of the United States reflect a more diverse cultural heritage. For instance, the U.S. Congress has estimated by 2010 nearly one quarter of all children living in the United States will be children of color (U.S. Dept. of Health and Human Services, 1985). Likewise, Zeller (1986) predicts that by the year 2000, one third of the U.S. population will be composed of minority populations. In a recent report by NEC*TAS, Edmunds, Martinson, and Goldberg (1990) suggests that in the 21st century, the population of the United States will be closer to the world balance of ethnically diverse populations. Thus, our Eurocentric concepts of health, disability, parenting, intervention, and authority relationships within a family will not serve us well. As described by Kavanagh and Kennedy (1992),

> Concern by health care providers at the challenge of providing appropriate care to increasingly diverse consumer populations has prompted greater exploration of ways to tailor care to the client's needs. There is a parallel effort to eliminate practices and policies that require consumers of health care to adapt and conform to a limited set of norms and values in order to utilize resources. (p. 1)

Though a variety of terms such as cultural diversity, cultural sensitivity, and cultural awareness have been used to describe the need to address issues of culture in services, this volume uses the term "cultural competence." Roberts and colleagues (1990), for instance, defined cultural competence as:

> A program's ability to honor and respect those beliefs, interpersonal styles, attitudes, and behaviors of both the families who are clients and the multi cultural staff who are providing services. The use of the word "competence" has gained ascendance in the field because it has felt that competence applies more than beliefs, attitudes, and tolerance though it also includes them. Competence also implies skills which help to translate beliefs, attitudes, and orientation into action and behavior. (p. 1)

This construct is quite similar to that supported by the Minority Initiative Resource Committee of the Child and Adolescent Service Support project. Cross and colleagues (1989) define cultural competence as a set of congruent behaviors, attitudes, and policies that come together in a system, agency, or among professionals to work effectively in cross-cultural situations.

Importantly, however, culture is not the only variable to consider in constructing programs. Within an ecocultural model, the ecology of families is equally important. Culture is not expressed as a univariate theme within any one group. Weisner, Gallimore and Jordan (1993) have posited that the heterogeneity within cultural groups with respect to the practice of particular cultural stereotypes is more likely the norm than one homogeneous way that cultural stereotypes are expressed. For example, Weisner, Gallimore and Jordan (1993), in their work on sibling caretaking in Hawaiian families, described it as a strong cultural stereotype though the heterogeneity among individual families with respect to how this was practiced was quite broad.

Two examples are given in describing how ecocultural issues affect services. In the first example, an ethnographic study of disability has been conducted recently with Navajo families of children in early intervention programs on the Navajo reservation. In the second example, a model of providing services to young children in a culturally competent way is discussed using the traveling preschool concept that has been developed with native Hawaiian families.

Disability within a Navajo framework

Using a model of ecocultural assessment developed by Weisner and colleagues (1993) and adapted by Begay, Roberts, Weisner, and Matheson (1996), Navajo parents of young children with disabilities eligible for the Part C system under the Individuals with Disabilities Education Act (IDEA) on the Navajo reservation were interviewed. Clear patterns emerged from this discussion with families that suggested significant culture-specific ways that Navajo families in general viewed both the disability and their interactions with health care providers, whether they were traditional healers, Indian Health Service staff, or state employees of the early intervention programs.

Spiritual support was sought during times of crisis in which a child needed to be hospitalized, often off the reservation. One mother described her situation and the two kinds of spiritual support her family gave:

> He just got weak and we didn't know what to do, so we took him to the hospital over here [Indian Health Service] and I was up that night...they told me I had to go into Phoenix [with him].... Then my grandfather was down there and he helped me. He prayed for the baby and me, and about a week later he [the child] was sitting up. Then my side of the family left and I think they had ceremonies and all that done for the baby cause they asked me for his pictures and all that, and his little clothes.

In the above example, spiritual support is interconnected with family support, medical services, and the extended family's resources.

Spiritual support helped families in many different ways. Parents perceived that ceremonies helped their child to improve physically or developmentally. Another benefit mentioned was that all types of spiritual services helped the family to accept and deal with their child's disability. In addition to emotional support, spiritual services also worked to provide instrumental support for families, and helped them to feel better about complying with medical procedures.

As an example, ceremonial healing helped the family to relieve their misgivings and, therefore, increased their compliance with the medical system while their child was in a hospital. A prayer ceremony made them feel much better about the medical procedures, and they felt that the ceremonies helped to protect their child from harm during an operation:

> The next morning they [husband and son] took back off to come up [to the reservation] to have more prayers done traditionally. We [mother and child] stayed in the hospital and we told them [doctors] to go ahead [with the operation].

In another family, the mother avoided the service providers who had set up appointments for therapy with her son; the service providers could not understand why she did this. The mother explained,

> You know, to me he knows what he's doing like when he wants something, so sometimes I think that I don't really have a Down's and I'm just waiting for him to start walking and start talking. That's what I'm waiting for, you know. I always wondered when he's going to really start walking. At what age, you know. Two, three, you know. I know it's going to take time. I just have to have the patience for that.

This mother acknowledges that her child is delayed, but does not feel she can do anything to hurry him. She feels that patience is the best thing she can provide. She also feels that the outside service providers who come to her house mark her as having a Down's syndrome child. The mother talks about how her other children take care of her son,

> They're really enjoying him, you know. He gets all the caring and he knows when he's going to get all that attention too. The twelve-year-old, she really helps me out. She knows what he's going through. She does treatment. She helps me out with doing treatment on him sometimes. I'm proud of her you know.

Ecological supports are important as well. Examples of indigenous supports and services commonly found in all families are: baby sitting or emergency childcare, emotional support, financial and other instrumental help such as food gifts for ceremonies, wood chopping, coal and water hauling, meal preparation, livestock care including purchasing and hauling hay, and transportation to agencies for formal services and to shopping, as well as shopping for needed items such as dog food, diapers, or baby formula for family members.

In obtaining indigenous support, most of the families engaged in the same activities as Navajo families without children with disabilities. In examining indigenous support systems, we do not want to give the impression that these systems are inherently better than bureaucratic support systems, or that bureaucratic programs are unnecessary because indigenous systems already exist. Nothing could be further from the reality of the situation. In our interviews with families there are many, many examples of parents who said that they were grateful for services that existed, and that they would not have been able to manage without them. Positive comments about the bureaucratic system were echoed by nearly all of the families.

These findings have powerful messages for service providers from bureaucratic systems within health, social services, and education. Stated in simple terms, these messages are:

1. Indigenous systems are constructed in response to enduring cultural and ecological constraints. They are sufficiently forceful that they

are not easily altered without serious consequences to family well-being.

2. Bureaucratic systems will be most helpful to families when services they provide honor, respect, and support indigenous models of belief and interaction. To do otherwise creates conflict and necessitates further accommodations from families already experiencing high levels of stress. The goal of such programs should be to fit into the indigenous system and require as few accommodations as possible consistent with the mutually agreed upon goals of child and family well-being.

Traveling preschool in a cultural context

The second example comes from work reported by Roberts (1993a) in an earlier volume within this Advances in Applied Developmental Psychology series, *Coming Home to Preschool: The Sociocultural Context of Early Education*. In this example, a program was explicitly developed to assist native Hawaiian families in providing educational experiences for themselves and their children, prenatal to five. The model began prenatally with home visiting, moving to a traveling preschool for two- and three-year-old children, and then to center-based preschools for four-year-old children. Support provided to families should be congruent with their cultural beliefs and attitudes, sustainable within their everyday activities, and meaningful within the context of their goals for their families and their children. The goal was not to teach Hawaiian families how to raise their children. Rather, it was to provide activity settings that maximized good learning environments for young children and families within the cultural context of the family in normal everyday activities as opposed to separate institutional settings. At the same time, as Roberts (1993b) has said elsewhere, "It was neither possible nor desirable to mirror all the components of Hawaiian interactions in the school or intervention setting" (p. 527). The business of school and the business of a family were different. They had different goals and the means through which these goals were met were different as well. At a minimum it was important that they did not work at cross-purposes and the school or the learning activities were able to build on that which the home environment provided. Our work in the traveling preschool then was to create activity settings with families that honored this concept to its fullest. The traveling preschool was a two-day-per-week, two-hour-per-day, preschool that was set up in parks, churches, beach fronts, and any open space that could be used in a safe manner with young children. One teacher was present and the preschool came in a van driven by the teacher. As the van pulled up to the parking lot of the selected site, families helped the teacher set up the preschool on large mats in a confined area. Usually there were between 20 and 40 children at each preschool and as many as 8 to 20 adults as well. Each child needed to be accompanied by his or her caretaker for that day. That caretaker could have been an auntie, a mother, a babysitter, or childcare worker. It was important that these activity settings be set up in such a way that they did not violate the patterns of interactions familiar to families. However, at the same time, children would be exposed to new concepts and new learning environments. The adults became active participants in the learning process with children in particular ways that made sense within Hawaiian culture. An example is taken from Roberts (1993b) to described how this worked:

> A description of how a finger-painting activity worked out one morning in the traveling preschools is instructive. Five or six children, ages two to five, sat around on two large lauhala mats which contained all of the paper and painting materials. Three adults sat interspersed throughout the group of children. As the activity progressed, the children talked among themselves and got involved with the materials. The adults carried on a separate conversation while they watched their children play. The child-regulated conversation was mostly concerned with the how and what of the finger-painting activity. They shared materials and talked out loud about what they were drawing. The parents' conversation involved material unrelated to the preschool activity. It was apparent, however, that the adults were also aware of the children's behavior and would comment on the progress of the activity from time to time. One parent commented on the colors that her daughter was using while another said, "Nice fish you draw, Keani." It was clear that the children at quite a young age could interact with one another, decide for themselves how they were going to become involved in the task, share a limited amount of resources, and enjoy themselves without major adult-specific direction. At the same time, the presence of the adults may have kept the children on task and from wandering off to other activities. The parents were clearly engaged with their children from the short interchanges. Parents could see for themselves the skills of their children without becoming overly directive. (pp. 527-528)

In a more controlled study, Roberts and Barnes (1993) found a similar pattern of interaction within laboratory tasks between Hawaiian mothers and their four-year-old children. Thus, the activity settings that were set up within this construct incorporated information about parent and child scripts for interaction to provide a comfortable and culturally appropriate activity setting for learning.

The Navajo examples described above draw the issue of culture as a defining variable into high relief and point to the need for bureaucratic systems of care and support to *first* understand these important powerful issues before and during services development. The Traveling Preschool example demonstrates that both the activity setting model and culture are important elements to understand in the actual implementation of a program.

Both of these examples not only demonstrate the need to attend to Value Number 3, "Respect for Cultural Norms and Practices," but also show how each of the principles work interactively. Since cultural stereotypes do not predict individual family circumstances or beliefs, programs cannot ignore the need to be individually responsive or to involve constituents in the planning and implementation phases. Each principle is a part of the proverbial elephant described by the blind men as they are all needed and all part of a whole, healthy system.

Principle Four: Accessibility

Planning a community-base of services does not necessarily imply that the services that are available are accessible to families. That is, accessibility implies more than that the services are physically located within the community. It implies that the services are both psychologically available to families, physically available to families, and financially available to families over time. In addition, the services within the community must make sense and address particular needs that families have expressed in order for them to be relevant and used. An example of this accessibility issue can be demonstrated in work by Roberts and Wasik (1996) in which the Community Integrated Service System Programs were described and analyzed. These programs were developed by the Maternal and Child Health Bureau to help communities develop a more integrated system of care for families with very young children. In one particular example, a local hospital was concerned that though it was close to a series of migrant camps, mothers who worked in the migrant program did not avail themselves of free prenatal care and appropriate well-child primary care available through the hospital. Appropriately, as part of the grant activity, the service providers from the hospital visited and worked with parents from the migrant camps to better understand the needs of pregnant women as a way of starting to redesign their services. As the discussions ensued, it became apparent that though the services were quite accessible to families who had transportation, the services were not accessible to families from the migrant camp even though the distance between the migrant camps and the hospital was not great. The free, public transportation bus that passed through the migrant camps did not go anywhere near the hospital. Over time, the hospital worked with the transportation system in that community and routes were developed that routinely went from the migrant camps to the hospital. Miraculously, the number of migrant women who began to receive prenatal care and use the well-baby clinics improved dramatically (Roberts & Wasik, 1996).

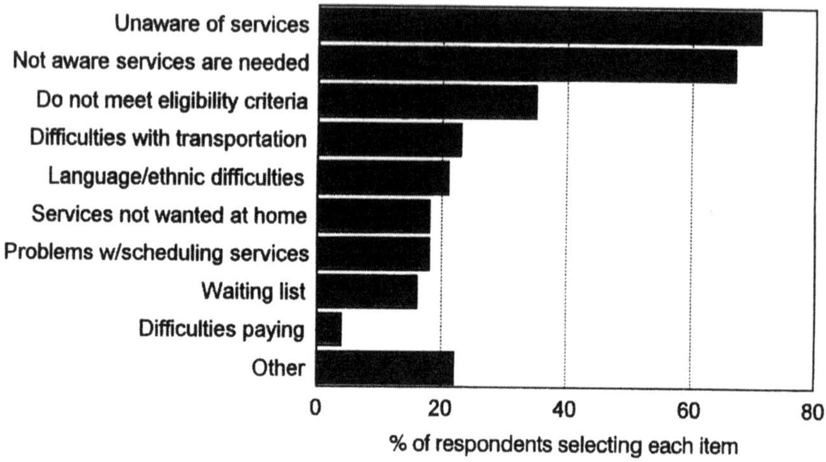

FIGURE 2.3. Major factors preventing families for using services. Reprinted with permission from Roberts, Akers, and Behl (1996).

Therefore, when we think about accessibility within the community context, we must think about accessibility as a function of family involvement, cultural competence of service providers, the meaningfulness, sustainability, and congruence of the proposed activities with families' lives and the differences among families' living conditions that may predict their ability to use one type of service or another. In a recent study of family-level service coordination efforts within early intervention programs (Part C-IDEA) (Roberts et al., 1996), agencies were asked to identify major factors preventing families from using their services. Figure 2.3 presents their responses. By far, the major factors were lack of public awareness with respect to availability of services and what those services might be able to do to help them with their children.

Principle Five: Affordability

The United States had developed a patchwork of private and public funding for services and supports for families with young children. With the continuing devolution of responsibility moving to the states and closer to communities, the promise of more rational, noncategorical funding models for public dollars has a chance of being tried in some communities and states. Block grant programs are increasingly popular, which can add flexibility to potential funding sources. In addition, new federal programs are being developed which have an impact on the affordability of services to families. For example, the recent Children's Health Insurance Plan (CHIP) now provides funding at the state level for families with children who do not qualify for Medicare/Medicaid, yet are also not eligible for private health insurance through their employers. In most states and communities, this program will provide a safety net for what has been known as the gap-group of children who have been uninsured.

At the same time, welfare reform at the federal and state levels has already had an impact on income levels for very poor families. Though many families are leaving the welfare roles through state reform efforts and the Temporary Assistance to Needy Families Program (TANFP), these families face additional challenges in affordability of childcare and other work-related expenses. Communities face many challenges with respect to welfare reform in developing appropriate funding sources for newly employed families. In addition to childcare and health insurance, other issues include transportation, job education skills, training, and sufficient stable jobs at a living wage above the poverty line as examples.

The combination of private and public funding to make the support network sufficiently available to all families in a community is a complex task which must be worked out at each level in the system. Families, for instance, in developing IFSPs, need to know where the funding will be coming from for each of the services listed. In some programs, this is more automatic (e.g., Part C IDEA) than others. In a recent study by Williams and colleagues (1991) many funding sources were identified as potential payers for Part C services. At the community level, the categorical nature of funding continues to thwart efforts to make services more affordable by allowing for some flexibility in providing exactly what a family needs rather than what a diagnosis requires. As noted earlier, some block grants assist in this effort but not very consistently. A recent survey of early intervention programs found that only 16 percent used blended or braided funding to make services more accessible and affordable to families (Akers, Roberts, & Behl, 1998). States continue to be challenged with federal regulations which require categorical funding streams as well. Though private dollars through foundations and community fundraising efforts help in providing services, the social contract requires that the state provide for its citizens' welfare at least at the level of coordination and insuring appropriate safety nets for its youngest citizens.

Principle Six: Collaboration and Coordination with Families and Across Service Agencies

The final principle to be discussed involves the basic issue of collaboration and service coordination. Almost every chapter in this book addresses this issue at one level or another. Rather than repeating many of the issues that are described in more detail throughout other sections, some of the basic concepts will be described here. The concepts of service coordination are used to describe a number of different but convergent ideas. Such terms as cooperation, collaboration, coordination, and integration refer to similar but somewhat different constructs. In the chapter on evaluation by Innocenti and Roberts, a continuum of service integration is discussed and suggests the inter-relationships among these terms. The differences tend to center on how formalized the relationships are among agencies and how autonomous each agency may be. The definition of service coordination is developed by Roberts, Rule, and Innocenti (1998) states that:

> Service coordination occurs at several levels within a system and refers to the ability of public and private agencies to work together with each other and with families in a manner that ensures that services are provided in the most effective and efficient manner possible by avoiding duplication and enhancing information exchange. (p. 49)

Though specifics of service coordination will be discussed individually within a variety of chapters, a model taken from Wood and Gray (1991) is used to describe the collaboration process. Wood and Gray suggest that collaboration "occurs when a group of autonomous stakeholders of a problem domain engage in an interactive process using shared goals, norms, and structures to act or decide upon issues related to that domain" (p. 146).

Obviously within the model that we present here, this collaboration process occurs both at the family level, developing individual services, and at the systems level. At both levels, all stakeholders must be involved in decision making, including families, members of the community, and service providers. Wood and Gray (1991) define a comprehensive theory of collaboration, which is suggested in Table 2.5.

The example given earlier of a group of mental health professionals learning to work together and with families at the systems level is an example of horizontal integration and collaboration. Agencies within a community, for instance, work toward reducing redundancy and making the system more efficient in the way that services are available.

Another example from the CISS projects referred to earlier in the discussion on accessibility (Roberts & Wasik, 1993) is an example of how vertical integration can be either helpful or problematic. Community agencies discussed their relationship with state-level agencies from two perspectives. Either the relationship was one in which information

TABLE 2.5.
Toward a Comprehensive Theory of Collaboration

- "Convening power," that is, the ability to induce stakeholders to participate
- Legitimacy among the stakeholders, who must perceive that the convener has the "authority to organize the domain"
- An unbiased, even-handed approach to the problem domain, to prevent the convener from losing credibility in the eyes of the stakeholders
- Appreciative, envisioning, and process-oriented skills, meaning that the convener must "appreciate the potential value of collaborating" and must be able to "envision a purpose to organizing the domain" and establish a collaborative process and context
- The ability to identify all relevant stakeholders, who must have legitimacy and thus "be perceived by others to have the right and the capacity to participate" in the collaboration

Source: Wood and Gray (1991).

flowed easily in both directions and the community level programs felt a great deal of support from their state level sponsors in being able to suggest creative solutions and try new approaches or the opposite was true. Some programs reflected the theme that they were only able to be creative and get their jobs done if they never told the state-level agencies what they were doing. It was only through reducing contact to a bare minimum that they could move forward in systems development because the state system was felt to be more likely to throw up road blocks and regulations that made it difficult to change systems. From the perspective of the community base of services, the roles of bureaucratic bodies at other levels of the administrative structure are to assist and support the activity at the most proximal level to the family and child—that of the community. Top down strategies, to the extent that they are helpful, help to formulate policies that ensure some fairness and equality in how systems operate and that outcomes are being achieved that reflect the social good.

Much has already been said about collaboration at the family level in the earlier description of family-centered care. Other chapters such as those by Akers and Behl (Chapter 10) and Boyce and colleagues (Chapter 11) elaborate on the issues of collaboration in much more detail.

CONCLUSION

When applied psychologists and other human service providers begin to work with families with young children, we frequently design programs that match where we live as professionals as opposed to where children and families live as people. This chapter has illustrated some of the issues that need to be addressed as we more closely consider the need to work in collaboration with families in communities. As we do so, we are more able to foster the supports families can use based on the reality of their present circumstances.

This transfer from professional-dominated to community-focused supports is a movement that has promise but a considerable way to go before becoming a reality. First, to step back and listen to family stories in the manner suggested in this chapter and by other work exemplified by Weisner and colleagues (1993) as well as Dunst and colleagues (1998) is an important first step. A second step is to examine our knowledge about what works in a more logical and systematic way. As an example of this strategy, over the course of the last several years, staff at the Early Intervention Research Institute (EIRI), in collaboration with staff at other universities and families across the country, have been developing and testing models of intervention that address the issue of the relationship among background variables, intervention variables, and outcome variables (Guralnick, 1997; Roberts, Innocenti & Goetze, 1997, 1998; Roberts & Wasik, 1993). Figure 2.4 presents the schematic that outlines the suggested relationship between these variables. In brief, the background variables, which include child, family, and community character-

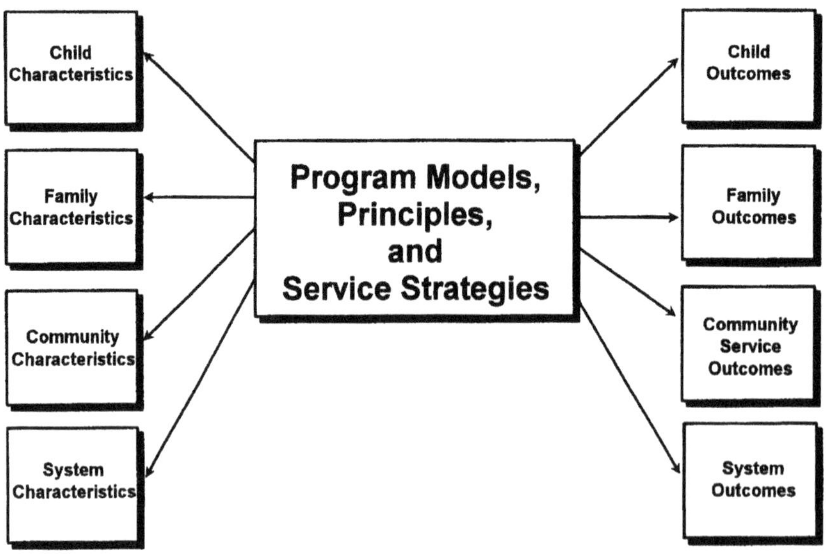

FIGURE 2.4. Conceptualization of relationships for program projects. Reprinted with permission from Roberts and Wasik (1996).

istics, should predict the type of treatment or support suggested, which should in turn be related to the outcomes for children, families, and community.

Surprisingly, even in some of the more sophisticated published studies, these relationships are not apparent in the rationale for the intervention or the reason that the target population has been selected. As an example, in a recent meta-analysis of home visiting programs, the primary selection criterion for including families as subjects in the studies was the income level of the family based on family size for a subsample of 50 of the 150 studies in the overall meta-analysis. The dominant focus of treatment, however, which was provided for these families, was a once-per-week home visiting program aimed primarily at providing child development information and family support to prevent child abuse and neglect. One of the most frequently occurring outcome measures for the 50 studies was the cognitive growth scores of the children whose families were involved in the studies. As an overall pattern, no logical connections were typically found within the introduction nor the subject selection sections of these articles with respect to the presumed relationships among poverty, gaining knowledge on child development and child abuse prevention, and cognitive gain scores of young children (Roberts & Morris, 1994). With respect to these studies, one is reminded of a favorite quote of a friend of children who once said, "I've never heard of anyone being serviced out of poverty."

Though these studies tell us much about the effects (or lack thereof) of home visiting programs, they tell us relatively little about creating programs in partnership with constituents, which can make a difference within the ecocultural worlds in which families live. As we document system reform efforts throughout early childhood programs, it is hoped that this next generation of programs more closely honor the principles set out here and in a number of the chapters in this book. For the stories and the knowledge that can be gained as families allow human service providers into their world is worth its weight a thousand times over in our ability to provide supports where and how children live.

REFERENCES

Akers, A. L., Roberts, R. N., & Behl, D.D. (1998). The use of blended and flexible funding in Part C programs at the community level. *Infants and Young Children, 11*, 46-51

Bailey, D., & Simeonsson, R. (1988). *Family assessment in early intervention*. Ohio: Merrill Publishing Company.

Begay, R. C., Roberts, R. N., Weisner, T. S., & Matheson, C. (1996, April). *Indigenous and informal systems of support for Navajo families who have children with disabilities*. Address presented at U.S.-Mexico Symposium on Disabilities, University of Arizona, Tucson.

Bernheimer, L. P., Gallimore, R., & Weisner, T. S. (1990). Ecocultural theory as a context for the individual family service plan. *Journal of Early Intervention 14*(3), 219-233.

Bernheimer, L. P., & Keogh, B. K. (1995). Weaving interventions into the fabric of everyday life: An approach to family assessment. *Topics in Early Childhood Special Education, 15*(4), 415-433.

Brofenbrenner, U. (1979). *The ecology of human development*. Cambridge, MA: Harvard University Press.

Coleman, J. S. (1988). Social capital in the creation of human capital. *American Journal of Sociology, 9*, S95-S120.

The Council (1998). *Your organizational systems at work*. Townson, MD: The Council on Quality and Leadership in Supports for People with Disabilities.

Cross, T., Bazron, B., Dennis, K., & Isaacs, M. (1989). *Towards a culturally competent system of care: A monograph on effective services for minority children who are severely emotionally disturbed*. Washington, DC: Georgetown University Child Development Center.

Denzin, N. K., & Lincoln, Y. S. (1994). *Handbook of qualitative research*. Thousand Oaks, CA: Sage Publications

Dunst C., & Bruder, M. B., Trivette, C. M., Raab, M., Hamby, D. W., & McLean, M. (1998). *Natural learning environments for infants, toddlers and preschoolers with or at-risk for delays*. Unpublished manuscript.

Dunst, C., Johansen, C., Trivette, C., & Hamby, D. (1991). Family-oriented early intervention policies and practices: Family-centered or not? *Exceptional Children, 58*(2), 115-126.

Edmunds, P., Martinson, S. A., & Goldberg, P. (1990). *Demographics and cultural diversity in the 1990s: Implications for services to young children with special needs*. Chapel Hill, NC: NEC*TAS. (ERIC Document Reproduction Services No. ED 325 565)

Furstenberg, F. F., & Hughes, M. E. (1997). The influence of neighborhoods on children's development: A theoretical perspective and a research agenda. In R. M. Hauswer, B. V. Brown, & W. R. Prosser (Eds.), *Indicators of children's well-being* (pp. 328-345). New York: Russell Sage Foundation.

Gallimore, R., Goldenberg, C. N., & Weisner, T. S. (1993). The social construction and subjective reality of activity settings: Implications for community psychology. *American Journal of Community Psychology, 21*(4), 537-559.

Gallimore, R., Weisner, T. S., Bernheimer, L. P., Guthrie, D., & Nihira, K. (1993). Family responses to young children with developmental delays: Accommodation of activity in ecological and cultural context. *American Journal on Mental Retardation, 98*, 185-206.

Guralnick, M. J. (1997). *The effectiveness of early intervention*. Baltimore, MD: Brookes.

Jencks, C., & Mayer, S. (1990). The social consequences of growing up in a neighborhood. In L. E. Lynn & M. G. H. McGeary (Eds.). *Inner-city poverty in the United States* (pp. 111-186). Washington, DC: National Academy Press.

Kavanagh, K. H., & Kennedy, P. H. (1992). *Promoting cultural diversity: Strategies for health care professionals*. Beverly Hills, CA: Sage.Kotlowitz, A. (1991). *There are no children here*. New York: Doubleday

Maslow, A. H. (1954). *Motivation and personality*. New York: Harper & Brothers.

O'Donnell, C. R., Tharp, R. G., & Wilson, K. (1993). Activity settings as the unit of analysis: A theoretical basis for community intervention and development. *American Journal of Community Psychology, 21*, 501-520.

Roberts, R. N. (Ed.) (1993a). *Coming home to preschool: The sociocultural-context of early education*. Norwood, NJ: Ablex.

Roberts, R N. (1993b). Early education as community intervention: Assisting an ethnic minority to be ready for school. *American Journal of Community Psychology, 21*, 521-535.

Roberts, R. N., Akers, A. L., & Behl, D. D. (1996). Family-level service coordination within home visiting programs. *Topics in Early Childhood Special Education, 16*, 279-301.

Roberts, R. N., Barclay-McLaughlin, G., Cleveland, J., Colston, W., Malach, R., Mulvey, L., Rodriguez, G., Thomas, T., & Yonemitsu, D. (1990). *Monograph and workbook: Developing culturally competent programs for children with special needs*. Logan, UT: Early Intervention Research Institute, Developmental Center for Handicapped Persons, Utah State University. Prepared by Georgetown University Child Development Center, Washington, DC.

Roberts, R. N., & Barnes, M. L. (1993). Quality and quantity of maternal-child interaction. In R. Roberts (Ed.). *Coming home to preschool: The sociocultural context of early education* (pp. 145-166). Norwood, NJ: Ablex.

Roberts, R. N, Behl, D., & Akers, A. (1998). *Opening Doors into Rural Communities* (# 5 H02 MC 00047-02). Rockville, MD: Bureau of Maternal and Child Health and Resources Development.

Roberts, R. N., & Calkin, R. (1989). *Planning and establishment of family-based education centers (FBEC)* (Grant Final Report. Rockville, MD: Bureau of Maternal and Child Health and Resources Development.

Roberts, R. N., Innocenti, M. S., & Goetze, L. (1997). *By what outcomes should Part H be evaluated at the state level?* Prepared for the Subcommittee on Service Integration and Continuity of Services of the Federal Interagency Coordinating Council, Washington, DC.

Roberts, R. N., Innocenti, M. S., & Goetze, L. D. (in press). Emerging issues from state level evaluations of early intervention programs. Manuscript accepted for publication in *Journal of Early Intervention, 22*.

Roberts, R. N. & Morris, C. H. (1994, December). *Community integrated service systems: Issues in theory and practice*. NCCIP, Zero to Three Conference, Dallas, TX.

Roberts, R. N., Rule, S. & Innocenti, M. S., (1998). *Strengthening the family-professional partnership in services for young children*. Baltimore, MD: Paul H. Brookes.

Roberts, R. N., & Wasik, B. H (1994). *Initial evaluation of 1992 funded community integrated service systems projects* (Grant #: HRSA 93-410 and HRSA 93-506). Rockville, MD: Bureau of Maternal and Child Health and Resources Development.

Roberts, R. N., & Wasik, B. H. (1996). Evaluating the 1992 and 1993 Comunity Integrated Service System Projects. In J. M. Marquart & E. L. Konrad (Eds.), *Evaluating initiatives to integrate human services* (pp. 35-50). San Francisco: Jossey-Bass.

Tharp, R., & Gallimore, R. (1988). *Rousing minds to life*. Cambridge, England: Cambridge University Press.

Tolstoy, L. (1960). *Anna Karenina*. New York: Bantam Books.

Tribe, C. (1982). *Profile of three theories*. Dubuque, IA: Kendall/Hunt Publishing Co.

U. S. Department of Health and Human Services (1985). *Report of the secretary's task force on Black and minority health* (Vol. 1: Executive Summary). Washington, DC: U.S. Government Printing Office.

Weisbourd, B., (1994). The evolution of the family resource movement. In S. L. Kagan & B. Weisbourd (Eds.), *Putting families first: America's family support movement and the challenge of change* (pp. 28-47). San Francisco: Jossey-Bass, Inc.

Weiss, H., & Halpern, R. (1990). *Community-based family support and education programs: Something old or something new*? New York: National Center for Children in Poverty.

Weiss, H. B., & Jacobs, F. H. (Eds.). (1988). *Evaluating family programs*. Hawthorne, NY: Aldine de Gruyter.

Weisner, T. S., & Gallimore, R.G. (1994). Ecocultural studies of families adapting to childhood developmental delays: Unique features, defining differences, and applied implication. In Leskinen, M. (Ed.), *Family in focus. New perspectives on early childhood special education* (pp. 11-25). Jyvaskyla, Finland: University of Jyvaskyla.

Weisner, T. S., Gallimore R., & Jordan C. (1993). Unpackaging cultural effects on classrom learning: Hawaiian peer assistance and child-generated activity. In R. N. Roberts (Ed.), *Coming home to preschool: The sociocultural context of early education* (Vol. 7, pp. 59-90). Norwood, NJ: Ablex.

White, B., Kaban, B., & Attanucci, J. (1979). *The origins of human competence*. Lexington, MA: Lexington Books.

Williams, S., Kates, D. A., Bettenberg, A. F., Black, T., Kaufman, R., & Walsh, S. (1991). *NEC*TAS financing workbook: An interagency process for planning and implementing a financing system for early intervention and preschool services*. Chapel Hill, NC: The National Early Childhood Technical Assistance System, Frank Porter Graham Child Development Center, The University of North Carolina at Chapel Hill.

Wood, D. J., & Gray, B. (1991). Toward a comprehensive theory of collaboration. *Journal of Applied Behavioral Science, 27*(2), 139-162.

Zeller, D. (1986). Demography: Real numbers–Real changes. In C. Moore (Ed.), *Reaching out: Proceedings from a special education symposium on cultural differ-*

ences and parent programs (pp. 5-28). Eugene, OR: Western Regional Resource Center. (ERIC Document Reproduction Service No. ED 284 408).

section II

Issues in Defining Community Support for Programs

Within the ecological models described in Section I, strong community-based systems of care must be supported through the larger ecosystems in which they exist. In Section II, examples of three critical support elements are described in more detail. First, Suzanne Bronheim and Nancy Striffler, in Chapter 3, demonstrate how coalitions of community-based programs form a solid support network to enhance the efforts of each of the individual programs. Similar to the concept of a developmentally appropriate context for families and children to connect families into other networks that can facilitate their growth, communities need a similar support network. The Communities Can Coalition (CCC) is an example of such a national support effort, working at the community level. Such a network serves: 1) to facilitate communication of ideas; 2) as a forum for discussion of common issues; and 3) as a support network and a conduit to help individual communities locate other communities confronting similar concerns. Such a coalition provides another important service in highlighting issues of concern to communities through a more unified rational voice rather than through individual programs only.

A critical support issue for any community base of services is the need to fund programs in ways that are creative while meeting the needs of families in natural contexts. Chapter 4, by Linda Goetze and Susan Mackey Andrews, provides a description of funding models for community services and describes a case study of how these models have been applied in Indiana's early intervention program. Unless models of funding are developed that move beyond categorical and program-specific requirements, the ability of communities to create local solutions to problems and challenges is severely restricted. These issues from the state to the local community level are explored here.

In an experimenting society, the use of evaluation as a tool to both inform and guide program growth is critical. Mark Innocenti and Richard Roberts, in Chapter 5, describe evaluation in this context as "participatory realism." The need for evaluation support at the community level is ever present but increases as federal and state mandates for performance measures and indicators of goal attainment require more systematic attention to this potential source of support. The development of community capacity to participate actively in and structure such evaluation efforts so that their needs are met becomes even more critical.

chapter 3

A National Coalition of Communities

Suzanne M. Bronheim
Nancy Striffler
Georgetown University Child Development Center

Humans are social animals. Interacting with each other and forming groups—families, tribes, communities, working groups—is a critical part of our nature. The importance of social interaction is seen in our very survival and development. We are now learning how critical interaction with others is to the neurological, physical and social development of young children—it is as much a basic nutrient as food (Greenough, 1991; Rymer, 1993). Without social interaction, infants can literally languish and die (Bowlby, 1969). Cooperative behavior and the effective ability to work in groups and support one another has been a key to the survival of our species and allowed us to survive in a broader set of environments than most other complex species—through connecting and working together, we are now even able to survive in the hostile environment of outer space. Our most successful endeavors are those in which we band together to share our expertise and that more intangible ingredient—social support.

THE NEED FOR SOCIAL SUPPORT

The literature that examines the role of social support in our lives is extensive. Suffice it to say for understanding the issues facing communities, that social support is found to have a key role in many realms of human functioning. It is seen by many as key to actual survival of serious illnesses and disabilities (Berkman, 1985; Ganster & Victor, 1988). It has been shown to improve the outcomes for those facing the challenges of disability or other life challenges (Dalgard, Bjork, & Tambs, 1995; Kessler & McLeod, 1985). Social support is seen as an element in enhancing the ability of professionals to serve their clients (Raiser, 1987). Clearly connecting with each other is a potent force in human life.

In the past, most social groups and cooperative work groups have been made up of people who were geographically close and knew each other through naturally occurring connections—family, membership in local institutions such as churches or schools, common heritage, and so forth. They have been based on the commonalities of members and their common needs and experiences. In the past 30 years, however, several phenomenon have expanded our horizons and have supported the development of a new type of social support phenomenon—the issue-specific support group. First, with greater ease in transportation and communication, we have become a mobile nation—thus individuals and families no longer necessarily live close to other family members or in their communities of origin and can be disconnected from natural support systems. People have become more inclined, out of need, to turn to strangers, whom they perceive as sharing some common need or goal, to find the social connections and support they need to thrive. At the same time, this greater ease in traveling and communicating over greater distances has enlarged the definition of potential "community" or support group. As social commentators decry the decline of community in general, human social animals have been busy creating synthetic groups to meet their needs, particularly when faced with difficult and unknown challenges. The enormous popularity of connecting with others on the Internet is testimony to this creativity in fulfilling our needs for social connection. In relation to young children with or at risk for disabilities, there has been a steady growth of such support groups and organizations.

Communities Need Support Too

Communities or, perhaps more accurately, the groups of people in communities working to build a system of services and supports for children, including young children with disabilities and their families, are also very much in need of the types of support that banding together can bring. The networking they need, however, is different—it is not person-to-person, but community-to-community. Yet the reasons they need to network for support and the benefits they gain from such networking are identical to those that have driven the development of issue-specific support groups and networks for families, for professionals, for government officials and consumers. To understand how a support network for communities works, it is helpful to first understand the concepts of how support groups work for individuals. Then one can apply these same principles to support communities that are trying to build integrated systems of services and supports for young children and their families.

Why Support Groups And Networks Form

There are several functions that support groups or support networks provide for their members that may go beyond the typical benefits of being part of a work or social group. These new synthetic support groups arise when natural supports are not sufficient to meet the needs of the members. This failure of natural supports can occur for a number of reasons including:

1. *The problem being faced is new or relatively rare and few others within the natural support system have any experience or expertise to lend to the effort.* For example, when families began taking home very sick children who were technologically dependent, there was no common wisdom to offer them and experiences of other parents were in many ways not related to nor applicable to the experiences these families faced. There might be only one child in a community with these needs, so that nobody within that child's extended family, their religious institutions, social network or even professional support network had any experience or expertise to offer.
2. *There is some characteristic about the individuals needing support that puts them outside the naturally occurring group.* Families who are not from the dominant cultural group in their community, or who do not speak the dominant language of the community, may find it difficult to access many of the possible supports and groups within that community. As a result, they may often seek to develop their own networks of support. Another example might be single fathers of children with disabilities who are often not naturally included in the groups of mothers who may meet and support each other at special programs or clinics (May, 1991, 1992).
3. *The problem faced is in some way caused by or a by-product of the behaviors, attitudes or institutions of the natural community or support group.* A classic example of this type of issue is that of inclusion of those with disabilities within our communities. Policies and architectural barriers as well as prejudices about people who were seen as needing protection rather than inclusion left individuals with disabilities needing

support and connections to help them change the naturally occurring social institutions and groups within their communities and throughout the nation. In the early days of the women's movement, special support groups were a common mechanism.

So strong is the human need for social support and having a group within which to function and work when facing challenges, that the phenomenon of the synthetic or special-issue support group has blossomed. It is the modus operandi for family members who have a member with some special need or circumstance—parents of children with special needs, siblings of children with disabilities, children of older parents who now must become caretakers of family members who are disabled or demented, or parents of children who are adopted here or overseas (Gibbs, 1993; Shelton & Smith-Stepanek, 1994). There are even support groups for people who face a challenge so unusual that there may not be enough other people in the world to build a support group, such as the National Organization of Rare Disorders (NORD). Professionals serving children with disabilities and their families or other specialized groups also band together in support groups. There are formal national organizations that provide general support and advocacy for professions, but there is a plethora of specialized groups within those groups to create a support for professionals dealing with very specific and sometimes unusual challenges. For example, there are special organizations for minority members of particular professions; psychologists who serve children with chronic illnesses or other physical problems; and so forth. On the informal level, professionals create support groups as well—for example special education teachers within an area creating a support network to help them address the teaching challenges that they face in their community that other teachers may not (Raiser, 1987). Even agencies and government officials find this need to create special groups to help them meet their challenges. There are special organizations for State Directors of Special Education, for county executives, for state Maternal and Child Health Directors, and there is even an organization of organization directors, the American Society of Association Executives.

How Do Support Groups and Networks Function?

What do support networks and groups provide that is so compelling? This process of connecting provides a number of functions that are important to individuals, families or communities facing new, unusual or particularly difficult situations. The functions served by support networks address emotional needs, informational needs and empowerment needs. The ways in which special support groups and networks address emotional needs include:

1. *Decreasing a sense of isolation*: Since those seeking these synthetic groups are typically facing an unusual circumstance, there is a strong sense of "I am alone and the only one in this situation." Given the strong drive to be part of a group that is key to human existence, these feelings of isolation can be overwhelming and add to the despair of facing a difficult situation. This sense of isolation is well articulated by a parent of a young child with a very rare neurological disorder seeking support in the newest incarnation of the support group—the World Wide Web. "Thank you for your Web pages. So often we find that we are on our own....We still feel unique, no one understands or can comprehend the problems" (Fisher, 1998).
2. *Encouragement and inspiration to keep going in the face of great challenges*: when times are difficult, we all need "cheerleaders" and it is most helpful if those urging us to find the strength to persevere have been in a similar situation. Twelve-step programs such as Alcoholics Anonymous utilize this strength of groups—hearing another person's story of struggle and triumph can renew the spirit and give one strength at low moments.
3. *A place to express frustrations and feelings of wanting to give up*: this function is the companion of number two above, but equally critical. It may not be socially acceptable or politically expedient for individuals or even governmental agencies and officials to ever admit publicly that they are tired of the struggle to meet challenges and they really want to give up. Parents of young children with severe disabilities who require constant special care that seems to make any semblance of a "normal" life impossible, may only feel comfortable sharing their feelings of wanting to quit or escape with others who have lived that experience without fearing being labeled an uncaring or bad parent. The ability to express negative emotions and garner support is another important function of specialized support groups.

We are said to live in the information age and we talk about travel down an information highway. For individuals—family members, professionals or agency/government members—facing new or unusual challenges, that highway of information may seem more like a small country lane. There may be limited experience with the challenge and thus little information has been generated or disseminated or there may be such a limited audience for the information that the mainstream institutions that provide information are not interested in working with it. Thus, special support groups provide the critical function of:

4. *Sharing of information and skills that will improve the situation that is not readily available elsewhere*: for example, parents in conversations and books written for the general public naturally share tips and information about how to make it through the challenges of children's needs—what is best for diaper rash or teething, and so forth. For parents of children with special problems, however, there may be no one in their usual support network who has any information about their particular problems and no books on the ever growing shelves at bookstores marked "Parenting." Even professionals who have not had the 24-hour care of a child with a special need may not have the types of information families need—the best place to purchase special equipment, how to handle siblings' needs for attention during the difficult and perhaps time-consuming process of feeding a child with a severe neuromuscular disorder, and so forth. Learning from someone else who has walked the same path and discovered new wisdom related to a very special problem or situation is an invaluable aspect of special issue support groups.

As already noted, sometimes special support groups and networks arise to provide the participants with the sense that they can change the status quo that is not meeting their needs in facing particular challenges and to provide the power that groups have over individuals in advocating for such changes. Thus, two additional functions that support groups and networks provide are:

5. *Providing a sense of empowerment to bring the problems within the status quo to the attention of the general "community" or public*: by talking together and sharing experiences and frustrations, people with a wide range of disabilities developed a sense that they should have the same rights and access to community life that all other citizens enjoyed. They stopped accepting others' definitions of their abilities and roles and became convinced of their own different view. When individuals or groups want to make a change in the way institutions, laws, or communities work, they must first believe in themselves and their cause. Banding together with others enhances that sense of having and using one's voice.
6. *Advocacy to change the system through the strength of a group "voice"*: by joining together families of children with special health care needs from across the country that have become knowledgeable and that articulate about their particular needs within the general world of health care reform, the Family Voices organization has become a highly effective voice to make changes to or build protections into any legislation or policies at the federal and state levels that may

have an impact on their children. By being a strong group voice they are heard in Congress, the White House and in legislatures and state houses throughout the country. At the community level, when a group voice raises concerns about the lack of effective supports for families of young children with disabilities in terms of daycare or recreation, there is a greater chance of that voice being heard than if one family at a time expresses concerns. Perhaps because humans are such social animals, a concern shared by a group is given more credence than that of any one individual. In addition, in a political system such as ours, when large numbers of potential voters are concerned, their voices are listened to more closely.

Why Communities Need a Support Network

Communities that are sincerely working to make all children and families welcome, supported and served within their neighborhoods, towns, counties, cities or regions are facing a set of issues and challenges that meet all the criteria for needing to create a special support network—there are new challenges that require new information, behaviors, attitudes and skills; there are no existing support networks for communities working to meet this challenge; and many of the policies of the federal, state and local governments seem to impede progress towards the goal of building inclusive communities with integrated, coordinated systems and services for families and children

Communities that care for its members galvanize resources to accommodate the needs of families and individuals, so that families can acquire the services that they need in order to be healthy and provide for their children, especially children with disabilities. Communities accomplish this by meeting a set of new and historically different challenges including:

1. Develop and foster *family-centered* services and supports;
2. Center the community around *culturally competent* practices;
3. *Integrate services* and supports;
4. Create an atmosphere where individuals with disabilities and their families are *included*;
5. Create *financing* structures that maximize all available resources;
6. Understand and effectively deal with the *complex and, at times conflicting, federal and state laws and regulations* that relate to community service system development; and
7. Develop and mobilize the *leadership needed to accomplish these tasks.*

Develop and Foster Family-centered Services and Supports

Family-centered care is the:

> philosophy of care in which the pivotal role of the family is recognized and respected in the lives of children with special health needs. Within this philosophy is the idea that families should be supported in their natural care-giving and decision-making roles by building on their unique strengths as people and families. In this philosophy, patterns of living at home and in the community are promoted; parents and professionals are seen as equals in a partnership. To achieve this, elements of family-centered care and community-based care must be carefully interwoven into a full and effective coordination of the care of all children with special health needs (Brewer, McPherson, Magrab, & Hutchins, 1989).

While the importance of this concept has been recognized for well over ten years (Koop, 1987), its implementation remains a challenge in most communities and there is a great need for support to make this new paradigm a reality.

Although the philosophical notion of family support is generally well-accepted among professionals, changing current practices and priorities is difficult (Bailey, McWilliam, Winton, & Simeonsson, 1992). The implementation of family-centered care has proven a challenging task for a number of reasons. First, educators, health care providers, social service personnel, and so forth enter their respective fields out of a desire to work with children and they receive training that is almost exclusively child-focused (Bailey, Simeonsson, Yoder, & Huntington, 1990). Thus many have neither the new information and skills nor the desire to work with families. Communities are also in need of road-maps toward this goal. There is great uncertainty surrounding the actual implementation of a family-centered approach and the how-to-do it. Second, a family-centered philosophy challenges the long-held view of the professional as the primary decision-maker in the management of young children with disabilities, since a fundamental tenet of the family support movement is family choice and a responsiveness to family priorities (Bailey, 1987). Relinquishing control of decisions about the nature and extent of services may be viewed as threatening. Third, professionals work in service-delivery systems designed to provide child-focused services. Finally, barriers may be systemic. They may be in the form of bureaucratic procedures related to scheduling services, the types of services permitted, the type and amount of paperwork required, fee schedules and billing practices, data collection and reporting, or any other number of rules imposed by those governing early intervention services and programs. A provider's efforts to provide quality services may be thwarted by an administrator's rules and regulations. If infrastructure variables are not considered in planning, then no matter how competent a provider is in his or her role as a service provider, the procedural constraints are likely to make quality service implementation impossible. A provider who fills multiple roles may have a clear understanding of the expectations associated with those roles, but may find it difficult to perform those functions due to time demands or other constraints (Saal, 1992). Thus, there are aspects of the existing system that thwart efforts to become family-centered—communities working toward that goal need not only the know-how, but the sense of empowerment and sometimes the advocacy to change the status quo.

Center the Community Around Culturally Competent Practices

"Cultural competence is a set of congruent behaviors, attitudes, and policies that come together in a system, agency, or among professionals and enables this system, agency, or those professionals to work effectively in cross-cultural situations" (Cross, Bazron, Issaacs, & Dennis, 1989, p. iv). Culturally competent communities recognize, respect, and value the uniqueness of individuals and groups whose cultures are different from those associated with mainstream America. Culturally competent services are those perceived by clients as relevant to their problems and priorities and helpful for achieving the desired outcomes (Dana, 1993). To develop such services requires that providers know the cultural norms for appropriate delivery of services to various ethnically and culturally diverse groups. It also requires the planners of services to be responsive to sociopolitical issues relevant to the needs of the various cultures represented in their community.

Communities seeking to develop services and supports that are responsive to all children and families face many challenges. These include: adapting services to differences in family structure, expectations, preferences, and help-seeking behavior; eliminating geographic, linguistic, and other barriers that restrict access to services by consumers of diverse ethnic and cultural backgrounds; avoiding the use of culturally biased diagnostic instruments and approaches; and providing ongoing cultural-competence training for providers. Communities need the support of other communities in sharing the information and skills to accomplish this goals, as well as the encouragement and support to persist in the process of becoming more culturally competent even when the progress may seem slow or difficult.

Integrate Services and Supports

One of the greatest challenges facing communities is changing the way in which services and supports are organized within the community. Too often there is fragmentation—one system or service provider does not communicate with another; families must go from program to program and agency to agency trying to piece together the services and supports they need. Families too often face multiple intake processes and find that eligibility rules make it difficult to consistently keep the services and supports they need. In addition, some communities may have too much of one kind of service and none of another because there is no coordinated and thoughtful planning process. The challenge to the development and implementation of comprehensive, coordinated services that work for all families in a community is great. Adding a program here or a service there will not be enough. To make a real difference, the service-delivery system must be fundamentally altered. "Child and family serving institutions must work together to change fundamentally the way they think, behave, and use their resources" (Melaville, Blank, & Asayesh, 1993).

Communities need to know they are not alone in facing this challenge; they need to be able to share successful and less successful approaches and encourage one another. They can also provide, for each other, the sense of empowerment it takes to significantly change the way a community and its members work together.

Create an Atmosphere Where Individuals with Disabilities and Their Families are Included

The transformation of national policy affecting individuals with developmental disabilities over the past two decades represents one of the great reform movements of our time. Laws and regulations are now in place at the federal level that affirm the rights and fundamental dignity of Americans with disabilities. States have been largely responsible for leadership in meeting the needs of individuals with developmental disabilities, within the context of federal programs and policies. The Developmental Disabilities Task Force of the National Conference of State Legislatures noted many innovations that have been developed at the state and local level. These innovations include supporting people to make personal choices about where and how they live, focusing specially on supporting people in natural settings (Wright, King, & the NCSL Task Force on Developmental Disabilities, 1991). As with the previous challenges described, communities need a great deal of help in having information and skills needed to make this concept a reality. They also need to become empowered as a community to move to inclusiveness. Communities can learn concrete approaches from other communities to plan and implement services and supports needed by children with disabilities and their families so that children and families feel valued, supported, and included in all aspects of community life.

Create Financing Structures that Maximize all Available Resources

Financing services and supports for children and families presents communities with a number of special challenges. The federal government is taking steps to shift responsibility for designing, and funding, supports and services for children and families to states. States, in turn, are shifting more responsibilities to local governments. This shift challenges communities to: build new fiscal, administrative, and management capacities; strengthen partnerships among state and local governments, businesses, and the philanthropic community; find ways to generate new sources of revenue; and develop effective strategies to maximize all existing resources. Strong leadership is needed at the state and community level to foster change and to build the necessary base of support to ensure the permanence of change. It is difficult for any one community to have the knowledge of all potential funding sources, creative ways to share and combine funds, and the best way to organize financing of services for children and families. While each community may develop its own unique approach to financing services, progress toward approaches that promote family-centered, culturally competent and integrated services can be greatly enhanced for communities if they share any knowledge or special expertise they have gleaned with each other. It is the old story of "not reinventing the wheel."

Understand Federal and State Laws and Regulations that Facilitate Community Service Systems Development

Communities across the country are adopting new structures to improve services and supports for children with disabilities and their families. For these communities, collaborative decision making holds the promise of shared responsibility and accountability for achieving results, and more effective use of public and private resources to design and deliver comprehensive, coordinated services that are responsive to all children and families in the community. If communities are to achieve this promise, federal and state governments must work to provide a supportive structure by creating opportunities for collaborative entities to develop, giving them access to resources, and establishing a reasonable system of accountability for results.

Historically, the bulk of public funding for education, health, and social services for young children and their families has been categorical. As pressure mounts for communities to meet the growing demand for comprehensive, coordinated services that are affordable, there is an urgency for federal and state laws that facilitate rather than impede these efforts.

The Balanced Budget Act of 1997, which amends the Social Security Act, provides an example of the potential impact of federal laws on state and community service provision. Title XXI of the Act outlines the State Children's Health Insurance Program (SCHIP) which provides block grants to states and territories to create and expand health insurance to uninsured children, States have great flexibility, whether they expand Medicaid or create new child-health programs. Not only did it create a new child insurance program, the new law gave states significant flexibility under Medicaid. For example, states no longer need waivers for managed care (except for children with special health care needs). This flexibility is enhanced by the federal government's willingness to grant waivers permitting Medicaid innovation, such as charging families premiums on a sliding scale. Similarly, a state choosing to adopt a new child health insurance program can determine payment levels, use managed care, charge families modest amounts, determine which health plans and providers participate in the program, set eligibility rules, and determine benefit levels. However, a state using federal funds to start a new child health insurance program must follow certain basic rules, set forth in new Title XXI of the Social Security Act. States are now facing many important decisions. Should they participate in SCHIP? If they do participate, should they expand Medicaid or create an entirely new program? If states choose to design a new program, how will they determine eligibility, the benefits package, and the delivery system? And how will advocates, families, and local communities become involved in the planning process?

A number of state legislative efforts are providing supports to communities to facilitate the development of coordinated service systems. In Kansas, the Developmental Disabilities Reform Act of 1995 culminated three years of consensus building on state policy. The Act states that it will be the policy of the state to assist people who have developmental disabilities to have

> Services and supports which allow people opportunities of their choosing to increase their independence and productivity, as well as integration and inclusion in the community; access to a range of appropriate services and supports; and the same dignity and respect as people who do not have a developmental disability. (Jaskulski, 1995)

This Act provided communities with legislative authority to redesign their community resources to include a single point of entry and service coordination supports in each region. These were critical steps toward increasing access and coordination of services for individuals with disabilities and their families in each region.

If communities are to truly be the place where policies are implemented and families are best served, then they must become empowered to make their voices heard in the development of the morass of federal and state policies that affect young children and their families. A strong support network of communities within a state can begin to have a voice and impact on how funding, administration and regulation of services for children are legislated and regulated to make sure that policies truly support communities in their efforts to best serve and support families. Just as families must have a voice in policymaking that affects them, so too must communities have a voice in making decisions that affect the way in which they work toward best serving those families. A similar scenario is critical at the federal level. With most legislation regarding services to children with special needs mandating community-based, family-centered, culturally competent, integrated services, it is imperative that communities come together to find a voice that says loudly what it is like trying to implement that vision at the community level in light of current federal laws and regulations. At all policy levels, there are voices for government and agencies, for professionals, now for families, but none for communities—the "organisms" that will be called upon to implement the policy and make it a reality for children and families.

Develop and Mobilize Leadership

In order to meet all the other challenges facing them, communities must identify, develop and mobilize leaders committed to serving families and children in new ways. While natural leaders exist in all communities, these leaders may not have the knowledge or skills to provide the kinds of leadership needed to meet the challenges just articulated here. Efforts are needed to engage and support leaders in communities across the country.

Community leaders in effective communities have learned to:

1. Recognize that the days of the standard one-size-fits-all model are over;
2. Believe in a new way of looking at community development;
3. Understand that community members want to make a meaningful contribution to their community; and

4. Recognize that community members can build upon each other's ideas and experience (Wellins, Byham, & Wilson, 1991).

Development of the special, collaborative type of leadership that it takes to build caring, inclusive communities with family-centered, culturally competent, integrated services and supports for families means that communities must share information and build a networking infrastructure within which they can develop and provide for themselves the formal training and informal mentoring relationships needed to build leadership.

COMMUNITIES SUPPORTING COMMUNITIES

Given the strong need to seek support, it is not surprising that communities have found ways to connect to help them better serve their young children and families. There are several ways in which communities have managed to connect for support, including:

1. Outreach to other communities to "share the wealth,"
2. Bringing in expertise from other "successful" communities
3. "Matchmaking" by state agencies charged with supporting community systems development to serve and support children and families.

By making these connections, communities can share information, learn new skills, and gain emotional support to continue the difficult work of systems and services development.

Sharing the Wealth

One impediment to successfully serving young children with disabilities and their families within the community is the lack of professional and other supports who have the specialized skills needed to deal with the families' and children's needs. Sharing skills and information is a key support network function that can help develop community capacity to serve families. One area in which communities, particularly small communities in more rural areas, are lacking, is the medical expertise and trained personnel to support children with special health care needs close to home. Even before birth, if there is a high risk of a problem, families may be forced to look beyond the community for maternity and neonatal services. Frequently, however, there are larger communities with a fuller range of medical services and expertise within the region. When these larger communities can "share their wealth" by providing training to upgrade expertise and capacity in small localities, then community-to-community support helps build community-based services for children and families.

Kearney, Nebraska, through its Good Samaritan health care system, has provided just this type of community-to-community support to the 18 rural communities whose hospitals feed into Good Samaritan Hospital, the U.S. government designated Regional Referral Center. They have established several outreach and training efforts and have more in the planning stage. Two examples particularly touch the lives of young children and their families. First, staff from the Good Samaritan system have done training for the personnel of the small, community hospitals in Neonatal Advanced Life Support (NALS) and Pediatric Advanced Life Support (PALS). This training has greatly enhanced to capacity of these hospitals to deal with the needs of families facing high risk births and for those with children with significant health problems. Without this type of capacity within the community, these families either have to seek care in distant medical centers or consider leaving their home communities, because local services cannot support their needs.

Kearney is now developing a new training program for the surrounding communities. In most small towns, emergency medical workers are volunteers with no professional training. In the recent past, personnel from Good Samaritan have provided them with training to deal with medical emergencies for adults, but the special needs of dealing with very sick children were still problematic. Families with children who were likely to have medical emergencies in these communities were lacking the supports they needed. There are now plans to develop and deliver a special training program for the volunteer medical emergency crews in these surrounding small rural communities to give them the specialized skills needed to stabilize and transport children with emergency medical conditions. This type of "sharing the wealth" is a good example of community-to-community support.

Learning from "Successful" Peers

Frequently, a community will identify an area of systems development for children and families that is not working well for them. Looking to other communities who have successfully dealt with that issue is a natural way to find the skills and support to improve the situation for their families. This approach provides both the support network functions of sharing information and skills and providing a positive inspiration to continue the hard work. Woonsocket, Rhode Island, has an active and effective effort that brings together agencies, providers and families within the community to plan and implement needed efforts to support children and families. Even in this well developed and organized community, however, new challenges bring the need to find new approaches. With the emphasis on community collaboration mandated by the reauthorization of the Individuals with Disabilities Education Act (IDEA), Woonsocket looked for a way to better bring together its continuum of integrated mental health services with special education services within the community to enhance resources and improve services for children and families. The lack of integration of mental health services and IDEA based services for young children as well as school aged children was a target for Woonsocket reaching out to another Rhode Island community that had worked through this issue.

Woonsocket is clearly not alone in facing this issue. In fact, a few years ago, this lack of collaboration was driven home at a statewide conference to bring closer collaboration between early intervention and mental health services. Each system was to present a family that exemplified its system and the needs families have. It turned out that each system was presenting the same family!

The Coordinator of Children's Services for the Northern Rhode Island Community Mental Health Center had attended a state meeting for special educators and heard an excellent presentation from a community in western Rhode Island that had developed a collaboration between special education and mental health. A panel consisting of the superintendent of the community schools, parents, a teacher, and a mental health professional presented their successful collaboration in relation to IDEA that led to an enhancement of services and supports to families. Seeing this presentation suggested to Woonsocket a resource to support its own desire to change. Woonsocket hosted an open house in the mental health agency for its school personnel to rebuild and strengthen connections. Although it was the mental health agency that initiated these efforts, the meeting was cosponsored by education and special education—mental health was the third host listed. The featured speaker was the superintendent from the western Rhode Island community, who quite eloquently told the story about his initial hesitations about increased collaboration and the tremendous pay-off he has seen for families of that collaboration. Choosing the right connections in other communities is often a key to success. As the Coordinator for Children's Mental Health Services in Woonsocket noted, "You have got to have club members talking to club members." Thus, she chose an educator to talk to educators about the benefits of collaborating more effectively with mental health services in the community. Learning how others have solved a community development issue and getting some inspiration from their successes is a second effective method of intercommunity support.

"Matchmaking" by State Agencies

Several state agencies that receive federal funds have a legislative mandate to support communities in developing integrated systems of services and supports for children with or at risk for disabilities and their families. One of the most effective mechanisms that these state agencies can use to help communities is to serve as brokers or matchmakers, pairing communities who have found successful approaches with communities who need help. In doing so, they create a support network that can allow for the functions of decreasing a sense of isolation in pursuing one's goals, sharing information and skills, having a positive model to provide encouragement, and having another group that understands how hard community systems building can be. Input from other community people who have faced similar challenges is often more easily accepted than that coming from state agency staff who may be perceived as not really understanding how difficult the tasks communities face really are.

In Colorado, the state Part C (of IDEA) agency used this successful approach to help a community that was not in tune with the vision, and expected roles of community interagency boards, in implementing early intervention services. The community board had taken on the role of being a provider of, or payor for, early intervention direct services, rather than working to develop more capacity throughout the community to serve young children with disabilities. If that community wanted to stay within the Part C program, it had to develop a different vision and the skills to implement that new vision. Rather than send state agency staff to the community to tell them "the right way" to do things, the state Part C Coordinator arranged to have a community that had successfully implemented the state-wide vision mentor the target community. Since Colorado has a statewide Part C network, these communities already knew each other.

Families comprise a large proportion of most of the local early intervention boards in Colorado, thus the initial contacts were between family members on both boards. Using state technical assistance funds, the mentor community was paid to provide 10-12 consultation days over two months to work with the target community. Initially, the new vision was presented to the community board and research to support that vision was provided. The consultants then helped the board focus on process—how they interacted—that would better support their new roles. Members of the board needed to learn to broker services rather than provide them and to keep people and new projects motivated and working effectively to increase the capacity to serve young children and families. The mentors helped them work on mapping within their community—understanding where services, supports and resources existed and what gaps they faced. They also worked on focusing on issues of inclusion, such as how to provide training to daycare providers so they could serve all children in the community. The target community now has a broader understanding of the mission of Part C and willingness to pursue that new mission has greatly increased, as has support for the parents in the community. There is still more work to be done and a formal, longer term contract is about to be implemented to continue this community-to-community support. State agencies have resources and knowledge about communities that can make community support a reality.

BUILDING A NATIONAL COALITION OF COMMUNITIES

While individual community-to-community support efforts are highly effective, they do not address the needs of the tens of thousands of communities across the country facing similar challenges in effectively serving young children and their families. There is a need for a more systematic and broad scale effort to support communities by sharing the wealth, seeking successful models and matchmaking among communities. There is also a need to bring large numbers of communities together to give them a credible voice in a broader world.

The Beginnings of a National Coalition of Communities

During the 1980s, there was a major shift in thinking about how children with or at risk for disabilities and their families should be served. A major component of that shift was to bring services and supports to the communities where families lived and for communities to take the responsibility for creating an integrated system of services and supports. This new way of thinking was formalized in numerous ways. In 1987, then Surgeon General Koop put out a call for action (Koop, 1987) to all states, communities, providers and families to make this shift in the way services were delivered. In 1989, legislation changed a part of the mandate for state Title V Maternal and Child Health programs—they were now responsible for supporting and ensuring that communities built integrated, family-centered systems of services for children with special health care needs (OBRA, 1989). This change in legislative mandate was quickly followed by other federal legislation that mandated or emphasized the importance of providing services and supports in a coordinated, integrated, family-centered way in the community. Most notable of these new legislative efforts to move to community-based service systems was Part H (now Part C) of the Individuals with Disabilities Education Act (IDEA) that instituted early intervention and supported interagency efforts at the community level.

While families, providers, and government representatives applauded this shift in emphasis in the service system, communities found themselves faced with new challenges and new pressures to meet the needs of children and families in very different ways. While this idea of developing integrated, family-centered systems of services in the community was readily accepted, communities often felt baffled and frustrated in trying to implement this abstract concept. Like individuals in need of support, communities found themselves with little experience in dealing with this new challenge; not part of any organized group state-wide or nationally that could help them meet the challenge; and trying to solve a problem that their own systems in the past had helped create. As each community tried, on its own, to build this model system of services, it often felt frustrated, alone, and lacking the information and skills to make the vision a reality.

In the early 1990s, the American Academy of Pediatrics and the federal Maternal and Child Health Bureau teamed up with the Georgetown University Child Development Center to provide the first organized approach to supporting communities in the hard work of systems development. The effort, called the "Communities Can Campaign," was designed to provide several key functions of a support network by identifying communities that had made good progress toward developing a community system of services for children with special needs and their families and sharing their experiences with other communities across the nation. The activities of the Communities Can Campaign were carried out by the Center for Child Health and Mental Health Policy at the Georgetown University Child Development Center. Initially 14 communities were identified and studied to identify what they had accomplished and how they had accomplished their goals. A monograph identifying the building blocks of a system of care was developed (Bronheim, Keefe, & Morgan, 1993), meetings for community and state teams were held, and a newsletter that shared information about how communities had successfully created some aspect of an integrated system of services was provided to thousands of interested parties. These initial activities addressed the first set of needs for individuals and, in this case communities, who need support:

1. A decreased sense of isolation: communities knew that other communities were struggling with the same challenges;

2. Encouragement and inspiration to keep going in the face of this challenge: seeing that other communities had actually succeeded helped a community persevere;
3. A place to express frustrations and feelings of wanting to give up: participants in the meetings of the Communities Can Campaign always commented that having a chance to talk about the problems with others facing the same challenges was invaluable; and
4. Sharing of information and skills that is not readily available elsewhere: the idea of community systems building was so new that professionals and families had no previous formal training in the "how tos;" new information was being created as communities attempted the challenge and they were the best, and in some ways, the only sources of information about how to build these new types of systems.

Communities Can Expands its Scope

In 1994, the Communities Can Campaign moved to a new level to encompass the other two key functions that support networks and groups can provide—empowerment and providing a strong voice for its constituents in broader arenas. At that time, national health care reform was being debated. There were, indeed, many strong voices being heard—professional organizations, health insurers, employers, and families also effectively organized to have a voice. As solutions that once again looked to communities for implementation were discussed, however, one voice was clearly missing—a voice for communities. At that time, Communities Can made the transition to a coalition of communities whose members pay no dues, but who receive not only the support from other communities and the information and skills needed, but also could become empowered to bring a voice for communities to state and federal policy making.

Today, Communities Can is a growing network of almost 2,000 members supported by multiple federal agencies. Its members look to the organization and each other for:

1. Links with other communities to learn from each other;
2. Information about how to best serve and support families;
3. Help to develop leadership to support systems development;
4. A voice for communities in policy arenas; and
5. A mechanism to recognize and publicize the achievements of communities.

Using the Internet, communities can look to each other for support and information through the listserve for members. Meetings, monthly electronic news bulletins over the listserve, offerings of training in leadership and collaborative dispute resolution and publications continue to help decrease the sense of isolation of communities and provide the support, information and skills they need to keep working at a difficult, but vital challenge—building integrated systems of services for their families.

More importantly, Communities Can has been recognized as a voice for communities. The Federal Interagency Coordinating Council (FICC) for Early Intervention—a group with representatives from the United States Departments of Education, Health and Human Services, Agriculture, Defense and the Social Security Administration as well as state agencies and families—has endorsed Communities Can as its connection with communities. One of its first collaborative activities with Communities Can was the development of a brochure, "A Community Vision for Young Children and Their Families," which puts forth a view from these diverse federal agencies on what should be happening in communities. Table 3.1 summarizes the FICC's vision for what comprehensive, coordinated services and supports in communities should entail. The FICC also now turns to Communities Can to get input on their activities—members of Communities Can were asked to provide feedback about what key issues the FICC should set as its priorities for the next few years. Members of Communities Can were also asked to comment on a proposed set of suggestions about inclusion of young children with disabilities to be used in drafting all federal legislation and regulations related to day care.

The activities and plans for Communities Can are developed by the Community Leadership Group. This council of representatives from highly successful communities understands what communities need and what they can offer to state and federal policy makers.

There are two types of membership in Communities Can—individual and community groups. Community groups (councils, task forces, committees, interagency groups, and so forth) who are developing a comprehensive, family-centered, integrated way to provide services and supports for children and families in their communities are encouraged to join and receive the full range of activities offered through Communities Can. Only Community group members are eligible for special recognition awards. The Coalition recognizes, however, that there are many individuals with a deep interest in community systems building who are looking for support and information to spark such efforts in their own communities—thus the Individual Membership category. All individual members who join are encouraged to develop the skills to make their own communities successful examples of Communities Can. To join

TABLE 3.1.
FICC Community Vision for Young Children and Their Families

Children Will...	• receive care, education, health, social services, and supports that relate to their everyday experiences and home culture • play, learn, and grow as valued and accepted members of their neighborhood.
Families Will...	• have the supports and services they need to nurture their children • be supported in their decisions • choose their services and supports • know where to get information they need • learn and receive support from other families
Communities Will...	• know that support is what a family says it is • make adaptations and accommodations so that children and families can participate in community health • respond when families tell them something is not working • respect the family's culture, values, and beliefs • be safe, friendly, and responsive • show that the supports and services they provide improve the lives of children and families
States Will...	• assure that policies and practices make it easy for communities to develop creative programs, services, and supports • support collaborative partnerships at the community level to hear the diverse voices of the communities • show that the supports and services they fund make a difference

Communities Can simply contact the Membership Coordinator at (202) 687-5095 or e-mail them at communities@gunet.georgetown.edu.

AN EXCITING FUTURE FOR FAMILIES AND COMMUNITIES

With the growth of Communities Can, the effectiveness of all communities to serve young children and their families will continue to be greatly enhanced. As community learns from community and effective practices in communities are recognized and publicized, the vision articulated by the FICC (Table 3.1) can become a reality. In addition, as federal and state agencies begin to hear the collective voice of communities, policy decisions may begin to better support the stated goal of integrated, family-centered, culturally competent systems of services and supports in communities. The community is the place in which the service systems set into motion by federal and state policy finally touch families and children. With an organized voice from those communities, one hopes that future policy will work better for young children and families.

ACKNOWLEDGMENT

The authors would like to thank Ellen Kagen, Center for Child Health and Mental Health Policy of the Georgetown University Child Development Center for her help in preparing this chapter.

REFERENCES

Bailey, D. B. (1987). Collaborative goal setting with families: Resolving differences in values and priorities for services. *Topics in Early Childhood Special Education,* 7(2), 59-71.

Bailey, D. B., Simeonsson, R. J., Yoder, D. E., & Huntington, G. S. (1990). Preparing professionals to serve infants and toddlers with handicaps and their families: An integrative analysis across eight disciplines. *Exceptional Children, 57*, 26-35.

Bailey, D. B., McWilliam, P. J., Winton, P. J., & Simeonsson, R. J. (1992). *Implementing family-centered*. Cambridge, MA: Brookline.

Berkman, L. F. (1985). The relationship of social networks and social support to morbidity and mortality. In S. Cohen & L. Syme (Eds.), *Social support and health* (pp. 241-262). Orlando, FL: Academic Press.

Bowlby, J. (1969). *Attachment and loss: Vol. I. Attachment*. New York: Basic Books.

Brewer, L. P., McPherson, M., Magrab, P. R., & Hutchins, V. L. (1989). Family-centered, community-based, coordinated care for children with special health care needs. *Pediatrics, 83*, 1055-1060.

Bronheim, S. M., Keefe, M. A., & Morgan, C. C. (1993). *Building blocks of a community- based system of care: the communities can campaign experience*. Washington, DC: Georgetown University Child Development Center, Center for Child Health and Mental Health Policy.

Cross, T. L., Bazron, B., Isaacs, M., Dennis, K. (1989). *Towards a culturally competent system of care. A monograph on effective services for minority children who are severely emotionally disturbed. Vol. I*. Washington, DC: Georgetown University Child Development Center, CASSP Technical Assistance Center.

Dalgard, O., Bjork, S., & Tambs, K. (1995). Social support, negative life events and mental health. *British Journal of Psychiatry, 166*, 29-34.

Fisher, M. (1998, July 19). The doctor is out; When illness struck, he plunged into the new medical reality—and discovered that the line between patient and physician is gone. *The Washington Post*, pp. W08.

Ganster, D., & Victor, B. (1988). The impact of social support on mental and physical health. *British Journal of Medical Psychology, 61*, 17-36.

Gibbs, B. (1993). Providing support to sisters and brothers of children with disbilities. In G. Singer, & L. Powers (Eds.), *Families, disability, and empowerment: Active coping skills and strategies for family interventions* (pp. 343-363). Baltimore, MD: Brookes.

Greenough, W. T. (1991). Experience as a component of normal development: Evolutionary considerations. *Developmental Psychology, 27*, 14-17.

Jaskulski, T. (1995). *The journey to inclusion: A resource guide for state policy makers*. Washington, DC: ACF, U.S. Department of Health and Human Services.

Kessler, R., & McLeod, J. (1985). Social support and mental health in community samples. In S. Cohen, & S. Syme (Eds.), *Social support and health* (pp. 219-240). Orlando, FL: Academic Press.

Koop, C. E. (1987). *Surgeon General's report: Children with special health care needs. Campaign '87*. Rockville, MD: U.S. Department of Health and Human Services.

May, J. (1991). *Fathers of children with special needs: New horizons*. Bethesda, MD: Association for the Care of Children's Health.

May, J. (1992). *Circles of care and understanding: Support programs for fathers of children with special needs*. Bethesda, MD: Association for the Care of Children's Health.

Melaville, A. I., Blank, M. J., & Asayesh, G. (1993). *Together we can*. Washington, DC: Department of Education.

Omnibus Budget Reconciliation Act of 1989, PL 101-239. (December 19, 1989). Title 42, U.S.C. 6501 (a)(1) et seq: *U.S. Statutes at Large, 103*, 2273.

Raiser, L. (1987). A teacher support network. *Teaching Exceptional Children, 19*, 48-49.

Rymer, R. (1993). *Genie: An abused child's flight from silence*. New York: Harper-Collins.

Saal, F. E. (1992). Finding room on the rack for more than one hat. In V. Vaux, M. S. Stockdale, & M. J. Schwerin (Eds.), *Independent consulting for evaluators* (pp. 21-32). Newbury Park, CA: Sage.

Shelton, T., & Smith-Stepanek, J. (1994). *Family-centered care for children needing specialized health and developmental services* (3rd ed.). Bethesda, MD: Association for the Care of Children's Health.

Wellins, R. S., Byham, W. C., & Wilson, J. M. (1991). *Empowered teams: Creating self- directed work groups that improve quality, productivity, and participation.* San Francisco, CA: Jossey-Bass.

Wright, B., King, M., & the NCSL Task Force on Developmental Disabilities (1991). *Americans with developmental disabilities: Policy directions for the States*. Denver, CO: National Conference of State Legislatures.

chapter 4

Financing Early Intervention Services: Perspectives and Practicalities from the Community Level

Linda D. Goetze
Utah State University

Susan D. Mackey Andrews
Solutions, Financing and Technology Consulting Services

Maureen Greer
Indiana Family and Social Services Administration

INTRODUCTION

This chapter summarizes issues and strategies that communities and states have considered in order to achieve early intervention outcomes by using financing as a vehicle for change. We begin with background information on Part C, including the history of the enabling legislation, and some of the changes that occurred within states and communities as a result of reauthorization of that legislation. Secondly, we will review some of the finance models that communities and states have adopted to solve the most critical problems they have identified within their early intervention system. Next, we examine *steps* that states and communities have found effective in achieving desired changes. These steps are described by Striffler, Perry, and Kates (1997) and have been voiced in discussions with key stakeholders in communities and states that have undertaken both minor and major restructuring of early intervention finance systems. Fourth, we discuss some of the many issues and areas of concern as we seek to refine various finance models focusing on topics that come up most often in finance discussions. We will discuss how these issues may be affected by using finance strategies as a catalyst for change or negotiation. Finally, we will describe one finance model in greater depth, looking at how stakeholders see effects on key issues in Indiana communities. Many tradeoffs inherent in setting goals and implementing policies make success in this arena a real challenge for those involved.

This chapter focuses on how changes in financing strategies can result in more optimum models of early intervention for families and children. Finance used as a tool or vehicle for change can result in a system of early intervention with greater benefits for families, children, and the community. We will discuss some of the issues that communities have identified as problems and targets for change, as well as some of the ways that finance can move people closer to their desired outcomes. As you will see, many issues overlap or have a direct influence upon the others.

All elements of early intervention are touched by finance. In an ideal world, individuals who need services will get them in a way that is timely and not contingent upon eligibility determination requirements, which may take weeks or even months to process. A state's finance system is like crews working behind the scenes in a major theatrical production producing something tangible—quality services for families—with invisible yet necessary support. In many respects, families may judge the success of a finance model in very different ways than they evaluate early intervention services. That is, the finance model may be largely invisible to families. If financing is working well in a community, there is greater likelihood that quality services will be available to address the needs of families and children in a timely manner.

The challenge with such an invisible funding model is the management and allocation of resources—people, time and money—in an efficient and effective manner. Consequently, the stakeholders in the system—families, providers, and administrators—must make decisions about where to spend the various resources most effectively. Not all resources will be apparent or accessible to all stakeholders; not all resources can be easily measured or quantified. Throughout each of the states' Part C systems, the access and allocation of resources is as individualized as is the development of each family's Individualized Family Service Plan (IFSP). State Part C systems vary considerably and have different resource "portraits"—histories and practices that have evolved over time. Assessing how these various resources are employed, their efficiency, and where improvements are possible within the Part C system is a difficult task for early intervention program administrators.

The purpose, design, and development of the federal Part C system differs substantially from other systems contained within the Individuals with Disabilities Education Act, or IDEA. It is often presumed that the Part C early intervention system is similar to Part B special education for children age 3 to 21; but, with the exception of a few components, nothing could be farther from fact. This presumption has contributed to some serious challenges to Part C systems, not the least of which is the application of the term "entitlement" or mandate (Brown & Conroy, 1999). While eligible children and families are "entitled" to receive needed services, the manner in which these services are provided and financed will vary greatly from state to state, and perhaps even from locale to locale within a state. Different from mandates or traditional entitlements, Part C financing may include the use of family resources including private or public insurance, co-payments, deductibles and/or sliding-fee scales. This assumption of "entitlement," coupled with the history of services to this population within each state, has resulted in many states assuming a greater level of financial responsibility for early intervention services than was anticipated by Congress.

Implications of Reauthorization

Certain federal regulations were enhanced under the Part C IDEA reauthorization that affect financial structures, availability and certain costs to Part C systems. These include:

1. Reinforcement of the federal requirement to utilize natural environments for Part C services, which challenges states to move from traditional center or clinic-based service settings to family-centered environments, including the home. Natural environments also challenge providers in the approaches they employ in the provision of services. Combined, this requirement is anticipated by most states to result in higher service costs and reduced personnel availability.
2. Enhanced transition planning and information to include the collection and reporting of exit data to describe why children leave Part C services, and where they go. This in part is an attempt to respond to Congress' question "What happens to children as a result of their participation in this program?"
3. Reauthorization increased the incentives for states to serve infants and toddlers at risk, including the development of tracking systems

as well as adjustments in eligibility criteria to be more inclusive of this population.

4. While not necessarily impacting financing, states are now required to offer mediation services as part of the procedural safeguards for Part C participants. Of more financial significance is the potential for regulations permitting "compensatory services" as a resolution to an individual family's complaint. Given emerging data that there are often significant differences between the services that are delivered through the IFSP as compared to those that are planned in the IFSP, the implications of payment responsibility for compensatory services pose serious financial, policy and systemic challenges.
5. In addition, there is the potential for changes in existing Part C regulations that permit states to use a variety of resources without regard to "cost" issues. Such changes could apply the "at no cost" Part B definition regarding use of private insurance to Part C.

Prior to the implementation of Part C in the late 1980s, most states had some level of services for infants and toddlers with disabilities. These services varied greatly, as did eligibility requirements for services and how these services were funded. Additionally, few states served preschoolers, ages 3 to 5, under IDEA at this point in time. For these states, the passage of P.L. 99-457 was a double challenge in that the Section 619 component of the law was a mandate to states as compared to Part C, which continues to be voluntary.

One of the statutory obligations of the lead agency under federal regulations is "to establish a statewide system" for Part C services. This assumes some level of standardization or consistency of the system throughout the state. This implies that access and availability to Part C services is equitable no matter where in a state the family resides, regardless of family income or education level, the nature of severity of their child's disability, or their race or ethnicity. There is a natural tension between this obligation and the manner in which many states have established their Part C systems. Few state early intervention systems are managed from a central location. The majority of states have implemented systems where the locus of control for a variety of functions—including financing—rests within a regional or county structure. These structures offer a great deal of variation in terms of their knowledge base, access to resources, and authority at the local level. Consequently, the system of services and financing options may vary tremendously and result in a patchwork of services, rather than a statewide system. The tension between state, regional and local responsibilities needs constant discussion and attention in order to ensure that local stakeholders have the necessary resources to cultivate early intervention systems, and that families have equitable access no matter where they reside.

Perhaps the greatest controversy to states in implementing Part C was the obligation of the governor to appoint a lead agency, different from Section 619 or other sections of Part B where the state Department of Education was statutorily the lead agency. Depending upon the history within each state, coupled with the politics, the designation of lead agency often proved divisive and political. The reality, that the lead agency can and does change over time, contributes an additional level of instability to state Part C systems. The physical relocation of the system from mental health to public health can signal a variety of system changes, including philosophy, terminology, personnel, and capacity—not to mention financing options and priorities.

As states elected to participate in Part C, few had the opportunity to start from a "clean slate," working to internalize and conceptualize the stated purpose, principles, and tenets of the law and design a system that met the criteria established by Congress: "to develop a statewide, comprehensive, coordinated, multidisciplinary, interagency system" of early intervention. Most states adopted the system at hand and have, over time, added improvements and services in an ever present desire to meet the federal obligations and intent and meet the needs of families and young children within their borders.

Consequently, states did not ordinarily plan their financing system or necessarily change their existing system with a planned, conscious focus. The fact is that few states have conducted thoughtful financial system analysis and change. Most states' finance systems are not systems, but are the structures that they inherited when they bought into Part C. Some states have cobbled additional financing changes onto this original structure, usually to solve an immediate problem. Years later, we are beginning to see some of the system implications of immediate fund maximization without attention to the "big picture," or the implications of these short-term fixes over time. For example, the early use of P.L. 89-313 funds by some states negated an early discussion of family cost participation because these funds, similar to Part B funds, required services to be provided "at no cost." These funds have since been blended with Part C and these historical rules no longer apply.

Family cost participation also affects access to other fund sources, such as insurance, where the fund source serves to protect the enrolled member from financial liability. And, to complete the link, if a child is dually enrolled in Medicaid and has private coverage, Medicaid has existing federal regulations that require tapping all other forms of coverage. Consequently, in order to garner increased fund sources to support early intervention services, some states are reinitiating the cost participation discussion and debate—sometimes with great angst and resistance from the provider community.

Only a few states have evaluated their financing system, understood their current financing arrangements as these relate to their service delivery system, or to their options to improve those systems. Few have made changes based upon their vision and values. In the rapid pressure to establish systems and provide services, many states have either been forced to fund Part C services with federal or state early intervention allocations in the absence of other, established funding. Still other states have entered into funding partnerships with Medicaid/Title XIX, for example, that restrict the provider or location of services and further compromise the integrity and compliance of the state's system with federal regulations.

Old ways die hard. The evolution of disability services through the United States has been largely the domain of the private, not-for-profit sector and have extended beyond infants and toddlers into services for adults. Special purpose agencies developed in local communities. As IDEA has been implemented throughout the country, these agencies have gradually lost clients to the public schools and are struggling to survive within managed care systems, reduced service needs, and increased costs. One of the key challenges to most state planners is keeping these valuable entities as service resources within their communities, while assisting them to modify their practices and come into compliance with Part C and the state's vision. Nowhere will this challenge be more evident, financially and systemically, than in the area of providing services in the natural environment using naturally occurring learning opportunities, routines and community supports based upon the individual nature of each child and family.

The integration of managed care into the financing quilt for Part C continues to challenge most states because managed care poses an inherent conflict to a key principle of IDEA—that services be based upon need, and not upon available resources (people, time, money) and that these services should be individualized. It further challenges the authority of service planning and compliance by placing this in the hands of a multidisciplinary team as opposed to the primary care physician.

Further challenges to the financing integrity of Part C are the obligations for payor of first resort (i.e., Medicaid/Title XIX and Title V). This may mean for some states that, even if the provision of these services is inconsistent or incompatible with Part C, the source of payment must be honored. Further, depending upon the location of the lead agency, relationships and communications may not be established, or necessarily cooperative, resulting in difficulty in accessing these resources even if federal law requires it. This has certainly been the history of Part B financing, dating back to 1975.

COMMUNITY VERSUS FAMILY INVOLVEMENT: DIRECTION IN RESOURCE ACCESS AND MANAGEMENT

In an ideal world, resources like money and the services that money can buy, are used to produce the greatest positive outcome for society. One of the dilemmas in early intervention involves providing services and using resources where they have their highest possible use, as measured by outcomes for families and children. In the private sector, businesses respond to the priorities, wants and needs of consumers of their products. Similarly, active and informed family member involvement in developing the plan for early intervention services is extremely important because this involvement can increase the efficacy of those dollars. By using the family's concerns, priorities and resources to determine service type, frequency and intensity, families learn to manage the various resources available to them. Why are so many states moving toward billing private insurance and families through parent fees? They are attempting to increase limited resources and improve the way resources are used by increasing the financial commitment of key stakeholders in the system.

Again, in an ideal world, resources would not be scarce, and funding would be adequate to meet the needs and support the provision of services in such a way that providers were appropriately and justly compensated. In reality, however, we aim for an optimal balance by developing funding models that maximize access for families and children, while at the same time, using funds for the best possible effects. The options for funding Part C vary substantially from state to state, and are influenced by a variety of factors including eligibility criteria, location of the lead agency, "competition" from other populations, or the level of understanding and time by program administrators to pursue fund expansions while simultaneously managing systems.

Accessing diverse resources to support IFSP services is complex and challenging. Some funds are accessible only through individual client application, such as the access to private insurance. Other fund access is facilitated at a systems or state level, as would be the case in establishing an Administrative Agreement with a state's Title XIX/Medicaid program. Still other funds, such as Head Start or childcare, may be accessed only at the community level through locally developed partnerships with other agencies and programs. One of the challenges in building early intervention financing is to ensure stability and equitable access to resources. Part C requires collaboration in fund identification, access and accountability at all levels in order to develop service delivery systems and appropriate infrastructures that comply with federal Part C regulations.

EARLY INTERVENTION FINANCE OPTIONS

States have used a variety of methods to manage the variety of resources available to support early intervention systems. In a case study, Russell (1991) described the primary methods used by six states that assessed the degree to which states had addressed financial issues like coordination, as covered under the initial P.L. 99-457, Part H legislation. A wide array of methods had been used, including the following:

1. *Unit Rate Financing*, with a rate schedule for service reimbursement;
2. *Contracting for Services*, with individual contracts between state and local providers, within which contract reimbursement may be a general lump sum, a flat grant, per child, per unit of service, or other negotiated rates for service packages;
3. *State Core Financing*, when the state relies largely on state funds to provide early intervention services, augmented with less reliable non-state funds;
4. *Local Funding Initiatives*, detailed in Clifford's (1991) study as important in localities with a history of local control of revenue sources for early intervention services.

Russell (1991) describes other funding variations like the use of formal and informal Interagency Agreements when funding representatives commit a variety of their funds to early intervention, either formally (with legislative backing or administrative support or backing) or informally (without formal legal status). Local and state coordination varies across funding models in that some states coordinate funding centrally and others fund localities that maintain primary financial responsibility.

Most states employ multiple approaches to financing early intervention services, based largely upon the source of the funds and traditional method of accessing these resources. The myriad of structures can make financing complex and confounding. The costs (again, people, time and money) involved in accessing precious resources is proportionate to provider availability, attitude and willingness to participate in the Part C system. These costs may unnecessarily compromise the availability and provision of services to families and children, sap valuable professional time, and serve as a disincentive to providers who are being asked to modify the way they conduct their practice to more closely conform with the spirit and intent of Part C.

Characteristics of Funding Models

A number of characteristics, as revealed by procedures, distinguish one type of funding model from another. One variable is how different agencies access revenue sources and whether states, localities, or providers tap different sources. How funds are accessed or distributed is another characteristic that distinguishes some funding methods and models from others. States have varied in the way they approach the responsibility for accessing financing for early intervention services. Some states have established the responsibility for accessing individual fund sources upon local providers with no assistance from the state lead agency; others have tried to consolidate fund access at the state level with a myriad of reimbursement strategies established to fund local providers from this "concentrated" pool of funding. In fact, communities and states may use a combination, where funds such as Part C and Medicaid are channeled through state agencies to local providers, and other revenue sources like parent fees and private insurance are billed and paid directly to local providers.

Another variation for states is the method in which funds are disbursed to providers. Some early intervention systems use a fee-for-service approach, similar to Clifford's Unit Rate Financing method, where reimbursement depends on the amount and types of services. This approach requires a rate structure for services that assigns different values for locations, credentials and types and amounts of service. This procedure presents a number of challenges to policymakers since the reimbursement rate may affect such issues as provider willingness to provide services developed in the IFSP. Differences may occur between the cost of providing particular services and the amount providers are reimbursed. These differences stem from efforts to manage precious resources in synchrony with the vision and philosophy of the state Part C system. Further, state Part C systems must often comply with the rate structures and reimbursement approaches that exist in other state agencies and entities, which can further confound the development of an attractive, competitive approach to reimbursement.

One example of this is the challenge in developing an appropriate administrative or overhead rate. Traditionally these rates have incorporated buildings and grounds in the early intervention service rate. If the state's Part C system has placed a high value upon the provision of services to families and children in their natural environments, utilizing the normal family routines and "props," these additional costs to the provider agency will not necessarily be used or needed by the early intervention system. Consequently, some or all of these costs may not be incorporated in the rate but they remain a fixed cost to the provider agency.

When contemplating "fair and equitable" reimbursement, one of the more challenging factors of early intervention service delivery is the presence of extrinsic versus intrinsic rewards for those who provide services. Typically these provider systems are dominated by women with needs and priorities for benefits that differ substantially from traditionally male dominated employment fields. There are reasons why individuals pursue certain fields or avenues of practice that extend beyond wage and benefits, which are less tangible and more personal. These values tend to extend themselves into the way that people work within their roles, and it is not uncommon for traditional early intervention providers to work "beyond" the scope of their practice. They are simply trying to do what needs to be done and have a high degree of human empathy for the families that they serve. How is "good will" then measured for the purposes of reimbursement? And, should it be reimbursed? How do systems accommodate to the special needs of their provider group, where access to childcare and support for nontraditional hours may be more valued than employee health benefits, which are already accessed by the family through spouse or partner employment?

If the provider cost is higher than what they are paid, say, for a physical therapy visit in the family home, then shortages of physical therapists who will visit in the home may be a common occurrence. In fact, providing services in a clinic or center-based model often shifts transportation costs, especially time costs, to families. Even though families are reimbursed for mileage, those dollars do not cover the full cost of transportation, that is, the family's time.

If rate schedules are low for particular services or locations, providers may not work at those rates or vice versa, thus giving policymakers a strong tool to achieve other program objectives, such as those related to family choice and home services. Setting rates for natural environments at higher levels than traditional clinic or center rates creates an incentive for greater amounts of services in those environments. Fee-for-service is just one way that funds may be allocated. Many states allow localities to decide location and service priorities, each locality adopting its own rate structure or lump-sum contract with one primary contractor to serve the community. In other words, those who receive and distribute the money make the decisions.

Eligibility is another important finance model variable whether determined at the state level or determined locally. Does eligibility for funding drive services or does need drive services? States may opt for a "pay-and-chase" method of funding services, where services are provided locally, regardless of eligibility for categorical funding sources, after which a bill for services is sent to the state. The state pays for those services and then collects from funding sources for which the individual family is eligible and covers the difference in out-of-state funds. This makes funds or reimbursement invisible at the local level meaning eligibility is less likely to drive content, services, and location of services in the IFSP.

Program Components and Administration

Another important issue to a successful funding model is ensuring adequate funds for child/family early intervention services, system components, and administration. Figure 4.1 depicts the full array of components necessary to a healthy system that functions at a high level. The bottom line is that early intervention dollars must support all valued and desired early intervention components. This includes direct services such as Child Find, evaluation and assessment, eligibility determination, and IFSP services. For services to function well, however, other components must be in place as well. The left-hand side of Figure 4.1 shows system components that also require financial support. These components, combined with administrative structure, are what make a *system* of early intervention. This infrastructure is designed to maintain consistent, standardized procedures for personnel development and training; ensure procedural safeguards and complaint resolution for consumers; provide methods to resolve interagency disputes and agreements; respond to financial concerns such as rates, contracts, and payments; and manage a data system to obtain funds and to evaluate system strengths and weaknesses. While many of these components are unseen by direct consumers, they are necessary to generate and use revenues and other critical resources like personnel that are central to successful development and delivery of services. Some of these components, such as the state's data system, are critical to the ability of the Part C system to survive by providing information to decision makers including legislators, funding sources and advocates.

Responsibility for the various Part C program components is generally divided between the State Part C Lead Agency, the Local Lead Agency, and Early Intervention Service Providers, as shown in Figure 4.2. Adequate support, including financial support, must be included with responsibility if we hope to achieve success with respect to each component. Administration and less tangible system activities, such as data collection, procedural safeguards, and Child Find, may be undervalued and underfunded because these processes are not visible as direct services to families and children. Without an accurate view of the entire system, we cannot develop funding models that effectively support key

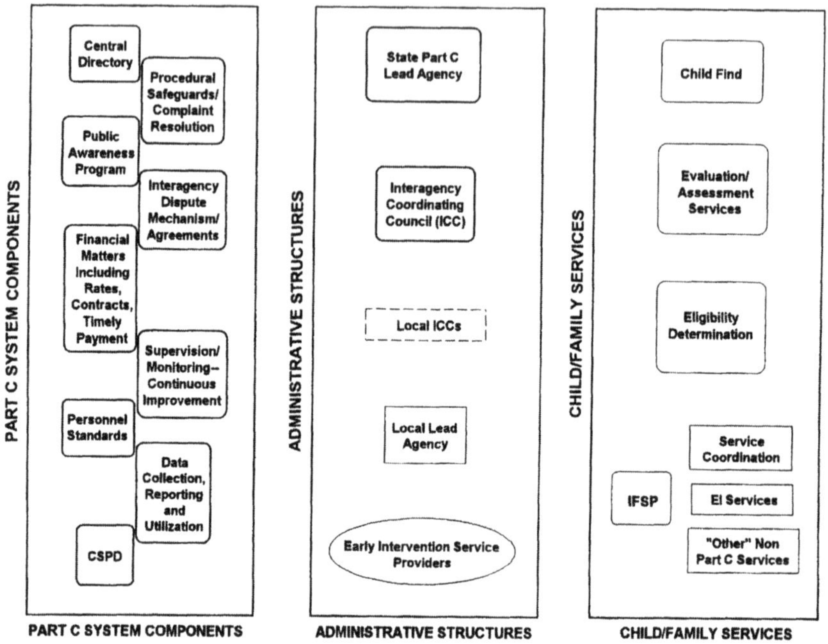

FIGURE 4.1. Early intervention program components.

components of early intervention. Many components of Figure 4.2 are often viewed as wasteful bureaucracy, using up funds better used to provide direct services. Rather, these facets provide a support system for early intervention pivotal to the success of the system or network—not simply individual services separate from the greater system.

In all models presented, we assumed the local lead agency was funded to perform child find, receive referrals, facilitate intake, and determine eligibility. These services are not invoiced on a per-child basis and are usually funded through a contract or grants mechanism.

Figure 4.2 shows responsibility for various early intervention components, depicted by the State Part C Lead Agency, the Local Lead Agency, and Early Intervention Service Providers. Many responsibilities overlap or are shared, such as data collection and Child Find, while state and local lead agencies each have responsibility for financial matters, procedural safeguards, public awareness, and supervision/monitoring. Such interrelationships illustrate the resource need at different levels in the system and the cooperative need as well. Figure 4.2 describes the options available with respect to funding, including variables that distinguish different funding models: how funding is accessed, where it is

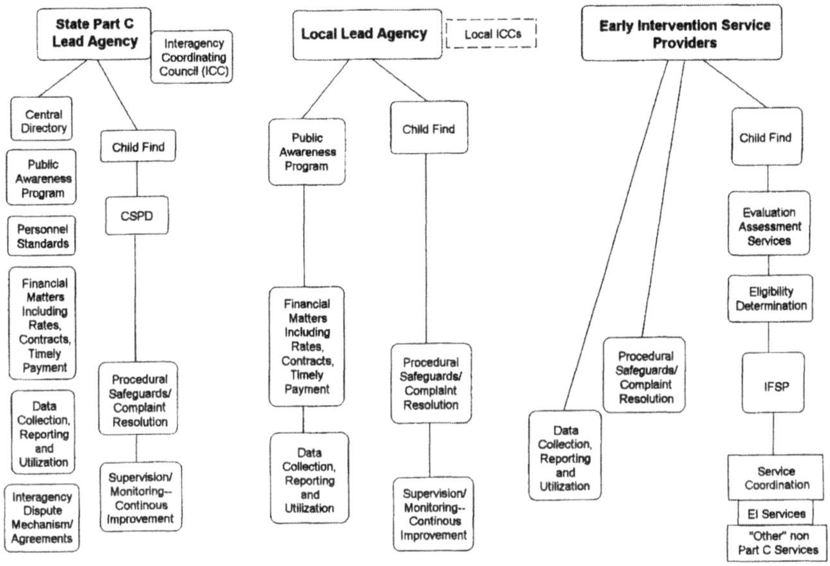

FIGURE 4.2. Locus of accountability for various Part C program components.

accessed, how it is distributed, and how and where eligibility for funding sources is determined. Many of these differences relate to which of the three entities—state lead agency, local lead agency, or providers—has which financing responsibilities.

Three Finance Models

Three examples of early intervention finance models will illustrate some tradeoffs inherent in model options that states and communities may consider as shown graphically in Figures 4.3, 4.4, and 4.5. One primary difference between the models is the extent to which the Part C State Lead Agency, rather than a local lead agency, is involved in financing early intervention. Models A and B depict a stronger state leadership role than Model C, in which the state lead agency has no direct role in finance which is left to the local lead agency.

Model A, as shown in Figure 4.3, combines grants/contracts and fee-for-service approaches to funding. The Part C Lead Agency collects state and federal funds available for early intervention and channels them to a local provider for referral/intake, evaluation/assessment, service coordination, and IFSP services. This creates a direct financial relationship between the state lead agency and local providers, who may be private

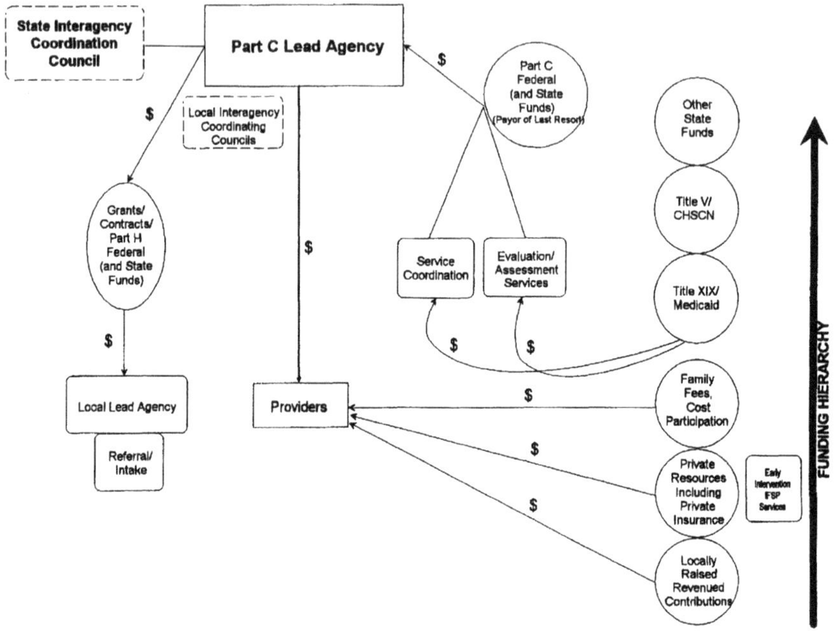

FIGURE 4.3. Model A: Combination approach of grant/contracts and fees for service structure.

or public entities that compete for the local Part C early intervention contracts/grants. Funds may be distributed to providers before or after services have actually occurred, and are reimbursed in one of two ways. Reimbursement may be based on the amount of services, or it may reflect a capitated "per child" amount. In this model, Part C dollars available through the grants/contract structure may only be used as "last dollar" (i.e., after all other funding sources are accessed). Additional funding sources may include other state funds, CSHCN, Medicaid, or other third-party billing sources. The local provider is responsible for collecting reimbursement for services provided from all sources, including parent fees, private insurance, and local revenues. Once all of these resources have been exhausted, the funds available through the grant/contract mechanism may be tapped to complete the reimbursement process and cover services that weren't paid by any other resource.

Model B, Figure 4.4, illustrates a centralized finance office for the state system under which funds are managed by one fiscal intermediary. The central finance office pays providers for services and collects funds for those services from all available sources. This is a "pay-and-chase"

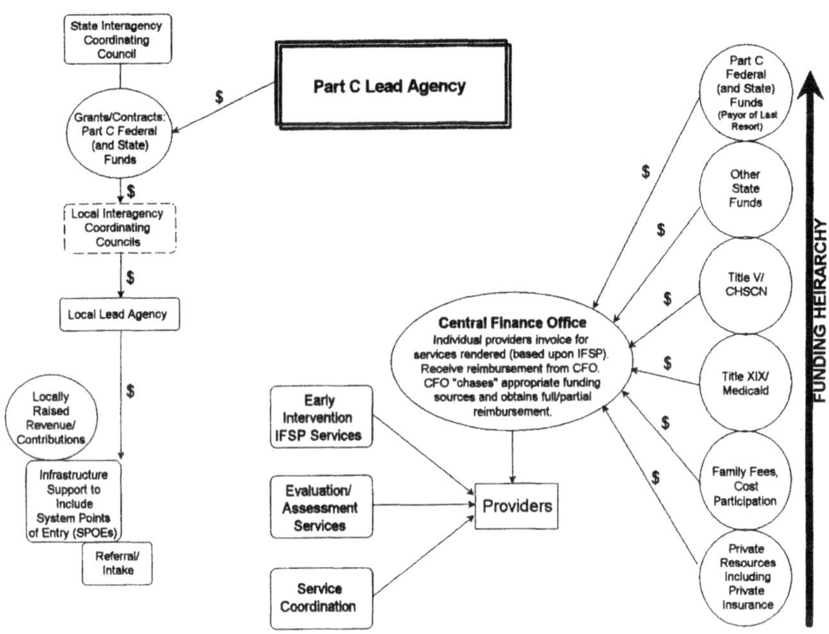

FIGURE 4.4. Model B: Central finance office (pay-and-chase system).

system, meaning that services are paid by a central finance office that then "chases" fund sources based upon individual child and family eligibility for services. Such funds may or may not include local sources or family cost participation such as family fees and/or insurance billings. Because fund sources are managed by a separate entity, neither the family nor the provider is immediately concerned with individual eligibility for different sources of funds. The state sets the rate structure for various services and locations, and all providers are reimbursed at these common rates. This common rate permits the lead agency to incorporate incentives to achieve desired Part C policies into the rate structures, such as promoting the use of natural environments through higher reimbursement rates for such services. This model combines central management of funds with a fee-for-service reimbursement structure, where the flow of funds to children is monitored with data to examine equitable fund access and statewide distribution.

Model C, as seen in Figure 4.5, depicts a locally controlled and managed finance structure with the primary financial relationship between the local lead agency and local providers. Here, a local lead agency receives funds from the state lead agency—primarily state and federal

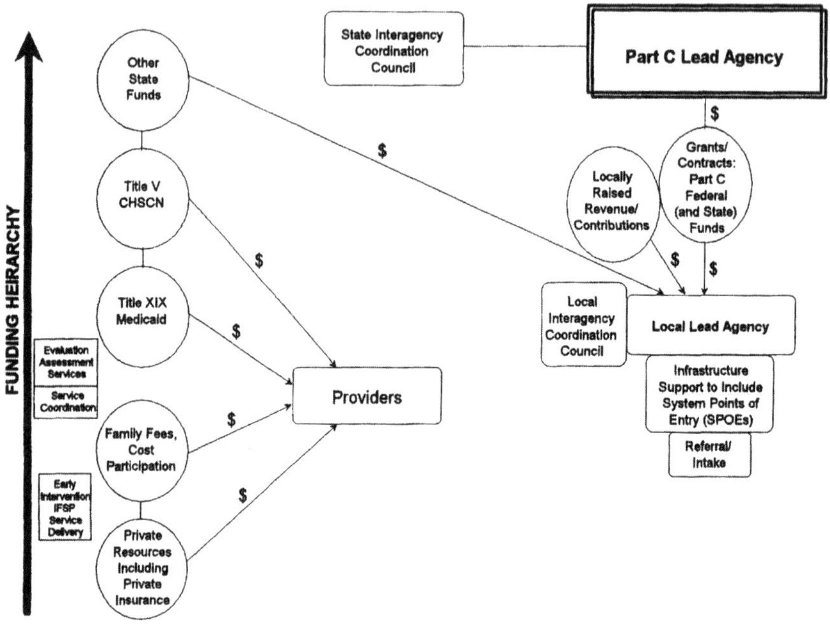

FIGURE 4.5. Model C: Local lead agency structure.

Part C funds—and parcels them out to local providers. Typically, providers contract with the local lead agency and are required to bill other funding sources, such as CSHCN and Medicaid, before billing the local lead agency. In this model, the provider may collect financial information directly from families, or they may relate to the system point of entry (SPOE), where the SPOE serves as the intermediary for family financial information passed along to the provider.

In Model C, the local lead agency has primary, direct responsibility for financing early intervention, whereas in Model A, the provider's financial relationship is directly with the funding sources and the state lead agency. Model C may result in large differences in expenditures between communities—since funds that the local lead agency and providers generate depend on family eligibility in a particular community for those various sources. Services may be determined by funding eligibility rather than the IFSP. The local lead agency may elect to structure Child Find (including evaluation/assessment), service coordination, and IFSP service provision in different ways depending upon the local culture and resources. These responsibilities may be maintained by the local lead agency or contracted to service providers. Table 4.1 summarizes charac-

TABLE 4.1.
Model Characteristics

Model	Description	Fixed components	Variable components	Comments
Combination Approach				
A	1. Grants/Contracts coupled with fee-for-service reimbursement 2. Part H accessible in one of two ways: (a) advance grants/contracts with routine, ongoing settlement and adjudication before additional funds distributed, or (b) payment made to providers "after the fact" with documentation that all existing third-party resources have been accessed.	Part H funds are: 1. "Last dollar" 2. Accessed only after all existing fund sources have been accessed. 3. Primary payment relationships involve provider and family. (a) Complex system to manage given rates that vary between funding sources. (b) Often little incentive to use third-party resources. 4. Providers encouraged to access other state and local resources and are responsible for collection of family fees, insurance billing, and recovery.	1. Some funds governed or directed at local level by LICC. 2. Grants/contracts may be established in advance of services and adjudicated routinely through finance reports or documentation by provider, with amount of third-party reimbursement obtained and balance due.	1. If advance grants/contracts not made to providers, they must plan adequate cash flow since reimbursement not made until ALL fund sources have been accessed, denials or partial payments documented. 2. Often results in reduced use of third-party resources.

(continued)

TABLE 4.1.
(Continued)

Model	Description	Fixed components	Variable components	Comments
Centralized Finance Office Approach				
B	1. All available state and federal funds are managed by fiscal intermediary external to state government.	1. Specific fund sources "invisible" to providers and families. 2. System works from encounter data obtained through the IFSP and invoices based on authorizations. 3. All EI providers bill CFO directly for services provided to eligible children, are reimbursed at common state EI rate for services. 4. CFO pays in advance, then "chases" available funding sources based on individual child eligibility. 5. Receipts from third-party billing recycled into CFO.	1. Fund sources contained with CFO individually tracked and reported but vary considerably. 2. CFO may or may not include local funds, family fees, and/or insurance billing proceeds. 3. Options for claims payment separate from central billing functions and located at individual funding agencies/state comptroller's office for provider reimbursement. 4. CFO acts as third-party billing intermediary for provider.	1. Model based on a fee-for-service structure, units ranging from traditional 15 minute unit to "episodic" unit of one month or one encounter, like evaluation/assessment services. 2. Funds distributed on per child basis, using data to monitor equitable distribution of resources and use.

Local Lead Agency Structure				
C	1. All funds for services managed by local lead agency, on receipt of grant from state lead agency. 2. Locally raised revenue (taxes, fees, fund raising) or historical efforts may be added to the "pot." 3. Providers invoice local lead agency for services not covered by other fund sources, are paid directly. 4. Documentation of third-party billing, denials, and claims adjudication required.	1. State lead agency plays no direct role in financing services. 2. Local lead agencies must be adept at projecting need on annual basis since no additional grants/contracts guaranteed.	1. Local lead agencies may become providers and use third-party resources and grants/contracts to provide EI services. 2. Funds can "float" between state and local levels, unused funds from one region being redistributed to where need exists.	1. Can limit Child Find by creating a financial "ceiling" of expenditures. 2. Individual nature of funds may drive service delivery (frequency, location, etc.) not IFSP.

teristics of the three different models, including general description, fixed components, variable characteristics, and additional comments.

CRITICAL STEPS FOR CHANGE

Researchers like Striffler and colleagues (1997) and Kates (1991) have identified some critical steps they have found effective for states and communities as they move to refine their finance systems to accommodate the needs of all stakeholders in the system. Striffler and colleagues collected data in three states that used "an interactive process model" to plan and implement goals and objectives for early intervention funding models. Evidence that states following this model achieved measurable success in desired outcomes included increased Medicaid funds, amount of service provided in natural environments, and variety of funding sources and interagency activities. Some of the steps that communities and states take to change a finance model are included here because they correlate with desired funding outcomes and because they illustrate experiences and challenges that key stakeholders have faced as they revamp early intervention funding models.

Identify and Involve Key Stakeholder Groups

Although all key stakeholders may not see eye to eye, key leaders in early intervention should be involved in any planned or anticipated changes. Those who work for change must have the political will, information, and power to facilitate change. Strong, committed and informed individuals who can withstand challenges should be recruited.

Involvement entails different levels of intensity and energy. Families want to be reassured that they will not be left out or lose services. Change may cause confusion or stress for providers and families alike. Disruption or loss of services, fear of job loss and the challenges of doing things differently are some of the key negative influences. Families, in one state where parent fees were recently added, expressed concern about the continuity of services. "I have insurance and my insurance may or may not pick up the bill....I have contacted insurance, and they don't have any information about it. And I have contacted them at the center; and they say we are not set up to deal with insurance. Where does that leave me?" And where does it leave providers concerned about continuity of income, revenue, and financial solvency? Throughout the process of change, it is critical to have regular meetings to discuss what is changing and how individual stakeholder groups could be affected. Open communications through meetings, newsletters and stakeholder correspondence will reduce anxiety, ensure continued productivity and participation, and prevent potential opposition to changes.

Empower Local Stakeholders

One way to conceive and implement change from the beginning is to shift some power about key decisions to local councils or other local stakeholder representatives, thus, ensuring valuable information and suggestions. Providers are empowered when they are able to meet the needs of specific families with information and support that allows them to say, "At least you feel like with more information you've got what little control you did have." Empowering local stakeholders helps build a successful foundation for future work, such as developing the vision and revisiting the system, because the people who know become involved in the plan for change. Success is more likely when changes come from representatives who have earned credibility as part of the system of early intervention and who have learned the importance of adaptability to change down the road. Empowering local councils, for example, creates a greater incentive for people who are affected most by early intervention to become involved in creating a practical system that will really work for diverse communities. As one local provider said about the process of major funding reform, "People who use it should be a part of its development." Involving local, diverse representatives in a meaningful manner makes them invaluable partners for progress. According to one respondent, "The bottom line is that parents need to have more power in the program, not just for The Council, but in everything. Anyone is more likely to make something a success if he/she has input."

Indeed, *political will* may be key to success or failure in changing the system. Informing and involving those who have power and show willingness to adopt change in the system is critical. Ensuring that these determined individuals develop an agreement on the direction for change based upon factual, accurate and timely information is imperative and offers yet an additional opportunity to educate and deepen individual appreciation and commitment. A core group may be critical to "divide and conquer" potential opposition efforts to proposed changes. Having local, respected individuals who will state their commitment to change in the face of adversity or challenge may well be key to the success of reform efforts.

Anticipate Possible Conflicts of Interest

A review of goals and power may reveal areas where interests of families and service providers diverge, for example, over a power shift such as that described above related to local councils or other stakeholders. Those who have traditionally made the decisions will either share power, fight to maintain power themselves, or withdraw from the process. Another area where interests may conflict relates to where services are provided. One goal of reform may be to establish or increase family choice, which may decrease provider choice. Using natural environments requires that providers leave their clinics or centers in order to provide services. Serving more families with new, alternative service approaches may result in an increased need for service provider capacity. Historical early intervention providers may be fearful of competition with emerging new providers; competition is a reality which business and industry have faced for years, but is not necessarily a condition that has affected the disability provider community.

Increased competition from a broader base of service providers may increase choices for families but decrease options for traditional providers. Shortages within specific disciplines shifts the power of choice to providers who can say where, when, and how they will provide services and schedule a full calendar of families for a higher wage rate. Changing reimbursement rates or ways to access providers may help to alleviate service shortages, but providers may see such changes as threats to income, financial security, long-term solvency, or method of providing services. Such changes might create an inherent conflict between the interests of families and other stakeholders, including providers who strongly oppose such changes. This may be a particular problem in states where providers have traditionally controlled where they provide services or what they charge because demand for services exceeds supply.

Conflicts may also arise if stakeholders attempt to reform the finance model by removing historical controls or restrictions that have been employed for various management purposes—often, most particularly for managing finances. One such example that is common is the assignment of defined geographical boundaries for individual provider entities. Loss of the security of these boundaries coupled with competition may create provider anxiety that translates into provider resistance to change. Families may feel uncertain about their ability to make sound selection of providers in light of the historical delivery system that didn't previously offer provider choice. These changes can fuel conflict and further resistance if families feel that services will be negatively affected by change—even if they agree with the desired outcome. It is difficult to manage conflict and affect positive outcomes in an arena where families and their interests come into such direct conflict with those of the providers who serve them.

Revisit the System

As earlier stated, it is impossible to manipulate the financing structure for Part C without affecting all facets of the delivery system. Planners should use this opportunity to review the existing system in comparison to federal requirements, identify strengths and needs of their system, and examine and use other state model options to create system enhancement and improvements supported by fund expansions. Understanding the history and evolution of the system is valuable in order to assess positive and negative traits of the system, the reasons why things evolved as they did and to clarify who holds power and why.

In addition to federal regulations as guidance in this systems evaluation, stakeholders need to identify what is working well and less well within the current system, thereby revealing the issues that will be the focus for change. A variety of information beyond personal opinion must be gathered to ensure that this review is conducted effectively. This may include review of a variety of extant data as well as surveying key stakeholders through written questionnaires, forums, or targeted meetings. This comprehensive process helps to not only validate the desired changes—local, state, structure, and system, but serves to provide documentation and support for change in specific target activities that are thus more likely to succeed.

Shifts in power are often the most challenging change. Since money and funding are key elements of power, identifying who has control over which resources becomes a critical step to successful achievement of state and community finance goals. One way to challenge the existing distribution of power is to work toward consensus among stakeholders about the priorities, visions, and steps to change the current system. This builds upon the earlier step of involving representatives of all key stakeholders from the beginning to work together toward the vision, agreeing as a unified group on targets for change and methods to get there.

Build Consensus About the Vision

Reaching agreement about broad issues and goals will set the stage for action and for successful achievement of the vision and goals. This is the time for consensus building in order to focus efforts on some goals that use specific steps and yield tangible results. Developing a list of areas needing improvement or change starts the process. Stakeholders should spend time grouping areas for improvement, and establishing priorities while also identifying those areas of change that will have some linkage or domino effect together. This approach to strategic planning for change will allow focused achievement of tasks, and help to prevent stakeholders from becoming overwhelmed. This approach also helps stakeholders to celebrate their "wins" and encourages a realistic workscope that helps to ensure success by making certain that the "to do list" is neither too long nor too difficult, yet concrete and realistic enough to be valuable and within the abilities of stakeholders to achieve. One example of such a vision is to develop a finance system that supports family choice; maximizes all funding sources; blends and coordinates sources; funds services efficiently and consistently for families; and assures easy, noninvasive, and confidential access to the system.

Target for Success

People respond well to tangible, positive changes. Setting specific objectives with activities that create immediate, positive changes builds support for continuing the process. Demonstrating successful strategies and activities will win commitment from stakeholders who are already involved and may even bring key people on board for the achievement of a broader vision. Long-term goals may be more difficult to achieve and require more time. However, separating more difficult goals from short-term goals will increase the probability of success.

Plan to identify in advance strategies that will lead to immediate success and those that will take more time and effort, thus anticipating any elements of surprise. One state identified new funding sources that were used specifically to promote systems change efforts. This money supported the vision and strengthened the efforts of stakeholders. The combination of resources and efforts is critical to successful change, which is why no single person or resource can explain the success or failure of finance reform efforts.

ISSUES AS TARGETS FOR CHANGE

All elements of early intervention are touched by finance. Certainly, increasing revenues or increasing the number of sources are good, obvious reasons to rethink a state or local early intervention funding system, but there are many others. Money causes people to change their behavior with many different results. It is a careful balancing act to use financing to drive meaningful and important system change and helping key stakeholders to view money as a tool for change, rather than the outcome.

Disability services—early intervention in particular, have not had a history of using family resources (including direct fees or co-payments). Providers of these services are resistant to discuss finance matters with families and have little history of asking for family income information, for example. This is important because the majority of fund sources available to support Part C are based upon income as compared to other variables such as disability type. For families, privacy may be an issue. "...All of a sudden everybody wants to know everything about you and what you bring home and what you make and where you spend your vacation money..." On the other hand, families who come together because of their needs related to their child's disability, are quoted as feeling "really equal, we feel like they're good friends, and it was a real support group." Money may actually be the quickest, easiest tool that community participants can use to change behavior. Finance can also be used to promote family choice. Changes in the way money is distributed may cause people to change the service approach, data collection, and family centeredness of services. Finance is a major factor that supports, directs, and influences what is done in early intervention, where it happens, and how it takes place.

Maximize Funds for Services

One obvious goal for various finance models is to maximize revenues to fund early intervention services; a more complicated goal than it might at first appear because of costs inherent in tapping new revenue sources or changing to use potential sources. One of the tradeoffs is actual cost in terms of staff time, money, equipment, and paperwork that may be involved in accessing new revenue sources. Will additional revenues exceed the cost of obtaining those funds? Communities must first identify and compare the costs and benefits inherent in particular funding models. Economies of scale may be found, whereby increasing the amount of service or the numbers and types of families, contribute to reducing costs for those families. The additional money realized by system improvements may make stakeholders wonder why they didn't think of this years ago!

Local or State Access to Revenue Sources

One of the major decisions in developing a finance model is to decide how best to access revenue sources—either at the local or state level. Funds may be greater if they flow through the state lead agency, yet such funds may not yet have a history of supporting local priorities and values. Decisions about where and which sources to access involve equity tradeoffs, which may be complicated by "linked" funding sources. This situation occurs when one fund source may not be accessed without another, for instance, Title XIX and family insurance. Procedures for parent fees developed as a local option may in reality create inequities for families throughout the state. Such decisions may also influence other funds that states and localities may access, like Title XIX.

Families with similar needs may pay very different amounts for services because of sliding fee scales or other participation rules. Local programs may spend different amounts on families with similar needs because they have obtained additional funding for their local early intervention services. As a result, families receive different amounts of service even though they have the same needs as those in a neighboring area. A family may drop out of early intervention or decrease service because of fees. One example of this was a family who withdrew from Part C because their only source of funds for the parent fee was a stepfather who refused to participate because he was not the child's biological father. Such dilemmas are common because early intervention, as a system, focuses on the individual needs of the family and child as reflected in IFSPs. Fund source decisions are crafted largely by regulations developed to address common social problems, or the needs of a common group, as compared to the individualized approach found in Part C.

Minimize Bureaucracy

Funding model reform should include streamlining the system wherever possible to minimize bureaucracy and paperwork. It is important to avoid unnecessary rules, regulations, and paperwork that result from blended financing efforts. The Part C system is a complete, self-contained system that has tremendous "marketability" to potential fund sources. Where else can these revenue sources find a system that has a clearly defined mission, a well articulated set of regulations and expectations, clear eligibility, defined services and personnel, and a supportive infrastructure that provides training, technical assistance, monitoring and procedural safeguards—all under one roof! Clearly, "selling" the Part C system as a package can help to reduce the potential for duplicate auditing, provider enrollment, and documentation, simultaneously reducing many provider costs as well.

Another approach to minimizing cost is to consider the existing protocols within each individual fund source and compare this documentation, etc. with the Part C system requirements. Where are the similarities and commonalities? How can one piece of documentation serve to address both systems? How significant are the modifications that need to be made by either system, and what is the ultimate outcome/benefit for families and providers? One state successfully developed a "combined enrollment form" that consolidated the paperwork for up to six state sponsored programs. While the enrollment form is considered "long," its six pages now replace the collective 47 pages required to be completed by families to establish various program eligibilities.

Equity of Service Delivery

A workable funding model should offer similar access to early intervention for all families, regardless of home address, economic status, race or ethnicity, or a child's presenting developmental concerns or program eligibility status. Sometimes funding sources serve specific individuals, such as the availability of Medicaid for families with low incomes. One example of how a specific funding source can affect equity occurred in a state where Medicaid reimbursement depended on a specified amount of service. In this state, a minimum of three face to face visits per month were the threshold for billing. As a consequence, families funded under Medicaid received three visits even though they often needed less. Conversely, non-Medicaid funded families receiver fewer services because reimbursement for their services were not tied to the three contact requirement. Rather than individually defined services in this state, service frequencies are being driven by funding which—in at least some instances—is excessive against the identified needs that families have defined, and inadequate for others.

Data Systems

States and localities struggle with the issue of what data or information to collect in order to make more informed decisions and access various funding sources. Families and service providers often feel burdened by paperwork, especially when they have to complete different forms that ask for similar data. For example, many providers are not comfortable asking families for information related to income because they feel that such information may alter their relationship with the family. As one parent said, "The kid is what matters, not what the tax return says." A recent study of the impact of family fees (Goetze, Akers, & Judd, 1998) found that over 95 percent of families either disagreed or strongly disagreed with the statement "it changed my relationship with my service coordinator when she told us about the possibility of a fee." The same study found that over 82 percent agreed or strongly agreed that the procedure to decide the family's eligibility to pay a fee was respectful of the family's privacy.

Training may help service coordinators and other providers better handle issues related to financial responsibilities and to deal with their own, personal feeling and understanding about this process. However, depending upon who is responsible for the information collection, completing forms may decrease time spent with the child and/or family on other matters.

How to achieve a data collection system that efficiently satisfies reporting requirements of revenue sources while not consuming providers, families, and administrators is a dilemma faced by most early intervention stakeholders. Van Dyck (1991) has recommended training *staff whose sole responsibility would be financial counseling.* This would alleviate provider concerns about direct-service time, concurrently increasing staff comfort level for those who work with finance information, and leading to more skilled individuals in this area of specialization. This kind of dedicated task assignment also helps to keep financing separate from the planning or delivery of direct services, which further supports and facilitates the individualized planning requirement of Part C services.

Which funding sources we access and where they are tapped influence the type of information we need to collect and where we send it. In a state-centralized finance system, the same data may be collected from all families and sent to the state. Sources that vary by locality mean more local variation in what, how, and from whom we gather data. Local providers in some states have tried to develop common documentation forms (including eligibility) so that one form satisfies needs of providers and funding sources.

Family-Centeredness

One critical goal for many programs is to provide a family-centered system of early intervention services; a system to be evaluated by how well early intervention responds to family needs based upon their unique needs. The degree of success in achieving this goal depends to a large extent on finance issues. To achieve family centered services requires development of the IFSP and resultant services based upon *what the family states are THEIR primary concerns, priorities and resources*. How financing is structured and accessed greatly influences whether services are individualized, or whether they reflect a routine "cookie-cutter" approach to meeting family and child needs.

In many communities and states, there are two obvious, related examples where improvement may be possible: *service shortages* and *service settings*. Where shortages exist, we are not meeting primary needs. How many of us remember criticizing the former Soviet Union because of long lines for goods where consumers waited to buy food? Similarly, we have queues for many goods provided by the public sector, including respite care, childcare, clinical therapies, therapies in home settings, and Medicaid waivers.

In fact, service patterns show that services provided in the home, as opposed to a center or clinic setting, are provided generally with less intensity or frequency (Escobar, Barnett, & Goetze, 1994; Perry, Greer, Mackey-Andrews, & Goldhammer, 1998). Whether such differences stem from family preferences or resource issues (such as provider choice or funding constraints), home visits are generally more expensive to the provider for each hour of service since transportation time cost-shifts from family to provider. Irrespective of who bears what piece of "cost," all costs combine together in the total cost of the system. Again these costs reflect "people, time and money" in the sense that there are visible and invisible costs that affect the total delivery system and serve as incentives or disincentives for participation by providers and family members.

Service Shortages

Service providers and families in communities we have visited in various states, with different funding models in place, have all reported some type of service shortage for families, most frequently in the areas of specialty therapy services. Changing or increasing resources and funding is one way to reduce shortages. Ideally, we would design funding models to maximize family choice with respect to services and providers; however, some models provide services with limited staff who are employed by particular agencies, and consequently provide no "choice" for family members. In fact, choice is not reflected in the Part C regulations. The only way that choice comes to legitimately bear upon a state's early intervention system is through financing partnerships with those funds—such as Medicaid/Title XIX—that require consumer choice.

Subcontractors—employees who receive no agency salary, but are paid hourly for the amount of service provided—are an additional cost to the local contractor. These organizations contract with the state lead agency to provide early intervention services to a specific geographic area in the state. These potential subcontractors may not be included in the IFSP even though the family could benefit from such service. For example, a state administrator in Part C told of difficulties in obtaining psychological services for a particular family and child. She had to intervene with the contractor to hire a psychologist consultant to properly assist to achieve the family's IFSP outcomes.

Service shortages, which occur in both rural and urban areas, are most often attributed to physical, occupational, and speech therapists. These shortages may be reduced by increasing the service supply, that is, by increasing wages to attract additional providers; however, this means either increasing funding or cutting other services to offset increased wages. In addition, restricted personnel requirements or credentialing obligations for Part C may also increase wage rates and create service shortages.

Another issue is whether all qualified providers who could serve a particular geographic area are actually being used. Several states have developed a broad service matrix that lists all qualified providers who are willing to provide services in a specific region. This model does not limit providers to traditional early intervention agencies but includes independent providers and hospital or home-health workers. A service coordinator who works where the service matrix has been adopted told us their provider list increased from 10 pages to 150 pages as a result of changes in the finance model. She jokingly said that the matrix made it easy to respond to a request from a parent who told her, "I want somebody old like you." Age, in this story, may equate with experience from the family's definitional point of view.

Expanding the provider base by removing artificial geographic boundaries may improve services and choices for families without requiring more funds. Such ideas challenge traditional local providers to compete, as earlier discussed. In establishing choice for families, there are concurrent challenges to systems that affect how providers are marketed or made available to families. These provider issues become more complicated because of questions about how monitoring or supervision of personnel occurs to establish and maintain a high degree of quality providers for families to choose from.

Service Setting

Changes in finance may influence services. One very salient example of this is the current movement to provide services in homes or other natural environments to support the routines and activities of families and children in their daily lives. Many local service providers say that the cost of providing services in a non-clinic or center-based location like homes or childcare facilities is sometimes prohibitive, particularly if local provider shortages continue to exist. Increasing the reimbursement rate for home visits can decrease shortages and support higher location costs by appealing to hospital or clinic providers. Higher reimbursements may also offset negatives such as travel time, weather-related travel issues, and absenteeism (by either the family or provider). It is imperative for each state to balance appropriate reimbursement with their mission to achieve good practice.

Absenteeism or the presumed "failure" of the family to "comply" with the service schedule is one of the most controversial elements of early intervention. Who fails to "show" for services? How does the service detail "match" what a family needs? Do those services reflect what the family values? While simple calculations can address the travel issues—distance and time—they fail to accommodate for episodes of services that are not provided due to either family or provider failure to "show."

Barriers to higher reimbursements for natural environments may exist when fund sources limit or restrict the site of service, thus reducing the options for families and communities as they expand the base of providers. In some instances, the fund source may not have location restrictions, but also is not willing to adjust their reimbursement because the site of service is not of concern to them. This is a barrier, however, that some states and communities have tackled with measurable success.

RELATIONSHIP OF FUNDING MODEL TO FINANCE ISSUES: THE INDIANA SYSTEM

This section illustrates how Indiana's shift from finance Model A to Model B influenced the state's vision and goals for early intervention and how achievement was accomplished through changes in the finance model. Indiana's experience demonstrates some of the tradeoffs and tangible effects of a particular model on target variables within early intervention, such as provider capacity or family choice.

The primary goals for the Indiana financial task force of family and service provider members were to maximize revenues, minimize bureaucracy and cost of accessing various revenue sources, and continue to focus on service goals, particularly family-centeredness and choice. Another primary change that was happening simultaneously was the shift to dedicated or independent service coordination. Organized system changes were two-pronged.

1. Indiana shifted to a system point of entry (SPOE) for intake, evaluation/assessment and initial IFSP development, which resulted in 59 SPOEs in 92 counties statewide.
2. The state implemented a central finance office model similar to that illustrated in Model B, Figure 4.4.

The major change in the way early intervention was financed moved from a system similar to Model A, Figure 4.3 (contracts/grants and fee-for-service) to a central finance office (pay-and-chase system).

One major step that defined changes surrounding the SPOEs was that the decision about specific SPOE selection was left to Local Planning and Coordinating Councils (LPCCs). The state established common "job descriptions" and offered model options to LPCCs. In some cases, the SPOE remained with the DD Agency, or went to the LPCC, or the contract went to some other agency like Workforce Development, a local hospital, or the United Way sponsor-agency.

Such a shift in decision-making created the opportunity to redistribute authority and power over critical SPOE issues to a more diverse group of stakeholders represented by LPCCs, resulting in more neutrality in decisions about services. This structure was designed to remove the potential for conflicts of interest that exist when one provider develops the service plan—the who, where, what, and amount of services—and that same provider delivers the services. Indiana implemented SPOE changes, along with other new developments like the CRO and statewide dedicated or independent service coordination, intending to achieve the vision of a family-centered system of care. This system of care was designed not only to expand the capacity of providers and services provided in natural environments, but to more effectively and efficiently use and coordinate available resources. The primary focus of stakeholders in this initiative was to increase family options and choice regarding the specific service provider, the location, and timing of services.

The central finance office model of funding and reimbursement—the central reimbursement office (CRO), as it is known in Indiana—was another major source of change. As shown in Figure 4.4, this central office collects funds for early intervention services from all potential funding sources and serves as a chase-and-pay system in which the CRO pays providers and then chases or collects the funds. Payment remains separate from the family's eligibility for service, thus increasing equity in service delivery. Since financial eligibility becomes invisible, there is no incentive to develop the IFSP to provide actual services based upon a child or family's eligibility for particular funding sources. This removes financial barriers to develop IFSP services, which are incentives based upon individual fund source limitations.

This system also increases the family focus of early intervention since the CRO pays providers based on a statewide rate schedule for services, regardless of a child or family's eligibility for funding. In addition, the rate schedule was designed to provide additional financial incentives for providers to serve families and children in home or natural environments. Rates for services outside of the center or clinic are set higher to compensate providers for travel time in order to alleviate service provider shortages, especially in natural environments.

The CRO/SPOE model also enrolls all available providers in the service matrix, this removing historical issues related to designated providers by geographical areas. The intake service coordinator at the SPOE uses a service matrix that includes a broad base of service providers, from various agencies, hospitals, home-health companies, and independent providers. The matrix describes characteristics of various providers—their experience, specialties, type and settings provided, hours of service, and additional notes such as a provider who is also the parent of a child with special needs. The family uses the matrix to select providers with characteristics that best meet their needs for their IFSP.

Two relevant, tangible outcomes of the Indiana model have been: (a) billing statements mailed to families and (b) a rich database. Billing statements describe the type, dates, amount, location and cost of services received for the month and boldly state THIS IS NOT A BILL. Families receive a summary of the services that are reported by their providers that helps them monitor their services. Some families have called the state lead agency, FSSA, to tell them when services and payment costs are greater than what they actually received from providers. Even though some families complain of increased time to complete paperwork, the resultant database provides rich information to communities and the state about what is actually happening in early intervention in Indiana. Every visit to each child and family is described in the database, along with information on time between referral and intake, number of referrals by locality for Child Find efforts, and differences between the IFSP and actual services.

Families and service providers in various communities gave generally positive feedback related to the new model now in place in Indiana.

1. Families said that they generally received the services that they value and need and that they usually had choices about where services were provided. *They described wonderful choices of services and settings.* Some families expressed concern about access to funds, enormous paperwork requirements, and time to obtain adaptive equipment. On the other hand, one family said that got a new, $3,000 purple wheelchair for their daughter. As one family member said, there is "red tape hassle, but I get what I need." The question remains is this "red tape" contained in policy or paperwork, or does it reference to the abilities, training and skills of the service coordinator in processing the document required to access the equipment?
2. Families also said that early intervention makes you more aware of what you can get, although in some cases the process was evolutionary. "Before we realized we had options, you had to fight for options, and how you fight against somebody who is giving you

something free that you're so grateful for... just like the seat that [our son] sat in for feeding. If we hadn't asked, we never would have had the seat. We asked and they accommodated and we were thankful..." Many parents learned from the provider the valuable child development information they needed to ensure their child's continuing services.

3. Families liked the billing statements because they summarize what the family gets and from whom they receive it. Some families said that this helps them when they transition to preschool because they know what to include for potential funding resources. For some, however, billings were confusing because they did not always notice the "THIS IS NOT A BILL" statement printed at the top and were confused by the bottom statement which reads "Balance Due."
4. Many felt the new system removed geographic barriers for service providers and increased incentives to provide services where needed.
5. One family said, "the program comes to the children instead of the children going to the program." Concerning home visits, another explained: "We sat around my kitchen table, and everybody I have worked with from the very start has been so incredible. My service coordinator... calls me when she hears of a focus group... sends me articles in the mail, and I can tell my therapist about my concerns with my child..."
6. One provider said that people get paid, they get paid on time, and that makes them happy.
7. As a drawback, some communities continue to report service provider shortages in areas such as service coordination, speech, occupational, and physical therapy.

Indiana's CRO/SPOE model is currently under active evaluation to examine its strengths, tradeoffs, and areas for improvement. Personal comments from knowledgeable families and providers are used to understand the consequences of change for the various early intervention stakeholders whose values and concerns matter: families, children, other consumers such as childcare providers, service providers, and administrators. These changes in Indiana illustrate the financial effects on issues that are important to any early intervention system. As one parent summed up the importance of early intervention: "Then the day comes when you have to realize that not only is she not going to catch up. She's going to start to fall further and further behind...if she hadn't had that early intervention. If we had waited until she was five or six, she would be ten years behind where she is now. It was so important for her to get all the things that she got and the help that she got when she got it."

CONCLUSIONS

As stakeholders move to change the way they finance early intervention in their communities, the experiences of communities and states will provide a base of knowledge to increase the probability for success. The issues that we target for finance reform are diverse and complex; and the relationship of issues to finance models is even more challenging to understand and predict—because of the many variables that can influence outcomes. In particular, this chapter was designed to show the various pieces of the finance puzzle, a puzzle that has more than one solution. The pieces that contribute to the puzzle may vary across communities or states, resulting in different pictures when completed.

This chapter has also described some of the vision or beliefs that may be the target of finance efforts. Funding, money, and other resources that flow to early intervention are key components in how we develop the system of early intervention, and whether we achieve the vision and objectives. Understanding the tradeoffs, options, and experiences of others with respect to the finance puzzle is a big step toward achieving an early intervention system and vision that are at the center of our efforts.

We began by examining the context of early intervention financing as it has developed through the Part C legislation, reauthorization and the state early intervention systems. Next, some of the finance models that have developed within early intervention in various states were described, along with the variables that distinguish one model from another. The steps that state desiring changes in their early intervention finance system, and some of the goals that are targeted with different funding models, were also described. Although not comprehensive, this list is meant to use funding models creatively and is intended, along with other changes, to solve some of the problems that communities face in designing a comprehensive system of early intervention that is family centered. We also examined some of the tradeoffs inherent in choices about goals and funding models. Some tradeoffs, such as equity and efficiency, were examined within the context of various funding models. Finally, we looked at one state that went through the process of change that was described. Stakeholders in this state faced many of the issues, tradeoffs, dilemmas and goals that were described; they struggled through some difficult challenges as they shifted from one finance model to the CRO/SPOE model in order to develop an early intervention finance model that encourages and supports more positive outcomes for families and children.

As one parent summarized her experience, "At first you think you can love them out of it (the disability) and then the reality sinks in. The support and services of early intervention are making a difference." Given the diversity of funding systems, eligibility and access to services, issues of financing services to children with special needs extend to include the life span for these parents. In addition to making services available to families during these early years of life, early intervention offers the first opportunity for information, education, and support to families regarding the wide range of issues—including financing—related to accessing and maintaining services for their child. This experience serves to lay the foundation for informed family involvement in what will be complex service delivery systems throughout their child's life.

ACKNOWLEDGMENT

The author would like to thank Deborah C. Gessaman for her work in editing this chapter and giving it the "human element."

REFERENCES

Brown, W., & Conroy, M. (1999). Entitled to what? Public policy and the responsibilities of early intervention. *Infants and Young Children, 11*, 27-36.

Clifford, R. M. (1991). *State financing of services under P.L. 99-457, Part H.* Chapel Hill, NC: University of North Carolina at Chapel Hill.

Escobar, C. M., Barnett, W. S., & Goetze, L. D. (1994). Cost analysis in early intervention. *Journal of Early Intervention, 18*, 48-63.

Goetze, L. D., Akers, J. F., & Judd, D. R. (1998). *Utah Parent Participation Impact Study (UPPIS)* (Final report submitted to the Utah State Department of Health). Logan, UT: Early Intervention Research Institute, Utah State University.

Kates, W. S. (1991). *NEC*TAS financing workbook: Interagency process for planning and implementing a financing system for early intervention and preschool services.* Chapel Hill, NC: National Early Childhood Technical Assistance System.

Perry, D. F., Greer, M., Mackey-Andrews, S. D., & Goldhammer, K. (1998). *Utilization of early intervention services by a population of infants and toddlers with and at-risk for disabilities.* Unpublished manuscript, Johns Hopkins University, School of Hygiene and Public Health, Washington, DC.

Striffler, N., Perry, D. F., & Kates, D. A. (1997). Planning and implementing a finance system for early intervention systems. *Infants and Young Children 10*, 57-65.

van Dyck, P. (1991). *Use of parental fees for P.L. 99-457, Part H.* Chapel Hill, NC: University of North Carolina at Chapel Hill.

chapter 5

Participatory Realism: Defining the Role of Nonevaluator Stakeholders in Evaluation

Mark S. Innocenti
Richard N. Roberts
Early Intervention Research Institute

Although the term evaluation is used generally to indicate a process by which we gain information on some topic of concern, the activities that constitute evaluation can vary along a variety of dimensions. It is the goal of this chapter to help stakeholders to understand how they can become more involved in the evaluation process, and for researchers and program designers to consider ways to more systematically involve the full spectrum of stakeholders in their work. Stakeholders may be policymakers, legislators or administrators who need evaluation information to make decisions about goals and objectives for ongoing planning, to gauge the effectiveness of programs, or to justify expenses involved in program delivery to a cost conscious constituency. Stakeholders are the people who work within programs, who are concerned about their effectiveness, and how to become better at reaching program goals. Likewise, stakeholders are the consumers of services; families whose children receive services and are equally concerned that they both have a voice in how services are delivered as well as ensuring that those services that are provided are effective in meeting their goals for their children and families. At the broad level, stakeholders are all those impacted by a program and its activities.

The first step to this understanding of evaluation is the knowledge that evaluation is a process that occurs along a continuum. This continuum is anchored on one end by research and on the other end by action evaluation. Evaluation at the research end of the continuum is characterized by studies that are frequently referred to as summative evaluation. The goal of this type of evaluation is to provide a specific answer to a specific question. Evaluation at this end of the continuum might seek to answer questions such as: How much do children's IQs increase as a function of being in a comprehensive preschool program? Do children receive more immunizations as a result of being visited by members of the community action team? Here, the focus is to answer a specific question raised and not necessarily to examine the process or the means by which the end event happened.

On the other end of the continuum are action-focused evaluations. These evaluations are characterized by their focus on evaluating the effects of using different activities, structures, or contexts in reaching a goal of improving a particular set of agreed upon outcomes. Making the decisions about both the outcomes and the strategies to achieve them are part of the evaluation effort. An example of this type of evaluation is an attempt to answer questions such as "What would make our community-based teams of professionals more satisfied working together?" The evaluation activities would consist of interviews, focus groups, or surveys from which the information obtained would be quickly used to effect change in procedures. The outcome, satisfaction, would be informally evaluated.

These examples are, of course, extremes on the continuum. In reality, most evaluations, especially those focused on community-based initiatives, attempt to do a number of things from answering summative type questions to determining the process involved. The history of evaluation has moved through phases that began as experimental and moved to a more action-oriented or pragmatic focus. Next were evaluations that developed within the process of evaluation itself—constructionist evaluations. Current evaluations tend to mix the best aspects of these approaches depending on the evaluation goal (Pawson & Tilley, 1997).

Our approach to evaluation is that there is not an inherently right or wrong approach to evaluation. A person trained in evaluation should have at his or her disposal a toolbox of evaluation strategies, methodologies, and techniques. Depending on the nature of the question asked, any or all of these techniques may be appropriate. At the same time, participation by stakeholders also occurs on a continuum moving from active to passive participation. It is our argument that active involvement makes for a better evaluation for a number of reasons that will be discussed throughout the chapter. Briefly, it can be said that active

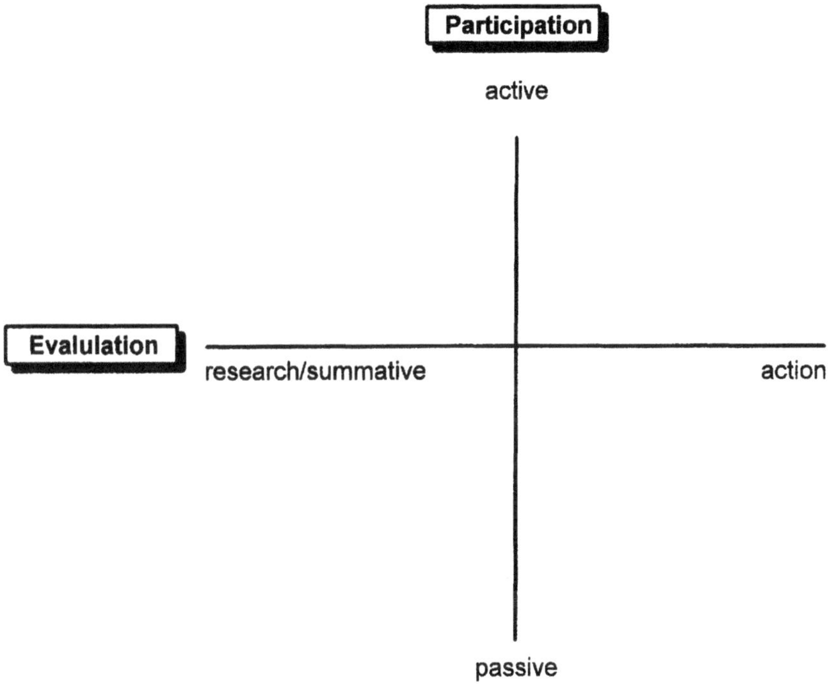

FIGURE 5.1. The evaluation-participation continuum.

involvement by stakeholders has the effect of making the process and products of an evaluation more ecologically valid. It does so by grounding the evaluation activities in more real-life situations and makes it more likely that procedures and evaluation tools are appropriate, family-friendly, and sensible at a consumer level. It also provides a context in which results and interpretations of data can be tested on an audience that has a stake in the findings and for which the phenomena have an everyday reality. Further, active involvement of stakeholders can occur anywhere along the evaluation continuum. The nature of the participation may vary, but opportunities for awareness exist regardless of where on the evaluation continuum the evaluation activities fall. This evaluation/participation continuum is presented in Figure 5.1.

Though some may argue that participatory action research can only be used when all of the stakeholders are involved in all aspects of the process, in the present model this is only one important point on the continuum. There are many obstacles (e.g., funding, time, legislative mandates, etc.) that impact this level of participation in the vast majority of evaluations. While still viewing full participation as the preferred option, understanding these varied factors leads to participatory realism and allows the needs of many stakeholders to be met.

WHY BECOME INVOLVED?

In this age of accountability, programs funded by federal, state, and local governments are in competition for a shrinking pool of resources. Since all programs may argue the benefits of their efforts for families, programs that are able to support such claims with documented effects are better able to claim they are worthy of continued support. As evaluation becomes more of a given, there is an increased need to understand different types of evaluation to make better decisions about the knowledge being obtained. Fetterman (1996), for instance, suggests that the understanding of evaluation must be a basic skill in the repertoire of any educated citizen in society. One of the best ways to better understand this process is to become an active participant.

The second point concerns the role evaluation plays in informing policy. There are some (primarily in the academic community) that believe evaluation data drive policy. Unfortunately, the history of politics and evaluation proves evaluation has relatively little impact on policy (Roberts, 1993). Policy is more often than not driven by beliefs and values. An extreme example of this can easily be illustrated by the relationship of auto speed on highways and accident death rates. There is a clearly established relationship between increases in automobile speed and increases in deaths as a result of crashes. However, these data seem to have no impact on policies governing speed limits.

This analogy is repeated in many instances in a variety of areas when one looks at the relationship between what is known about a phenomenon and the set of political practices that govern that activity. In some respects, policy decisions precede research and evaluation, and resulting evaluation is used to support or not support the decisions that were made.

Since policy frequently precedes evaluation, subsequent evaluation may serve to modify or create improved initiatives over time. In this respect, participation in the evaluation will allow stakeholders to clarify issues, specify more clearly the objectives of programs, and increase their awareness of political issues regarding the area to be evaluated. In so doing, stakeholders have increased their ability to make informed decisions about the appropriate outcomes for programs. This understanding of the relationship between values, politics and evaluation is critical to understanding the whole process of change in community-based initiatives. It is only through a participatory process, however, that one's values can be transformed into outcomes and the outcomes can be assessed.

A third rationale for involvement in the process is related to the nature of the phenomenon with which our community-based initiatives are dealing. At the most basic level, the goal of most community-based initiatives is to enhance family and child well-being for all members of the community. Many community efforts are faced with the increasing burden of poverty in addressing this issue. Poverty and the gaps between the ends of the economic continuum have been increasing for the past 30 years despite the efforts of the federal and local governments to deal with the issue. Community-based initiatives have arisen out of the view that community involvement is a more effective way to have an impact on outcomes for families and children. However, these initiatives as a group present a challenge in implementation and evaluation because they have broad based, multiple goals; are flexible; concentrate responsibility at the community level and develop over time (Brown, 1995). These qualities of the community initiatives clearly present challenges. These challenges cannot be met in the design or practice by one individual nor can they be met in evaluation by one evaluator. Stakeholders are important sources of information that can serve to make or break an evaluation effort.

The final rationale for participation is based on the belief that at the most basic level we are in the business of helping people and it is important to know if goals are being met at the family, program, and bureaucratic levels of service and support. Systematic evaluation is the only reliable way we have to gauge the effects we may be having. The recent emphasis on public program accountability, as evidenced in the Government Performance and Reorganization Act, has changed this landscape directly at the federal level and indirectly at the state and local levels. These changes strengthen the need for systematic evaluation to provide evidence of effectiveness in meeting goals.

The biases in this chapter are that evaluation is needed and stakeholders need to be involved in the evaluation. A number of evaluation models have been developed that include participation by stakeholders. These approaches are variously known as participatory research, action research, participatory action research, participatory evaluation, and empowerment evaluation, to name of few (Brown & Tandon, 1983; Hall, 1993; Pawson & Tilley, 1997; Whyte, Greenwood, & Lazes, 1991). These approaches differ in their relative emphasis on action compared with research and theory building, the role the researcher plays in the action, and in their political orientations. However, they constitute a group of approaches that recognize the role of the stakeholders in the process. The goal of this chapter is not to specifically endorse one particular approach, but to help the stakeholder be a more informed partner in the evaluation process. The next section will directly deal with the types of questions that can be asked to help participants better understand the process and to increase their role in the evaluation process.

DEFINING THE PROCESS FOR THE NONEVALUATOR PARTICIPANT

Table 5.1 contains 10 questions that can help guide stakeholder non-evaluators in becoming involved in the evaluation process. At the same time they raise issues that evaluators should address with stakeholders in realistic evaluation efforts. This list is not all inclusive as there are other questions that may arise as you participate in a specific evaluation. Similarly, the questions listed within the table overlap. This overlap will become clearer as some of the issues behind each of the questions are further explained.

Knowledge of the historical involvement of the family as stakeholders helps put stakeholder involvement into perspective. Historically, families played relatively little or no role in evaluations that sought information regarding the impact of interventions focused on children and families (Roberts, Rule, & Innocenti, 1998). The family typically had no role in the design of the evaluation process, may or may not have been involved in delivering intervention, and was not typically used as a source of information regarding the impact of the program. These evaluations were typically developed by researchers and disseminated primarily through academic outlets (e.g., journals, conferences). The evaluation frequently used a traditional, experimental design methodology (summative in nature). These types of evaluations were not necessarily bad evaluations and in fact some of these early evaluations have had a profound impact on policy toward children and families. For example, the Perry Preschool Project (Weikart, Bond, & McNeil, 1978) exemplified this type of program that found very positive effects of their intervention. It is essentially this program and its longitudinal successors that have helped develop and maintain Head Start in America. Although the immediate comparison of the Perry Preschool Project to Head Start is not direct, the relationship between the two has benefitted a number of children and families.

The next step in this progression was the involvement of families in the evaluation process, but most frequently this involvement focused on parents perceptions of what occurred as a result of some type of intervention. That is, families were typically used as a source of data. These evaluations tended to be more academic in nature or were broadened by

TABLE 5.1.
Questions for Stakeholders Participating in Evaluation

1. What is the purpose of the evaluation?
2. Who is paying for the evaluation?
   a. What requirements have been imposed that are unalterable?
3. What do you intend to do with the results (who are you trying to impact)?
4. Who are the stakeholder groups?
   a. What is their level of involvement?
5. How much funding is available for the evaluation?
6. What techniques (methods) will be used as part of the evaluation?
   a. Why were those chosen?
   b. Contrast this approach to other approaches?
   c. What is the relationship of these methods to the purpose and impact?
7. What are the outcome measures?
   a. Are these realistic measures (given the program or intervention)?
   b. Are they based on theory?
   c. Are they obtainable?
   d. Do our measurement techniques allow us to see changes on the measures if change does occur?
   e. Are the measures short or long term? (Do we have time to reach them?)
8. How will information be obtained?
   a. Can we use extant data?
   b. Can we use or modify existing forms?
   c. What are the time commitments of those providing information?
   d. How can we be sensitive to work/privacy/cultural issues?
9. How will we clarify the interpretation of results?
   a. Who is empowered to interpret data and their meaning?
10. How will evaluation information be disseminated?

an understanding that the changes in the child may affect family functioning (and vice versa) and they sought to measure this outcome. Families and other stakeholders were not actively involved in designing the evaluation or in disseminating the results of these types of evaluation. However, as in the previous level, many of these studies have had impacts that have benefitted children and families.

The next level in this progression represents a significant shift in which designing the evaluation more closely involves policymakers and service providers along with the evaluators. Families did not necessarily participate in the design of this study but they and other stakeholders served in advisory capacities that provided input on the evaluation process. Families became recognized not only for how the intervention may affect them and how they will affect the intervention, but also as a source of advice regarding intervention. There is a greater recognition that others need information from the evaluation and more active efforts are made to get information to stakeholders in the process of social change.

The final level includes the active involvement of all stakeholders in all stages of the evaluation process. Potential participants include all people for whom the results of an evaluation may have an impact. Within this model, representatives from each stakeholder group would be involved with the evaluator in determining the purposes of the evaluation and the types of data that represent outcomes of importance. With this historical perspective, we return to the questions for stakeholders. The next section provides a rationale for Table 5.1 questions and defines issues that drive the questions.

WHAT IS THE PURPOSE OF THE EVALUATION?

Since evaluation is not a unidimensional entity, information resulting from an evaluation can affect different audiences in a variety of ways. Jacobs (1988) stated several assumptions regarding evaluation that suggest the integral role evaluation must play in any ongoing program as a systematic collection and analysis of data to be used for a variety of legitimate purposes and audiences. The overall effect should be to enhance rather than detract from service delivery. Cohen and Ooms (1993) provide a detailed listing of different purposes of evaluation and potential audiences for them. These purposes may range from assessing the extent to which existing services in a community (or state) adequately meet needs or respond to problems (community or statewide needs assessments, cross-system data matches), to determining which of a number of similar programs or policies achieves the best results in dollar terms (cost effectiveness).

This awareness of the purposes of evaluation is not new. Jacobs (1988) discussed the purpose of evaluation within what she referred to as a five-tiered approach to program evaluation. This framework, presented in Table 5.2, helps clarify how the various purposes for an evaluation may interact with the methodology selected and audiences affected.

Neither the purposes nor the hierarchy is meant to imply that one tier or one purpose is superior. It is only meant to exemplify the different purposes for which evaluations may be used. An evaluation project may focus on a single tier or may incorporate aspects from multiple tiers. The purpose of evaluation will vary depending on the community initiative being evaluated. Cohen and Ooms (1993) described a community service initiative that systematically progressed through the five tiers described by Jacobs (1988). Other communities may begin evaluation of a service initiative, only to recycle back to questions raised in earlier tiers as new information is identified and incorporated into the service initiative as a result of the evaluation process.

TABLE 5.2.
Jacobs (1988) Five-Tiered Hierarchy of Evaluation

Tier	Evaluation objective	Audience
Preimplementation	1. Document need 2. Document fit between community and program	Funders, policymakers, community groups
Accountability	1. Document use of program 2. Justify/change funding levels	Funders, community leaders
Program clarification	1. Clarify program's mission, goals and objectives	Program staff and participants
Program objectives	1. Determine how to improve program 2. Document program effectiveness	Program staff, policymakers, community groups
Program impact	1. Contribute knowledge to field 2. Examine differential effectiveness 3. Identify replicable programs	Policymakers, academic community, program developers

Potentially, there are many purposes for evaluation and as noted these purposes may overlap. However, identification of this general purpose serves to influence the information obtained as you ask other questions and as you receive information from the other questions. The information from the other questions in Table 5.1 should be used to return to the issue of purpose to help define your purpose more clearly as you progress through the process of evaluation.

WHO IS PAYING FOR THE EVALUATION?

Knowledge of who is paying for the evaluation may directly impact on the purpose of the evaluation. In the vast majority of cases, the primary stakeholders are not the people funding the project. Funding typically comes from federal, state, or agency resources—whether planned as part of the implementation of a program, legislatively mandated as part of a program, or considered as part of a process to obtain information that is typically funded through grants.

Including all stakeholders at all levels is not always possible, nor is it always the evaluation method of choice. In some cases, the evaluation may be best served by a more traditional evaluation. The evaluator must be sensitive to the reality that someone is paying for the evaluation, and the needs of the "buyer" must be addressed. It is not uncommon for legislative groups or other government groups to ask that very specific outcomes be evaluated. If evaluators accept the evaluation contract in that situation, they are then expected to provide the information as requested. Having done so, however, does not preclude input from stakeholders. For example, it still may be both necessary and desirable to involve stakeholders in a number of preevaluation activities. The prevaluation process, or coming to understand which questions should be asked and how they would best be answered, should still be interactive among the contractor, the evaluator, and potential stakeholders. The purpose of attempting to conduct more collaborative evaluations is to make the identification of purposes and outcomes more of an inclusive process, ensuring that the evaluation addresses relevant needs. In doing so, these components must remain rigorous and valid for the evaluation to be acceptable to the very stakeholders who collaborate in the design process.

The needs of the contractor must be considered. As noted earlier in the chapter, both evaluation and participation lie on a continuum. Knowledge of who is paying must be included to locate the evaluation and the resulting participation in the appropriate places on the continuum.

WHAT DO YOU INTEND TO DO WITH THE RESULTS? (WHO ARE YOU TRYING TO IMPACT?)

Historically, information from evaluations was either directed toward academic audiences (e.g., through journals) or to reports for whomever paid for the evaluation. Either of these methods of relaying information tended to be very technical and had a limited distribution. In a participatory framework, the role of information from an evaluation is changed. Depending on the purpose of the evaluation and the various stakeholder groups involved, information is targeted in formats most relevant and useful to the involved groups. Information needs to be presented in concise, readable formats (particularly for policymakers, who are most likely to digest information in one-page bulleted-format summaries). The same recommendations hold true for many agency heads and other people in agencies. If parents are stakeholders, then a brief letter to parents may be a preferred information route. If the goal of the evaluation is to impact the practice of people in agencies, information needs to be conveyed briefly and interactively on what was found, as well as how practices should be changed. In many cases, it will be the responsibility of the evaluator to have a more detailed report available, but the primary use of this may be for reference if questions arise in regard to what was done. This is not to say that the more traditional academic and report outlets may not be required or are not appropriate. Rather, evaluation formats must be used that allow stakeholders to interactively understand issues and results as they incorporate them into their planning and programmatic activities.

The information on potential audiences to be targeted should be considered early in the evaluation process. The following four questions may serve as a guideline to help those participating in evaluation think about impact issues:

1. What are the major issues to be addressed as part of the evaluation?
2. Whom do we need to influence regarding these issues?
3. What types of information do we need to influence these people?
4. How do we (what approaches) go about influencing these people?

Use of these questions or similar questions to develop an overarching perspective on impact may benefit participants in the evaluation process. The specific information to be disseminated and more detail on the method of dissemination can be decided as you progress through the process, but it is an important issue to making the evaluation more useful and having it serve a purpose.

WHO ARE THE STAKEHOLDER GROUPS?

The first phase is to determine the specific nature and purpose of the evaluation. Therefore, in a participatory model, the evaluator must ensure that all appropriate stakeholders are represented in the evaluation process. This stakeholder group should include those not traditionally involved in evaluations as stakeholders as well as those typically represented. There are no rigid formulae for determining who the stakeholders should be. One step is to identify through those most interested in the evaluation (the people who are contracting for the evaluation), who they believe to be the important stakeholders. Stakeholder issues to be addressed include the representation of cultural diversity within the stakeholder group from representatives of various communities in the region being served, and the perspectives of citizens impacted by the social program.

Once a stakeholder group has been identified, meetings to identify or refine the purpose of the evaluation need to occur. As noted earlier, Jacobs (1988) identified a number of approaches to evaluation in her five-tiered hierarchy. Each of these purposes and others can be considered for the evaluation. The role of the evaluator becomes one of facilitating the stakeholders while they elucidate their specific questions and the audiences to which the evaluation will be disseminated. All stakeholders need to be represented equally in the process. This means the policy maker does not necessarily have more influence in the evaluation process than the parent or any other stakeholder; although stakeholders need to be aware of and sensitive to the realities of program funding.

This phase of the process has the potential of being the most challenging for the evaluator. It is within this phase that you might encounter someone with beliefs that evaluation must be conducted in a certain way or that only one purpose is appropriate for evaluation. The evaluator needs to work with the stakeholder group to identify the purpose of the evaluation and tie that to the audiences for the evaluation and the methodology that may be used. Questions can be raised regarding different types of evaluation that may occur. Evaluability assessment (Rutman, 1980) can be included to look at the present level and needs of the initiative. These and other concerns need to be addressed. It makes no sense to look at efficacy issues if a program is still under development. It makes little sense to assess child outcomes if the program is focused on family issues.

It should be also clear that it will not be possible to have all representatives from all stakeholder groups present as part of the evaluation process. The goal is to identify the appropriate stakeholder groups and to have representation from people who are considered viable within the groups. This means, for example, that if you are working with a parent group you do not want your representative to be the one with the beliefs that are extremely different from the other people in the group. It will be critical that the stakeholders who are involved in the process be able to support the process when returning information to the stakeholder group. It becomes the role of the involved stakeholder to help present the information in such a way that the stakeholder group acknowledges that it did have a role in the process and that it was a valid role. This information is best relayed by the involved stakeholder.

Other issues also need to be considered when defining stakeholder groups and identifying participants. One issue is that of paying nonagency stakeholders for their participation. If we truly value the input of people such as parents and consumers, then the possibility of reimbursement for involvement should be considered. An agency issue that sometimes arises is the selection of a representative who is not empowered to make decisions. This impacts on the group process. These only represent some of the issues that may occur.

HOW MUCH FUNDING IS AVAILABLE FOR THE EVALUATION?

This issue is the one where the rubber meets the road. The reality of conducting an evaluation is the fact that it can be a very expensive process. Typically, agencies or legislators only include a small amount of overall budget for an evaluation. This directly impacts on the scope of the evaluation in terms of what can be done given the money available. It is the role of the evaluator to be able to discuss different approaches along with the costs of different approaches, and to provide information to the participants on what can and cannot be accomplished given fiscal limitations.

In many respects, the purpose of the evaluation will best be addressed by a set of methodologies that need to be discussed with the stakeholders. Within this, the evaluator needs to be sensitive to fiscal issues in conducting evaluation and to realistically relate to the stakeholders the pros and cons of various approaches to the evaluation. If the purpose identified by the stakeholders requires a large comparative study to address it adequately, but the funding for such a study is not available, then the stakeholders need to be aware of this issue and incorporate it into the process. Many evaluators experience this need for "reality checks" with stakeholders as part of this process. The range of questions, as well as the degree of specificity, are quite broad. Focusing the questions to the "doable" ones can be an involved process. Issues related to the next three questions impact this "doability" factor.

WHAT TECHNIQUES (METHODS) WILL BE USED AS PART OF THE EVALUATION?

The issue behind this question involves the specific methodologies and techniques that will be used as part of the evaluation. The methodologies tie directly into the purpose of the evaluation and relate to the types of outcomes that are desired. There are a variety of methodologies that can be used. The evaluator should have these various methodologies in his/her tool bag and ready to go. One of the issues that arise frequently in regard to methodology is the use of quantitative and qualitative methodologies. Qualitative methodologies are those that involve information obtained from the participants in a manner that does not immediately result in some type of numerical data. This approach seeks to obtain information on opinions, concerns, attitudes, and other aspects of a phenomenon that are not readily quantifiable. That collection of these types of qualitative data can be very rigorous procedurally (for example, see Miles & Huberman, 1994). Collection and analysis of qualitative data can be a time consuming process. This type of information could be obtained through focus groups, individual contacts, or other means.

Quantitative information is information typically obtained through methods that result in assigning the information a specific number. Examples of this type of methodology involve the administration of tests that result in a certain score or in interviews or questionnaires where respondents provide a specific numerical response on some type of scale. The rigorousness of this approach can also vary from a short questionnaire, which can be returned in the mail, to a measure that can only be administered by certified professionals.

These quantitative and qualitative methodologies need to be distinguished from the summative and formative types of evaluation discussed earlier. As noted, summative evaluation involves an interest in the outcome of the evaluation. Outcomes can be obtained either through qualitative or quantitative means. Similarly, formative evaluation is focused on the process by which an intervention or initiative happens. Formative events can be understood either through qualitative or quantitative means. It is important to keep in mind that types of evaluation do interact with the methodology involved. The goal is to select the mix of methods that best represent the needs of the evaluation. Indeed, the use of mixed methods has become very common in most evaluations focused on community initiatives. That is, some information is provided in numbers and some information is provided in a more descriptive manner. These different types of information can then be combined to provide a richer overall picture of what may be going on within an evaluation. Greene, Caracelli, and Graham (1989) provide a useful conceptual framework for mixed-method evaluations.

The evaluator should be able to discuss a specific approach and issues that may arise. These questions address the issues of why was a specific approach chosen? The evaluator should be able to provide reasons for the methods used and defend them. The evaluator should also be able to present different approaches to demonstrate what types of information will and will not be given as part of a different approach. Finally, there should be a logical relationship between the methods, purpose, and outcomes that relate to the impact.

WHAT ARE THE OUTCOME MEASURES?

Once the purpose and type of evaluation have been identified, the evaluator must work with stakeholders in identifying appropriate outcomes related to these purposes. Many times, the overall goal for a project is very encompassing (e.g., all children will enter school ready to learn; all mothers will receive appropriate prenatal care). These are appropriate as goals but they are not the same as outcomes. Cohen and Ooms (1993) discuss the identification of outcomes, indicators, and benchmarks. Each of these is used at different levels in an evaluation. *Outcomes* are the results toward which the initiative activities are directed. *Indicators* are measurable events that demonstrate the impact of an outcome. *Benchmarks* are incremental steps toward the indicators. Within this framework, outcomes can be either long or short term depending on the evaluation purposes. As an example (see Center for the Study of Social Policy [CCSP], 1993), an outcome may be to increase the rates of healthy births. Indicators would be lower rates of premature births, fewer low birth weight babies, and increases in prenatal care. Benchmarks would be reduced rates of unintended births and teenage births, higher rates of students succeeding at school, and increased use of family planning and information services.

The issue of outcome selection becomes more complex as one takes into account the purpose of the evaluation, which may affect the type of outcomes and where the information to address the outcome may come from. Depending on the evaluation, information may be necessary on the child or youth, adults (usually the parents), the family system, the service system or the community itself. Each of these sources of information interact with the purpose of the evaluation in the determination of the final outcomes selected.

Given these issues, selection of outcomes can be difficult for a variety of other reasons (Cohen & Ooms, 1993). Outcomes must be defined at different levels for different stakeholders. Many service oriented professionals see themselves as providers of expertise and are uncomfortable with being evaluated on their outcomes. One set of indicators and benchmarks may not be equally appropriate for all programs that purport to impact the same area. If stakeholders come from a variety of professional groups, each may see the priorities of their profession or discipline as primary. These are examples of types of issues that will need to be resolved. It is important for evaluators to facilitate the selection of outcomes that will be addressed in the evaluation.

Another pitfall to be avoided is the selection of too many indicators for an outcome. Once again, it is not uncommon for evaluations, especially those conducted by larger systems, to identify many indicators across a wide variety of areas, only to pick and choose among them after a social program is in place. Although this may be a politically expedient strategy, albeit wasteful of resources, it fails to provide a coherent indication of actual program impact.

Cohen and Ooms (1993) present a number of issues and challenges they identified as relevant to developing outcome-driven policies. If all these issues are considered in the early development of an initiative, they would facilitate evaluation. These issues and challenges are presented below.

1. It is important that outcomes be developed in a public forum. If communities can pull together a cross-section of people to agree upon a set of outcomes and indicators that will assess their progress, wider ownership of both the process and outcomes will result. Although there is no guarantee that line workers and consumers would agree on what the outcomes should be, establishing the dialogue is a great contribution. Issues about the specific use of the outcomes data and the consequences attached to success or failure in achieving the outcomes should be clearly spelled out during these discussions.
2. Political pressure for immediate results is a potential barrier to outcome-driven policies. To be successful, programs require much more than well-defined outcomes. Staff and programs who will be held accountable must have real authority to implement interventions and adequate resources to respond to the needs of multi-problem families. Few communities have all the services and resources needed, which has implications for both the extent to which defined outcomes are realistic and the degree to which managers and staff will accept what are seen as new and unrealistic expectations without sufficient support behind them.
3. There are serious concerns regarding the quality and availability of data from which the indicators of the selected outcomes must be derived. Comparisons are usually difficult because the definitions of terms and measures are not standardized, and often the process of data collection itself is flawed. Furthermore, evaluation shouldn't focus on outcomes alone. The experimental nature of many of these projects means that process evaluation will be critically important to the projects themselves and the wider community that is trying to learn from these early innovative endeavors.
4. While we have gained some information about "what works," little is known about why certain interventions work, or to which specific aspect of a program this success can be attributed. Much finer-grained research and analysis are needed to clarify the relationship between short-term outcomes (which are often the most easily measured and monitored) and long-term impacts (pp. 15-16).

The identification of appropriate outcomes for an evaluation is one of the most critical and most difficult aspects of the entire process. Facilitating the selection of appropriate outcomes with stakeholders is important and will affect all other aspects of the evaluation.

In addition to these variety of concerns, there are some questions that can be asked of the evaluator to make the information more meaningful to the participants. These questions are outlined in Table 5.1 as part of question 7. The first question is, "Are the measures realistic?" This first issue relates to the potential impact the program may or may not have. As was noted earlier in the chapter, we are working in a very difficult arena with less than powerful interventions. Selections of measures needs to be based on what seems reasonable for the program to achieve within the time frame of the evaluation. For example, it may be unrealistic to say that you're going to have an impact on children's development if you are measuring a home visiting program that occurs once a month and you only have a six month time frame to evaluate the program. Care needs to be taken to ask about outcome measures that are reasonable, or the resulting answers may not be useful to the program, and may actually have a negative impact.

A second subquestion is, "Are measures based on theory; that is, are the outcome measures used selecting based on some accepted theory?" Evaluation questions may or may not be based on a theory. There are ways to include theory within the development of community initiatives and these should be explored whenever possible (Weiss, 1995). The use of a theory in some respects allows the relationship to a larger body of knowledge that can be used when discussing the outcomes of the evaluation. Use of a theory also allows an individual evaluation to fit into a larger framework with other evaluations to provide more general knowledge to the field overall. For certain groups, the utility of theory is welcomed. If nothing else, the community initiatives are typically based on some underlying theory and these should help drive the purpose of the evaluation.

A third question is, "Are the measures obtainable?" This question ties in with the next section on how information is gathered but also relates to the identification of outcome measures. It is only logical to attempt to select measures where the information that will be provided is realistic and believable. In areas where information may be highly personal, the information that may be obtained may not be accurate because of people's reluctance to answer honestly on sensitive topics. Similarly, issues of culture impact the way questions are developed. When working in an area with people from diverse cultures, one needs to be sure that questions are appropriate to accepted cultural mores. Other issues also impact on obtaining information and will be discussed in the next section.

The fourth question is, "Do our measurement techniques allow us to see changes on the measures if change occurs?" This also relates to the purpose of evaluation and ensuring that we can demonstrate reasonable outcomes from the evaluation. For example, if our evaluation is attempting to impact on the birth of low weight babies and our data is being obtained from a city-wide health database, but the intervention is occurring in a small part of the community, does impact in one part of the community result in changes on the larger data base? In most cases, it would not. This would mean that our program may indeed have been effective, but that we were not able to "see" the impact. Another example may occur if we are trying to measure a concept such as stress in parents. Many of our measurement techniques for gauging stress are very global in nature. That is, they are assessing a person's stress makeup beyond daily stress. If such a measure was used as your only outcome to look at stress, you may not see changes in stress over a period of time when indeed changes in daily stress levels are occurring. Similarly, the first author of this chapter was involved in a program that was in part evaluating family support. However, the measure of family support being used was too global. Upon careful examination, it was found that the intervention was at best only impacting on one or two items within the overall measure. This made it difficult to prove that any impact had occurred on family support. Clearly, this issue needs to be considered in development of outcomes. It should be kept in mind that there are multiple ways to assess different outcomes and these need to be considered in depth.

The final question to be asked is, "Are the measures short or long-term?" In some types of interventions it takes a long period of time to impact on certain outcomes. If your evaluation is only short-term in nature, care must taken not to select measures that will only demonstrate impact longitudinally. As an extreme example, it does not make sense to consider school placement as an outcome if your intervention is focused on infant/parent relationships and the evaluation is only two years in length. The bottom line question to be asked is if there is sufficient time in the evaluation such that the measures will show change.

HOW WILL INFORMATION BE OBTAINED?

There are a number of data collection methods for obtaining different types of information. The stakeholders must determine what types of strategies will address the outcomes selected. The evaluator should have a large "tool box" of potential techniques for collecting data and be able to present these, along with the information on what is and what is not obtained by various techniques, to the stakeholders in an understandable manner. The stakeholders then need to consider the goals and audiences of the evaluation and provide input into strategies of data collection. The stakeholders may be the best judges of what information can and cannot be obtained, and data collection methods.

One of the issues to be considered in this phase is the use of extant data (data already collected). Most agencies already collect a great deal of information for a variety of purposes. In some cases it may be possible to use these various data sources to obtain some of the information that address identified outcomes. Although this use of extant data sounds appealing, it has been more difficult to use in actual evaluations (Cohen & Ooms, 1993; Roberts, Innocenti, & Goetze, 1997). Many of these data sets are very specific and to use them for other purposes often fails to meet the mark. Issues of confidentiality also arise when dealing with different data sets (see American Public Welfare Association, Center for Law and Social Policy, Council of Chief State Officers, & Education Commission of the States, 1992; Hobbs, 1997, for a discussion of confidentiality issues in using cross-agency data). Sometimes, what appears to be the same information is collected in different ways by different agencies, making the reliability of the information suspect. This does not mean that extant data can never be used, but it does indicate that the evaluator needs to critically examine the data bases that information comes from. On a more hopeful note, some initiatives are having agencies jointly develop data collection systems that facilitate their use for evaluation purposes. One role of the evaluator is to advocate for these types of changes.

In developing strategies to collect outcome data, many of the concerns relevant to any type of research are valid. The format by which information will be obtained (e.g., interview, norm-referenced measure questionnaire, and so forth) must have some indication that it is valid and reliable. Tools must be staff and family friendly and able to be completed within a reasonable time period. The key complaints by those providing information in an evaluation relates to the length of time and to the complexity of forms on which information is requested. It is critical that forms be kept as simple as possible and the time to complete the forms be minimized as much as information needs will allow. There is a tendency on the part of evaluators to collect more information then they need based on the theory "get it while you have them there." The need for information requires close scrutiny to avoid obtaining extra and unnecessary information. The possibility of paying people for completing forms and being involved in the evaluation should be considered.

This not only helps increase participation and completeness, it also provides an indication of respect for the time of those providing information. Some stakeholders in evaluation will react negatively to the idea of paying those who provide information. However, we have no problem paying evaluators for conducting the evaluation or paying interventionists for providing a service. This represents a type of work. Similarly, completing evaluation forms, especially those that may be lengthy, complex, or both, is also work and people deserve payment for their activities.

Other issues to be considered are those related to privacy and cultural concerns. It is important that the stakeholders providing advice in the evaluation be representative of cultural groups that may exist in the sample to be studied. This will help in the development of measures and techniques to obtain information. Similarly, the procedures for obtaining information should be field tested with a variety of individuals to ensure that issues of culture or privacy are not being impacted on. This is an important consideration and should occur early in the development of techniques to obtain information.

A final issue within this area is regarding the use or modification of existing agency forms. This may or may not be feasible depending on what types of information are currently being collected and the level and amount of detail that is being provided. Some evaluators have worked with intervention sites to develop forms that are useful both for the intervention program, to answer immediate questions about intervention, and for answering questions in the evaluation. For example, McCroskey and colleagues (McCroskey & Meezan, 1997; McCroskey & Nelson, 1989) describe the collaborative development of an instrument for use in a family support program that combines case assessment, reporting/recording, evaluation structure, and research data collection.

However, this approach is not always feasible. Different agencies within the same community may use different forms to collect information and selecting one form may not be expedient for political purposes. Occasionally, forms that purport to obtain the same information assess different aspects of the same phenomenon and may not be compatible in actual use. Sometimes, developing a new form allows staff to step into a different mental perspective of what is going on and helps in completing the evaluation. Similarly, a bad form or an excessive change in forms can sometimes negatively impact an ongoing evaluation. Questions regarding the use of modifications of existing forms can only be made when knowledge of the existing forms is available and with a perspective on what the purpose and outcomes of the evaluation are.

Even after decisions have been made regarding the collection of data, the evaluator and stakeholders need to be vigilant. The evaluator must be alert to potential problems and be able to alter data collection if the data are not addressing the needs of the evaluation. Again, this requires collaboration with the stakeholders. It behooves evaluators to establish a process for the orderly collection of data. This is true regardless of the type of data being collected. Quantitative data needs to checked, coded, and entered using a monitoring process. Qualitative data needs to be reviewed and incorporated into a format that allows interpretation. The first stage of this phase is the establishment of these monitoring systems.

The second stage requires that evaluators be intimately aware of the information being obtained and review the information in relation to the purposes of the evaluation. For example, it may have been part of the plan to ask community programs about certain activities that should be part of the initiative being evaluated. This information was to be obtained through questionnaires completed by the community groups. However, on reviewing the questionnaires, you find that certain information is being left incomplete. Phone contacts with the community staff suggest that these questions do not assess the concepts intended. The information provided by these questions is critical to one purpose of the evaluation. The question becomes, "What should happen next?" This stage implies that this feedback on the ineffectiveness of the evaluation method be viewed with the stakeholder group and a new strategy for assessing this information be developed.

An example of this process comes from an evaluation of family support systems in Michigan using an emergent design methodology (Thompson & Herman, 1996). In this type of evaluation, uncertainty emerges about the program, which may come from stakeholders' lack of consensus or clarity about the program being evaluated. This uncertainty may also arise as a result of having a program that continues to evolve as it is being implemented. In the Thompson and Herman study, their first phase was to identify and portray a family support system designed for children with disabilities in a comprehensive manner. This first phase helped in the development of a template used for interviewing families regarding their participation in the system. This in turn, led to the development of a survey to obtain quantitative data from program staff that validated the earlier findings and identified directions for change. In this study, each phase directly affected the evaluation activities that occurred during the next phase. The stakeholders participated in the different phases of data collection in various ways.

This emergent design may not always apply and may not necessarily be used in the manner described here. However, it does represent a process that can be used in certain cases. It exemplifies the need to be aware of the data being collected and what information it imparts. The concepts of this type of evaluation model need to be considered even when conducting evaluations with different purposes. The final process, however, will be tied directly to the purposes of the evaluation being conducted.

HOW WILL WE CLARIFY THE INTERPRETATION OF RESULTS?

Once data have been analyzed, they will be prepared into a report or some format for presentation to the stakeholders. Although the initial analysis of data and interpretation is usually the responsibility of the evaluator, this should not stand as the final level of data interpretation. Once the data are prepared, they need to be presented to the stakeholders for clarification and interpretation. It is not the intent of this meeting to alter unfavorable interpretations to a more favorable light, but to ensure that data obtained, analyzed, and interpreted are addressing the needs of the stakeholder group. In fact, having all stakeholders represented in this process should decrease the number of evaluation reports that are primarily self-serving (i.e., for agencies or other government entities).

These meetings also serve as a partial validity check on the data. If the information obtained does not appear relevant from the perspective of the stakeholders or is not consistent with other sources of information, then the evaluators need to reconsider the activities that occurred prior to this point in time. An additional goal in this phase is to ensure that information is in a form that can be communicated to the various groups represented by the stakeholders.

HOW WILL EVALUATION INFORMATION BE DISSEMINATED?

Activities within this phase have multiple purposes. The goal of the evaluator is to facilitate the use of information obtained in the evaluation process—information that will have an impact on targeted audiences as identified earlier in the process (e.g., that the program being evaluated uses the information to improve). Again, the preferred dissemination methods will be somewhat dependent on the target audiences. Some ideas for formats were discussed earlier. The stakeholders can provide information on the best means and ways to disseminate this information.

In some instances, it may be more appropriate for the stakeholders to identify and serve as their own means for dissemination. The evaluators in this situation would facilitate the presentation of the results in a way that is useable by different stakeholder groups. The evaluators may also work with the stakeholders to facilitate the identification of practices or service structures that could be changed to improve the program being evaluated. However, final decisions about system change can only come from the stakeholders.

Another activity that could occur in this phase is the establishment of a self-assessment system for the program being evaluated. However, if this is a desired outcome then it should be made clear to all parties during the earlier phases of the evaluation. As an example, one aspect of empowerment evaluation is to identify for the program being evaluated some way to use the evaluation results for establishing a system to regularly self-assess areas of concern and by so doing, empower the group being evaluated (Fetterman, Kaftarian, & Wandersman, 1996). Self-assessment strategies can include establishing strategies that assess process as well as product (outcomes). The stakeholders can then use the self-assessment on an ongoing basis.

APPLYING PRINCIPLES TO PRACTICE

What follows in this section, will be two examples of the participatory interactive processes in evaluation at the community level as described within this chapter. The first is of a statewide evaluation of the early intervention programs for children with disabilities birth through five in the state of Utah. The second is a participatory model implemented within a project entitled Opening Doors into Rural Communities funded by the U.S. Maternal and Child Health Bureau (MCHB).

Example 1: Utah Early Intervention Project

By 1991 in Utah, a system of services for children birth to five with disabilities had been implemented and was functioning statewide. Early intervention for infants and toddlers (Part C of the Individuals with Disabilities Education Act [IDEA 97; P.L. 105-17]), referred to as *Baby Watch*, was sponsored by the Utah Department of Health. Services for preschoolers with disabilities (Section 619 of Part B of IDEA 97) was sponsored by the Utah Office of Education. Although both programs developed somewhat independently, by 1994 the effects of these two programs as well as the transition from one program to another were high on the minds of a number of stakeholders within the state. These included parents of children with disabilities, early intervention staff from the Baby Watch and the Preschool Special Education programs, state level administrators within the Department of Health and the Office of Education, and state legislators who were investing state dollars, as a compliment to the federal dollars, in early intervention programs. A steering committee consisting of state level administrators and evaluators from the Early Intervention Research Institute (EIRI) at Utah State University met to develop a plan for evaluating the effects of early intervention programs throughout the state. Over the course of several meetings of stakeholders, several research questions emerged.

1. How have the Part H and Part B programs for children birth through five and their families been implemented across the state in accordance with federal and state policies?
2. What are the effects of early intervention services for children birth through five and their families in Utah?
3. What are the overall costs of early intervention services for children birth through five and their families as provided through the Part H and Part B programs?

Contracts were developed jointly between Utah Department of Health and Office of Special Education with the Early Intervention Research Institute to conduct this evaluation project referred to as the Utah Early Intervention Project (UTEIP). A longitudinal research design was employed in which children and their families who were enrolling in the Baby Watch and Preschool Special Education programs were to be followed over a three-year period. In doing so, a number of questions had to be resolved with respect to how this research would be carried out to answer the questions mutually agreed upon by the stakeholders. Each agency was interested in understanding:

1. The characteristics of children and their families who were involved in the programs as well as the characteristics of the programs themselves.
2. The contract between parents and service providers with respect to the quantity, type and range of services and supports a family could expect from the early intervention programs using the Individualized Planning Process (IFSP and IEP) as the contract document.
3. The actual services that were provided to children and families as a function of their involvement in early intervention efforts as well as the costs for the services provided.
4. The outcomes associated with these services at the child, family, and community levels.

5. The relationship among aspects of 1, 2, 3, and 4 above.
6. The transition of children between and out of programs.

As part of this design phase, a number of lessons have been learned both from the perspective of the researchers and from the stakeholders throughout this effort. The intent of using the UTEIP project as an example is not to give details of the results of the evaluation itself, but rather to talk through those concerns that emerged over time and how they were resolved. The relationship developed with individual programs, community providers, and parents is also important to understand.

Participatory design

First it was clear that since this was new territory for both the Early Intervention Research Institute and for the Baby Watch and Preschool Special Education programs' staff, a design that forced interaction throughout the time that all worked together would be important. The study needed to be conducted in such a way that the results were believable and understandable to the constituents involved, and yet held itself to high standards of evaluation rigor so that the results could withstand the questions that might be asked of it throughout the political process.

Another reason for such a participatory design was that the results had to be useable by the stakeholders who were involved. That is, this study was not one that was designed as an academic exercise, but rather would inform policy and program development in the years to come through inclusion of its findings in the state improvement plan. Thus, the stakeholders needed to both understand what would be possible, what could be collected given the financial constraints of the project, and what some of the limitations of our effort would be.

The need for longitudinal information

The stakeholders were clear from the beginning that they would like to understand the effects of these programs on individual children followed over time rather than simply take snapshots of children in the early intervention programs at any one given time.

Cooperation with state and community programs

Since the design called for studying children who were enrolled in two separate intervention programs in five districts, a number of issues about cooperation between the state and community programs emerged immediately upon beginning this study. Stakeholders agreed that not all children need be followed and that a sampling procedure could be used.

In order to do so, it was necessary to select children within programs that were representative of the range of participant families in programs and communities. At the same time, children would be followed longitudinally and would likely transition from an infant/toddler program to a preschool program. Since each program was run by different agencies, their catchment areas differed according to those of their lead agency (health or education). We therefore needed to develop a way of ensuring cooperation between Baby Watch programs, that varied widely in operating structure, and special education preschool programs, run by local school districts, as children transitioned from one project to another to follow them throughout the study.

Given the financial constraints of this particular study, we invited five community sites throughout the state to work cooperatively on the evaluation. Sites were defined by the Baby Watch catchment area and included at least one local school district. It soon became clear in order to work closely with programs at the state, regional, district, and community level, that we would need much more direct contact with community providers than we had anticipated. The state cooperated by providing us with "agent of the state" status that allowed us to obtain names of families enrolled and to talk directly both with parents and service providers. Informed consent from parents was still a requirement for involvement and was reobtained yearly. Direct parent communication about the study was important to enroll children in the study as they were identified as eligible for intervention services that allowed a more thorough assessment of parent concerns and satisfaction with programs. Even with the "agent of the state" status, parent contact procedures were negotiated individually with the community programs. The end result of this process empowered parents by allowing them to decide (or not) on participation without program screening; work for the individual programs was reduced; and the evaluation project was able to be implemented more quickly while maintaining more integrity regarding the parent data collected.

Diplomacy

The number of people who were involved in carrying out this evaluation required a significant amount of diplomacy to ensure that needs of each of the constituent groups were met over time. Teachers, early intervention service providers, parents, administrators, and state level staff all had different priorities with respect to the role of evaluation in their efforts. As we began collecting specific information, which could only be gleaned from particular constituent groups, relationships needed to be nurtured to ensure that they understood the rationale behind the data requests and the uses to which it would be put. Constituent feedback with respect to appropriate ways of collecting this information became critical in our ability to conduct the study.

For example, in collecting the cost data, one could imagine a number of constituencies becoming quite concerned in having this information become public. The way that we handled guarding the confidentiality of certain parts of the data and ensuring that the data were accurate so that all of the costs associated with running these programs were included in our analysis became a particularly delicate issue to negotiate with each Baby Watch and preschool special education program.

In working with parents, we recognized that parents' time was important and that their willingness to cooperate with us may well depend on our understanding of their conditions and their situations. We addressed this issue in several ways. We piloted with parents each of the tools that were used in collecting information from families. Secondly, in using parent feedback, we made the data collection process as painless as possible for parents in that much of the data was collected through phone interviews that were set up so that the information could be directly entered into the computer as the phone interview continued. Third, we paid parents for their time; both for filling out questionnaires and for being involved in phone interview so that we could give them some tangible recognition that we appreciated both their input and the time that they spent with us. Since staff in the early intervention programs who provided information to us did not receive additional pay for their efforts, this became somewhat of a difficult issue over the course of the study and we had to rely on good will and patience to gather all the needed information.

Satisfaction and quality assurance

One of the issues in early intervention research is the finding that parents are satisfied independent of the particular services that are provided to them (Roberts, Innocenti, & Goetze, 1999). Thus we were committed to finding a somewhat more informative way of understanding parent satisfaction. In doing so, we needed to find novel approaches to evaluating satisfaction that went beyond simply asking if parents were happy with services received. We wanted information that would help inform policy and inform practice on areas where improvement could be developed. This led us to consumer satisfaction studies from the business community as models for us to develop a more appropriate way of looking at satisfaction within the early intervention and preschool programs.

Measurement development

Questions we were asking were not included in many of the existing measures for early intervention. Examples included studies of the transition process and parents' concerns with respect to critical elements within those transitions. Other examples included information about the range of services provided and associated costs. As one outcome perspective was the kinds of experiences children who were in early intervention programs had within communities, we needed to measure children and family inclusion in a wide variety of activities outside of the early intervention program. Such measures were not available when we began and needed to be developed. The process of developing these measures included a participatory action research model in the sense that parents and families of children with disabilities served, as well as agency staff, acted as co-collaborators and developers of these tools with us over time.

It would have been impossible to have developed each of these measures without a continuous interaction between stakeholders and the evaluators in ensuring that the full range of issues were covered within each of the evaluation tools. This included the initial item selection, the piloting of tools, and the development of reliability indicators as the tools were implemented.

Some portions of our study could not truly be understood until we were well involved in them. One example was our understanding of the transition process that children experienced throughout the time that they were involved in early intervention. Naively, as the program began, we assumed that children who were in Baby Watch programs would be in that particular program for a period of time and, as their needs were met, would either no longer be involved in early intervention or would be transitioned to the preschool special education program within their local community. This naive understanding of how families operate was very soon shattered as we looked at how children and families were involved in programs, and the number of options that were available as children exited Baby Watch programs was considerably more diverse than we had ever anticipated. Our ability to follow these children and to continue to understand the impact of early intervention on them was important to tell the complete story of all the children enrolled in the original sample. It is our belief that we would have been unable to do so without the cooperation developed over time with staff at the various centers and the parents of children in the study. Given their investment in the process from the beginning, we were able to bring issues such as the need to track every child completely over time to them for solutions that could work for everyone.

Review of data

Stakeholders have played an important role in reviewing data collected by UTEIP. Information from the evaluation has been regularly presented at state meetings to allow feedback from those involved in or potentially impacted by the evaluation (i.e., program staff, administrators, and families). Brief letters detailing results have been sent yearly to involved families. Meetings with the primary stakeholders (the state agency staff) regarding the data being collected have occurred regularly throughout the evaluation. These meetings have helped project staff to identify concerns with the way data were being collected or being interpreted by program staff and to address these in continued data collection. Meetings with the primary stakeholders have helped to better define the data needs and the specific questions that they want answered by the evaluation, as well as relate the data to larger issues in the field of early intervention. Although it has not occurred yet, a variety of stakeholders will be requested to read and comment on an early version of the final report. These activities have served to involve stakeholders in the data interpretation aspect of the project and, in so doing, have helped to improve the believability of data collected and to structure the specific issues to be addressed with the data.

Summary

This example of participatory involvement within the UTEIP project helps to illuminate a number of the issues discussed earlier in this chapter and to illustrate this concept of "participatory realism." In this project, design issues were addressed by the contractors and the primary stakeholders (state agency staff). The primary stakeholders wanted specific types of information that they perceived as meeting their training and legislative needs. The involvement of other stakeholders in the design phase was not deemed critical by the contractors. Summative information on the impact of programs and process information on program implementation were desired outcomes. However, even the process information was initially viewed more as an outcome than data that could serve to direct later action. That is, process information was not intended to be immediately turned into action steps. These needs would fall on the research-action axis of Figure 5.1 toward the research end of the spectrum.

One could take the position that given the initial planning of the project, the remainder of project activities should continue along similar nonparticipatory lines. However, participatory realism suggests that regardless of location on the research-action axis of evaluation, participation by multiple stakeholders remains a valid goal. The desired outcomes of the project did not preclude other stakeholders from becoming involved in other aspects of the project. The issue becomes one of how does one involve stakeholders. In this project both the evaluator and primary stakeholders saw the need for involvement by other stakeholders in the running of the project with different stakeholders being involved in different ways at different times. Stakeholders were then involved in the instrument selection and development, in methodology issues, in procedural issues, and in data interpretation issues. This involvement, from our perspective, served to strengthen the implementation of the project and, in some cases, to insure that information, which may have been unavailable (either because of lack of cooperation or insufficient experience with the phenomenon [e.g., subject tracking]) became available. If one were to place this study on the research-participation grid in Figure 5.1, then the UTEIP evaluation would fall in the left upper quadrant; not at the top in participation but representative of "good" participation.

Example 2: Opening Doors into Rural Communities

Staff at the Early Intervention Research Institute have been involved in a project called *Opening Doors* for the past several years. Chapter 10 in this volume describes some of the findings of the first phase of research conducted with states and communities in this effort. The second wave of this research, referred to as *Opening Doors into Rural Communities,* assists communities and states in their efforts to integrate services for young children with special health care needs (CSHCN) and their families into a more comprehensive, coordinated early intervention system using a collaborative development model that includes parents, community providers, and state policy makers. A series of replicable procedures have been designed to guide communities and states in examining local service integration issues, and provide a framework for systems change at both levels. The model for the participatory evaluation of this effort is described below.

A recent initiative of the Federal Interagency Coordinating Committee (FICC) has been the adoption in principle of a series of recommendations on service integration. FICC recommendations encourage coordinated funding, coordinated eligibility and application procedures, shared data/information systems, and coordination of early intervention services with the medical home. A second FICC initiative involves a major campaign called the *Communities Can Coalition,* which promotes community-based solutions for more comprehensive early intervention systems, which is highlighted in Chapter 3 of this volume.

A living laboratory of communities has been created in which each community has targeted one of the FICC recommendations as a goal in continuing to refine their own systems, and develop self-assessment and systems change procedures for creating more integrated services in other communities and states. In this work, the definition of service integration as defined by Kagan, Goffin, Golub, and Pritchard (1995) is used:

> increase the efficiency and effectiveness of systems providing human services, through both infrastructural reform (e.g., improved training/professional development, regulation, financing, and other supports), and direct service reform (e.g., an increased number of services, more equitable distribution of services, and higher quality services). At the same time, the goal of service integration is to positively impact human outcomes, enabling children and families to experience a higher quality of life. (p. 12)

This definition equally emphasizes both the need for an efficient system of care as well as one that is effective from the perspective of outcomes for families and children.

Four rural communities have gathered under the umbrella of a consortium sponsored by *Opening Doors*, and are committed to supporting and informing one another as they work toward both individual and group goals. Through the Opening Doors Project, we have found that community integration efforts must be sustainable over time, connected to and supported by other levels (e.g., state systems) to be most effective in addressing systemic issues that affect service integration. The collective wisdom of several rural communities supporting one another and learning from each other's experience is a valuable tool in reaching individual and collective goals. The synergy created by this approach is effective, efficient, and productive in that it multiplies the lessons learned from each program and can assist in dissemination throughout the network.

Unique demographic, economic, and cultural characteristics create multiple health care delivery barriers in rural areas. Indeed, reference is frequently made to the crisis in rural health care in the United States (Armer, Forney, Berfield, & Price, 1996). Such barriers include low population density, great distances from providers, and scarcity of fiscal resources. Rural communities, such as those forming the consortium, share many positive attributes that make service integration more likely. Examples of such strengths include volunteer maintenance of many community activities and duties, leading to co-production of social services by public and private sectors.

We have based the evaluation model on four core outcomes that correspond to the needs of this population of children and families. These core outcomes being evaluated are as follows:

1. All children with special health care needs will receive regular, ongoing medical care within a medical home.
2. All families of children with special health care needs will have adequate private or public insurance options (or both) to pay for needed service and care.
3. Services for children with special health care needs and their families will be family-centered, community-based, coordinated, and culturally competent. Structures at the federal, regional, state, and local levels support such a service system.
4. Families of children with special health needs will be satisfied with the appropriateness, affordability, accessibility, and effectiveness of services received by family members.

As described by Kagan and colleagues (1995), the goal of service integration requires both more effective, efficient policies and practices within a system and improved child and family outcomes. Our evaluation plan attempts to capture both aspects of service integration in order to evaluate these outcomes. Figure 5.2 depicts the evaluation plan, outlining how the information related to service integration policies and practices relates to the outcomes. Phases I-V are detailed below.

Phase I: community assessment

Descriptive and quantitative data are collected to document the current level of integration and systems reform in each community with respect to the four FICC recommendations. A variety of methodologies, such as needs assessment data already collected by communities; document reviews of relevant state and local documents; interviews with key informants in the communities and the state level bureaucracies; and focus groups with parents of children with special health needs and providers are employed to develop an initial picture of strengths and collaborative activities that are already ongoing in the community. This synthesis process occurs in phase II. Examples of specific tools from which assessment data are drawn are included in the Appendix.

Phase II: matrix development and community buy-in

Information is reduced for each community using coding procedures field tested through the Opening Doors project. This information is then placed in a matrix based on a similar one developed by Konrad (1996). As shown in Figure 5.3, this matrix suggests how several dimensions of service integration may be described. For example, the *partners dimension* would include a listing of the key partners within the community effort and be listed with respect to the functions they perform both within the systems reform effort and the services they provide to chil-

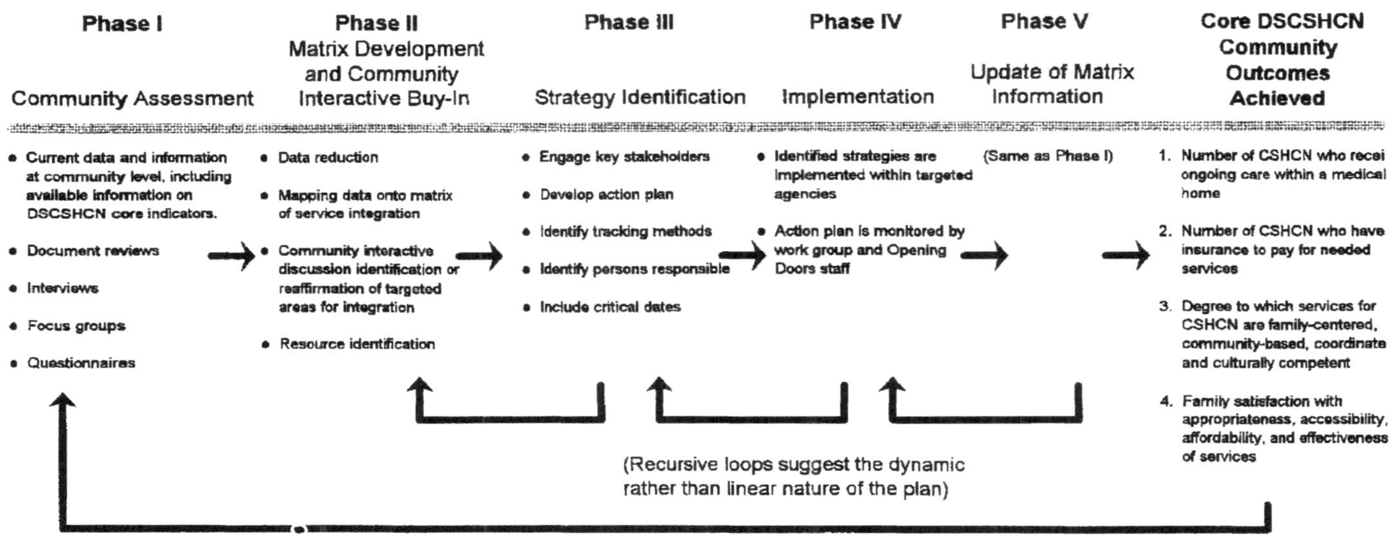

FIGURE 5.2. **Outline of evaluation plan for Opening Doors into rural communities.**

	Intensity of Integration Continuum				
	← Informal →		← Formal →		
	Information Sharing and Communication	*Cooperation and Coordination*	*Collaboration*	*Consolidation*	*Integration*
Partners					
Target population					
Goals					
Program policy and legislation					
Governance and authority					
Service delivery system model					
Stakeholders					
Planning and budgeting					
Financing					
Outcomes and accountability					
Licensing and contracting					
Information systems and data management					

FIGURE 5.3. Matrix of services integration dimensions and levels of integration. Reprinted by permission from Konrad (1996).

dren and families. The reduced data are mapped onto the horizontal axis by ranking the intensity of integration. The operational definitions of these rankings follow those suggested by Konrad.

Phase III: strategy identification

The completed matrix is used as part of the formative evaluation strategy in which the community stakeholders and the Opening Doors staff review and discuss the information displayed on the matrix and an accompanying report. Strategies currently in use as well as additional options are discussed in light of community priorities and existing resources. Strategies that address the top ranked community priorities are mapped on to the FICC recommendations and adjustments made as necessary to ensure that at least one of the priorities will receive significant attention.

It should be emphasized that there is no inherent good in formalizing integrative strategies if more informal systems are functioning according to the community desires and families feel that the services they are receiving are responsive to their needs. Thus, documenting a program as being in the consolidation (formal) level of integration is not better in an absolute sense than being at the cooperation and coordination stage. Rather a stage should reflect the product of the requirement of the system in order for it to be able to effect the outcomes it desires.

Phase IV: implementation

The implementation of these strategies along with the technical assistance provided by Opening Doors staff is documented through minutes of meetings held at the community level and scheduled phone calls/visits from the Opening Doors staff.

Phase V: update on matrix information

At the end of an 18-month period, a second round of data are collected, updating the information collected at the inception of the effort. Much the same process described earlier is employed with particular emphasis on areas in which change has occurred. These changes may be determined from several different sources: Examples include additional document reviews such as interagency agreements; or Maternal and Child Health Block grant data such as increases in numbers of children with special health care needs who have a secure medical home and reliable methods of payment for health care services. Other evidence may be in the form of perceptions of key informants on how interagency collaboration is working at the time. Evidence such as the refinement or reallocation of funding streams and dollars available for services are included as well. As the data are collected and reduced, the matrix is completed once more. The two matrices are compared to determine areas of change particularly regarding the FICC recommendations.

Experience to date with four communities suggests that this form of evaluation activity in which participation by the stakeholders in the ongoing evaluative process produces information that is both useful and important to the stakeholders and changes the way they interact with one another over time.

SUMMARY

This chapter has focused on an approach to evaluation referred to as participatory realism. The basic premise of this approach to evaluation is that most evaluations do not fit neatly into clearly defined compartments that match text book definitions whether the design be participatory or not. However, this approach recognizes the value of including stakeholders in the evaluation process at the most involved level possible given the demands of the evaluation context. These demands can be conditions by the contractor, time availability to complete activities, or a host of other factors. The end goal of this approach being an evaluation that has value and is used.

This belief in stakeholder participation in evaluation is not an empirically based belief. There are no clear data that suggest a participatory approach to evaluation will produce results that stakeholders more readily accept and use, or that will have greater impact on policy. In fact, it seems clear to those that engage in participatory approaches that it requires extra time on the part of all people involved and requires people to learn new skills. The participatory approach has both potential benefits and drawbacks (Turnbull, Friesen, & Ramirez, in press). The participation of stakeholders is a value similar to our value that people with disabilities should have access to jobs and activities, and be involved in communities. As a value, people accept participatory approaches in varying degrees. For example, some researchers see the value as being more applicable in applied research than in basic research. We would argue that participatory approaches apply in all evaluations and research, albeit in slightly different ways. It is necessary for evaluators and stakeholders alike to reframe their thinking to accommodate participatory approaches. Referring to our analogy to people with disabilities, it may not be possible to make all wilderness areas accessible, but we can make some parts of the wilderness accessible if planers are creative; the same thought process needs to apply with participatory approaches in evaluation and research.

Another rationale for participatory approaches is based on a philosophical approach to knowledge in evaluation. The use of participatory approaches acknowledges the view that no single method or paradigm allows for a final understanding of a phenomenon. This postmodern view is a key component of qualitative approaches which recognize that reality is based on the subjective experiences of those people who are involved in that reality (Denzin & Lincoln, 1994). Within evaluation, Pawson and Tilley (1997) have examined evaluation within the frame of philosophical realism. They note that social programs are social systems that can be understood only through examination of the social rules and institutions within which they are embedded. A given program embedded in different contexts (with different people, institutions, settings, etc.) will play out differently, with potentially different effects. A program is its personnel, place, past, and prospects. Pawson and Tilley suggest evaluators search for the causal mechanisms that lead to program outcomes while realizing the mechanisms may be context specific. The use of stakeholders in a participatory manner is one mechanism for gaining a better understanding of the social systems that impact upon an intervention and the impacts an intervention has on the components of the social system.

If we are to create a societal context, similar to that described by Fetterman (1996), in which evaluation becomes a skill with which all citizens are comfortable, then we need to establish a common value set around evaluation that is accepted by both those with skill in evaluation and by those stakeholder/citizens who are involved in or are impacted by the evaluation. The key value in this social context is the belief in establishing opportunities for participation by stakeholders and, secondarily, in making understandable information available to stakeholder citizens. There are other skills needed by both the evaluator and the stakeholder citizen. Brown (1995) presents an overview of some of these evaluator skills. This chapter attempts to present some of the skills needed by stakeholders. The behavior and values of many individuals needs to change to move to this new view of evaluation. This chapter has, hopefully, contributed to the process of making evaluation an ongoing and valued aspect of modern life.

APPENDIX
COMMUNITY ASSESSMENT MEASURES*

The following four measures have been developed in order to collect similar data across all consortium members of Opening Doors into Rural Communities (ODRC). The process is meant to assist the four communities to examine their current service system (Measures 1, 2, and 3) and consumer satisfaction (Measure 4). In addition to the methods described here, ODRC will help design community-specific measures to meet their unique needs.

1. *Community Service Mapping*

Each community will select a small team (3-4 members) to develop a draft version of the community service map. The center of each map may vary slightly based on the FICC strategy the community is developing. When filling out the map, in addition to typical private and public agencies, other groups should be considered such as, churches, consumers, civic groups, and other sources of formal and informal supports.

As an example, Jefferson County has tentatively identified the development of a common eligibility/application process. The map will provide an outline of the relationship among the providers and other key players in the community with which the common application process would apply. Which entity would be in the center needs to be determined. Other community agencies will radiate around the center and be woven among one another. The draft map will be shared with the larger community task force for additions and corrections. ODRC-facilitated discussions will be directed at focusing attention on possible gaps and overlaps in the community system.

2. *Community Self-Assessment Questionnaire*

ODRC staff have drafted a tool designed to target the four grant outcomes (medical home; adequate insurance; community-based, coordinated, comprehensive system of care; and family satisfaction and knowledge) so that core data can be collected across consortium communities on these outcomes, as requested by MCHB. The questionnaire will be completed jointly by a three-to four-member team representing different agencies or constituencies. A draft of the results will be presented to the larger group/task force for revisions and additions.

3. *Service Integration Matrix*

Following the completion and synthesis of Measures 1 and 2, ODRC staff will facilitate the completion of the service integration matrix with a small team. At best, we would schedule a two- or three-day trip to the site. ODRC would facilitate a large pre-scheduled group meeting to present a draft of the matrix, revise it based on group input, and then prepare an updated version.

4. *Family Survey*

While gathering information regarding community services, a telephone survey will be conducted with a sample of families who have young children with disabilities and/or special health care needs. The survey will provide a description of the services families are getting and their satisfaction with services in terms of adequacy coordination, and family centeredness. The survey will be completed by parents of children with disabilities hired by ODRC.

At the end of the 18-month intervention period, the four measures would be revisited.

1. Community Map—Assess whether linkages expanded or changed as a result of ODRC grant activities.
2. Community Self-Assessment—Assess changes in policies and practices related to the GIPRA outcomes.
3. Service Integration Matrix—Review the matrix and look for changes in forms of integration and achievement of grant-related goals.
4. Family Survey—Describe how families view the service system.

**Note:* These measures are available from the second author.

REFERENCES

American Public Welfare Association, Center for Law and Social Policy, Council of Chief State Officers, & Education Commission of the States (1992). *Confidentiality and collaboration: Information sharing in interagency efforts* (Document # AR-92-1). Denver, CO: Education Commission of the States Distribution Center.

Armer, J., Forney, D., Berfield, M., & Price, C. (1996). *1996 Missouri tri-county community health assessment: Chariton, Randolph, and Monroe counties*. Columbia, MO: Sinclair School of Nursing, University of Missouri.

Brown, L. D., & Tandon, R. (1983). Ideology and political economy in inquiry: Action research and participatory research. *Journal of Applied Behavioral Science, 19*, 277-294.

Brown, P. (1995). The role of the evaluator in comprehensive community initiatives. In J. P. Connell, A. C. Kubisch, L. B. Schorr, & C. H. Weiss (Eds.), *New approaches to evaluating community initiatives: Concepts, methods, and contexts* (pp. 201-225). Washington, DC: The Aspen Institute.

Center for the Study of Social Policy (1993). *Community services and support to improve outcomes for children*. Washington, DC: Center for the Study of Social Policy.

Cohen, E., & Ooms, T. (1993). *Data integration and evaluation: Essential components of family centered systems reform*. Washington, DC: Family Impact Seminar, American Association for Marriage and Family Therapy Research and Education Foundation.

Denzin, N. K., & Lincoln, Y. S. (1994). Introduction: Entering the field of qualitative research. In N. K. Denzin & Y. S. Lincoln (Eds.), *Handbook of qualitative research* (pp. 1-17). Thousand Oaks, CA: Sage.

Fetterman, D. M. (1996). Empowerment evaluation: An introduction to theory and practice. In D. M. Fetterman, S. J. Kaftarian, & A. Wandersman (Eds.), *Empowerment evaluation: Knowledge and tools for self assessment and accountability* (pp. 3-46). Thousand Oaks, CA: Sage.

Fetterman, D. M., Kaftarian, S. J., & Wandersman, A. (1996). *Empowerment evaluation: Knowledge and tools for self assessment and accountability*. Thousand Oaks, CA: Sage.

Greene, J. C., Caracelli, V. J., & Graham, W. F. (1989). Toward a conceptual framework for mixed-method evaluation designs. *Educational Evaluation and Policy Analysis, 11*, 255-274.

Hall, B. (1993). From margins to center? The development and purpose of participatory research. *The American Sociologist, 23*, 15-28.

Hobbs, L. J. (1997). Confidentiality requirements in integrated programs. In H. M. Wallace, R. F. Biehl, J. C. MacQueen, & J. A. Blackman (Eds.), *Mosby's resource guide to children with disabilities and chronic illness* (pp. 125-136). St. Louis, MO: Mosby.

Jacobs, F. H. (1988). The five-tiered approach to evaluation: Context and implementation. In H. B. Weiss & F. H. Jacobs (Eds.), *Evaluating family programs* (pp. 37-68). New York: de Gruyter.

Kagan, S. L., Goffin, S. G., Golub, S. A., & Pritchard, E. (1995). *Toward systematic reform: Service integration for young children and their families*. Falls Church, VA: National Center for Service Integration.

Konrad, E. L. (1996). A multi-dimensional framework for conceptualizing human services integration initiatives. *Evaluating Initiatives to Integrate Human Services, 69*, 5-20.

Individuals with Disabilities Education Act Amendments of 1997, PL 105-17. 20 U.S.C. § 1400 *et seq*.

McCroskey, J., & Meezan, W. (1997). *Family preservation and family functioning*. Annapolis Junction, MO: Child Welfare League of America

McCroskey, J., & Nelson, J. (1989). Practice-based research in a family-support program: The family connection project example. *Child Welfare League of America, 68*, 573-587.

Miles, M. B., & Huberman, A. M. (1994). *Qualitative data analysis: An expanded sourcebook* (2nd ed.). Newbury Park, CA: Sage

Pawson, R., & Tilley, N. (1997). *Realistic evaluation*. Thousand Oaks, CA: Sage.

Roberts, R. N. (1993). The family, the school, and the interface. In R. N. Roberts (Ed.), *Coming home to preschool: The sociocultural context of early education* (pp. 275-289). Norwood, NJ: Ablex.

Roberts, R. N , Innocenti, M. S., & Goetze, L. D. (1997). *By what outcomes should Part H be evaluated at the state level*? Prepared for the Subcommittee on Service Integration and Continuity of Services of the Federal Interagency Coordinating Council, Washington, DC.

Roberts, R. N., Innocenti, M. S., & Goetze, L. D. (1999). Emerging issues from state level evaluations of early intervention programs. *Journal of Early Intervention, 22*(2), 152-163.

Roberts, R. N., Rule, S., & Innocenti, M. S. (1998). *Strengthening the family-professional partnership in services for young children*. Baltimore, MD: Brookes.

Rutman, L. (1980). *Planning useful evaluation: Evaluability assessment*. Beverly Hills, CA: Sage.

Thompson, L., & Herman, S. (1996). Emergent design: Understanding and evolving measures of a family support system. *Evaluation and Program Planning, 19*, 235-252.

Turnbull, A. P., Friesen, B., & Ramirez, C. (in press). Participatory action research as a model of conducting family research. *The Journal of the Association for People with Severe Handicaps*.

Weikart, D., Bond, J. T., & McNeil, J. (Eds.) (1978). *The Ypsilanti Preschool Project: Preschool years and longitudinal results through fourth grade*. Ypsilanti, MI: High Scope Educational Research Foundation.

Weiss, C. H. (1995). Nothing as practical as a good theory: Exploring theory-based evaluation for comprehensive community initiatives for children and families. In J. P. Connell, A. C. Kubisch, L. B. Schorr, & C. H. Weiss (Eds.), *New approaches to evaluating community initiatives: Concepts, methods, and contexts* (pp. 65-92). Washington, DC: The Aspen Institute.

Whyte, W. F., Greenwood, D. J., & Lazes, P. (1991). Participatory action research: Through practice to science in social research. In W. Whyte (Ed.), *Participatory action research* (pp. 19-55). Newbury Park, CA: Sage.

section III

Developmental Perspectives on Community Programs

In this section, different examples of a developmental perspective are described. Community-level partnerships involve a developmental process both for families involved and the agencies at state and local levels. Roxane Kaufman and Amy Locke Wischmann, in Chapter 6, address the mental health needs of young children from a developmental, community perspective. "Developmental" in this sense refers to the child, family, and community as each continues to mature both physically and psychologically over time. A similar theme is incorporated in Chapter 7, by Gary De Carolis, in which the evolution of state-level supports for community-based services is described, using a state mental health system as an example.

chapter 6

Communities Supporting the Mental Health of Young Children and Their Families

Roxane Kaufmann
Amy Locke Wischmann
Georgetown University Child Development Center

The community's institutions, both public and private, are designed in ways that weave young children and their caregivers into the social fabric. (Carnegie Task Force 1994, p. 85)

INTRODUCTION

Strong and healthy neighborhoods and communities are essential in sustaining the positive physical and emotional development of young children and their families because human development occurs in the context of participation in joint activities with a wide array of people. Recent studies have illustrated the important role of neighborhoods and communities in molding the lives of families and children, and the overlap between the characteristics of the community and the mental health outcomes for young children are becoming increasingly apparent.

In addition to the existing research examining the positive and negative impacts of community on children and families, the past decades have seen an explosion of studies investigating how young children develop and thrive. Our understanding as a society about the affects of environmental and biological influences on young children's cognitive, physical, social, and emotional development has greatly increased (Meisels & Shonkoff, 1990, as cited in Knitzer, in press). It is an integrated understanding of *both* child development, as it applies to children's mental health, and community systems that will lead to implementation of effective community supports for the mental health of young children and families.

In our examination of how communities can support the mental health of young children and their families, let us first put forth a working definition of early childhood mental health. Early childhood mental health is built on developmental knowledge about young children and families, and enriched by clinical perspectives (Knitzer, in press). The aim is to improve the social and emotional well being of young children and families by strengthening relationships with caregivers, as well as promoting age-appropriate social and emotional skills.

Early childhood mental health has a strong preventive focus, reflected in a commitment to reach out to all children, particularly those at risk of developing emotional and behavioral impairments (Zeanah, 1993, as cited in Knitzer, in press). Knitzer further defined early childhood mental health as a set of strategies and perspectives to:

1. Promote the emotional and behavioral well being of all young children;
2. Strengthen the emotional and behavioral well being of children whose emotional development is compromised by biological or environmental risks, in order to minimize their risks and enhance the likelihood that they will enter school with appropriate skills;
3. Help families of young children address whatever barriers they face ensuring that their children's emotional development is not compromised; expand the competencies of nonfamilial caregivers and others to promote the emotional well-being of young children and families, particularly those at risk by virtue of environmental or biological factors; and
4. Ensure that young children experiencing clearly atypical emotional and behavioral development and their families have access to needed services and supports.

As this chapter discusses, a community-based mental health system for young children and families is a system that effectively achieves these goals and strategies.

Communities can play an important role in promoting and supporting a healthy start for young children. Through ensuring access to care,

Supporting parents and families of young children	Supporting caregivers/interventionists of young children
Increasing access to clinical programs, case consultation, and crisis intervention services	Fostering collaboration of services/supports and system-level integration

FIGURE 6.1. Building blocks of an early childhood mental health system.

education, health and social services; by encouraging neighborhoods to work together in addressing issues facing children and families; by fostering stronger connections between neighbors; and creating empowering opportunities and nurturing a sense of hope and responsibility, communities can positively impact the lives of their youngest members.

Perhaps most importantly, communities interested in promoting the emotional and behavioral well being of young children and their families must first recognize children as significant members of their communities. Children belong to a variety of communities, such as schools, clubs, peer groups, and the neighborhoods in which they live. Often, very young children are in group childcare, informal playgroups, and recreational programs. However, it is rare for adults to see the child as an integral and integrated part of the community. Even families of very young children are often overlooked while communities attend to the greater political power of their "working residents" (Carnegie Task Force, 1994).

Communities that acknowledge and understand the needs of their youngest citizens can move ahead in the development of a comprehensive, community-based early childhood mental health system that embodies the critical components shown in Figure 6.1.

These building blocks, which represent the ideas and experience of scholars and practitioners in the field of early childhood mental health, are essential in the creation of a truly comprehensive and effective approach to early childhood mental health (Arst, 1996; Stroul, 1996). Communities should work to incorporate all four of these building blocks as they build a system to respond to the needs of their youngest citizens. Through these mechanisms, communities will be better able to support *all* children and families, including those with or at risk for mental health challenges. In this chapter, each building block is conceptualized, examples of community efforts illustrate successful approaches, and a community checklist helps identify resources that promote good services and supports.

Supporting Parents and Families of Young Children

All families need support in balancing the demands of caregiving—a fussy new baby, the needs of jealous siblings—with the stress of the workplace and financial burdens. Often these responsibilities are met by a single parent or a young couple without the support of nearby extended family. Unfortunately, community services available to most families with children under age three are few and fragmented. The Carnegie Corporation Report (1994) identified four key supports that communities can provide to support young families: broaden quality childcare options; support parent education; guarantee adequate physical and mental health care; and strengthen community networks. In addition to making accessible the appropriate types of support, communities must work to ensure that mental health services to young children and families are delivered in natural settings, such as family homes and childcare programs, and are sensitive to the cultural and ethnic values of the families.

Supporting Caregivers/Interventionists of Young Children

Increasingly, young children spend large amounts of time in childcare settings and/or with non-relative caregivers. High-quality childcare helps children to become socially competent, intellectually curious, and emotionally secure. When the quality of care is inadequate, the group sizes too large, or caregivers overwhelmed by meeting the needs of increasingly greater numbers of children with challenging behaviors, all children suffer. Therefore, communities need to work diligently in establishing supports for staff who are often poorly paid, inadequately trained and undervalued. Childcare providers and teachers must have assistance in dealing with challenging situations, and communication between parents and caregivers should be facilitated.

Increasing Access to Clinical Programs, Case Consultation, and Crisis Intervention Services

Families, other caregivers, home visitors, family workers, and administrators working with infants, toddlers, and preschoolers should have access to clinical program and case consultation to strengthen their competencies in promoting emotional development in all young children. Mental health services have traditionally provided support to family and nonfamily members (e.g., teachers) only as a "collateral service." Nor are effective services to very young children with serious emotional disturbances provided in a 50-minute office session. Those conventional models are not appropriate for young children, where nurturing relationships with adults are central to healthy development. Family members and other caregivers need help in observing and understanding emotional and behavioral cues and in dealing with difficult situations in order to promote such development, and reduce the impact of unhealthy emotional development (Knitzer, in press).

In addition to clinical programs and case consultation, in some instances, more intensive services will be required. Young children, families, and programs experiencing violence, community disasters, or family-specific crises should have immediate and as necessary access to crisis intervention and support. An early childhood mental health system should help families and other caregivers cope with psychological, health and natural disasters. Primary care settings, particularly early care, education, and family support settings should have crisis plans in place, similar to those that many school districts now use (Knitzer, in press).

Fostering Collaboration of Services/Supports and System-level Integration

A truly effective early childhood mental health system encourages broad-based interagency collaboration at the child and family level as well as at the systems level. Unfortunately, there has been relatively little effort to build cross-system links around early childhood emotional development and mental health issues in a manner parallel to what is expected through the Individuals with Disabilities Education Act (IDEA), Part C. On a more positive note, recent analyses indicate that close to one-half of states are developing various types of community mobilization forums that could be a starting point for cross-system collaboration (Knitzer, in press). IDEA provides states with a foundation upon which to build a system of services for all vulnerable young children and their families. Mandated interagency collaboration at the state level and voluntary local collaborative initiatives can be expanded to include membership by all child and family serving agencies, parent organizations, and community partners.

Using these four building blocks as a foundation, this chapter will discuss the following:

1. the promotion of mental health for young children within the context of community;
2. some of the mental health issues specific to young children and their families;

3. factors that may contribute to the increased vulnerability of children and communities; and finally
4. specific supports communities can provide, including some best practice examples from the field.

PROMOTING CHILDREN'S MENTAL HEALTH IN THE CONTEXT OF COMMUNITY

> The neighborhood will mean different things to different aged children, but common to all of them will be a need for territory and belonging. (Henderson, 1995, p. 15)

The concept of community involves more than just discrete and separate programs or structures located in a general geographical area. It implies that the community is organized with a common understanding, shared values, a sense of identity, and some relational structures that are meaningful for those living within that setting. In the best case scenario, communities would be organized to provide supports and programs that encourage the healthy physical and mental development of young children and fulfill their need to belong. However, as Henderson (1995) argues in his book, *Children and Communities*, the very organization of children's services can have the effect of reinforcing a fragmented approach to working with children.

Children's services are often divided by differing policies and procedures and distinct disciplinary philosophies. Within the child-serving professions (e.g., social services, education, and recreational programs), there is evidence of involvement in the community aspects of children's lives. However, there is much work to be done in establishing effective and ongoing community-based connections between programs and disciplines. In addition to the fragmentation of services as the local level, there is no cohesive national public policy approach to serving the needs of our youngest citizens (Schorr, 1997). This lack of national direction with respect to children further enhances the separation of children's issues and community issues.

As the chapter introduction points out, communities interested in promoting the emotional and behavioral well being of young children and their families must first recognize children as integral members of their communities. Children are indeed a significant part of community life. It is not uncommon for people to recognize that they become most involved in their neighborhoods when they have children or are caring for children. As children grow and venture out into their neighborhoods, they seek a sense of belonging and respect, and deserve opportunities to play and develop as citizens. These first and formative experiences as children interface with their community have lasting impacts.

Obtaining a comprehensive picture of the role of the community and neighborhood in shaping outcomes for young children is critical. Chamberlin (1996) notes that:

> A greater understanding of the ecology of human development is leading towards an approach that stresses primary prevention and targets services to the community as a whole. This approach recognizes the interdependence of the individual, the family and the community, and understands that effective change requires modification of all three. (p. 117)

The habitats and contextual settings that envelop children play a crucial role in their healthy development. Indeed, ecological models are often used as a framework for community-level research as well as prevention and early intervention research. In studies on community, the term "ecological" suggests that a viable and sustainable environment is critical to the very survival of it's members. Applied to children's mental health, the ecological approach assumes that a family's effectiveness as a childrearing system is bolstered by the existence of supportive social networks that include people outside of the immediate family—relatives, friends, neighbors, coworkers, and other community members. "In short, it assumes that as we raise our children, communities count" (Carnegie Task Force, 1994, p. 87).

Chamberlin (1996) strongly suggests that communities develop programs and supports that recognize this ecological approach, asserting that "primary prevention works by keeping families or children at low and medium risk from becoming high risk" (p. 117). Recent research supports this understanding. A study of 160 families in 10 neighborhoods shows that when parents are more connected with other parents in their communities their children benefit. These larger networks of parents not only have a positive effect on the parents' ability to deal with stress, mothers' perceptions of themselves and their children, fathers' involvement in childrearing, and children's self-esteem and school success, but in some circumstances reduce the probability of certain mental and physical illness (Cochran, Larner, Riley, Gunnarson, & Henderson, 1990).

The importance of community support for promoting the mental health of young children and families is arguably more important now than ever before as children face tremendous societal pressures. Communities can mobilize resources and lay the groundwork for the necessary support systems for young children and families. And as more data becomes available on how young children develop and thrive, it becomes clear that these support systems must focus on prevention and early intervention activities.

MENTAL HEALTH ISSUES SPECIFIC TO YOUNG CHILDREN AND FAMILIES

In identifying community-based approaches to promoting mental health for children, there are a number of issues specific to young children that must be considered. The fields of infant mental health, early intervention, and child development have contributed a wealth of information that will assist communities in the evolution and expansion of activities and programs geared toward young children and families.

Brain Research

In the past decade, exciting new research into the physiology and chemistry of the developing brain has established that the first three years are more critical to the emergence of human capacities than any three that follow. Brain development occurs earlier and more rapidly, and is more shaped by babies' experiences and early relationships, than anyone had previously thought.

Child development researchers have found that the most ordinary daily experiences of young children shape their capacity to learn. While a developmentally appropriate level of stimulation leads to an efficient network of synapses in the brain, adverse environmental conditions, such as a lack of nurturing, stimulation, or stability, can leave the brain vulnerable.

Community policies and approaches that adequately reflect the emerging research on brain development would respect every new baby's immediate need for a very close and continuous relationship with at least one key adult (Henderson, 1995). Childcare would be upheld as the most important occupation in the world, and federal policies would reflect the notion that adults should be able to excel as both contributing citizens and caring parents.

RISK AND PROTECTIVE FACTORS IN YOUNG CHILDREN

Risk and protective factors for the young child are characteristics that could potentially serve as barriers or facilitators for healthy social and

TABLE 6.1.
Risk and Protective Factors Influencing Human Development and Functioning

	Risk factors	Protective factors
Child	male sex	Easy, responsive temperament
	low intellectual ability	High play involvement and initiative
	difficult, avoidant temperament	Receives positive recognition
	chromosomal abnormality	Good peer relations
	history of chronic illness	Secure attachment in early life
	communication disorder	High intellectual ability
	prolonged institutionalization	Good academic performance
	severe brain damage	Positive self concept
	perinatal complications	Internal locus of control
	developmental delays	Good sibling relationship
	history of abuse and neglect	Presence of a confidant
	inadequate nutritional intake	
Family	severe marital discord	Positive parent-child relationship
	maternal psychiatric disorder	Few prolonged separations from primary caretaker
	low parental education	Presence of supportive male partner
	maternal hostility or conflict toward child	Residential stability
	paternal criminality	Stable, high status employment
	overcrowding or large family	Close family
	family violence	
	poor parental social skills	
Community	many situational stressors	Support from adults in the community
	high exposure to toxic substances	Community involvement
	few alternative caregivers	High SES, increased family income

Note: For the purposes of this table, the heading "opportunity factors" was renamed "protective factors."
Source: Adapted from Grizenko and Fisher (1992, p. 718) and Dunst (1993, p. 147).

emotional development. These barriers and facilitators may be manifested at the individual, family or community levels. These factors represent a framework for identifying positive and negative influences, and should be viewed as just one component in a holistic assessment of the many risks, strengths, resiliencies, and competencies demonstrated by a child, family or community.

A wide variety of risk and protective factors affect young children and their families. Table 6.1 lists risk and protective factors that can be found at the individual, family, and community levels. Although the specific risk and protective factors are categorized as originating either in the child, family or community, it is important to remember that these factors *interact* to produce outcomes. While risk factors increase the *prob-*

ability that a particular negative outcome will occur, they do not necessarily cause the outcome to occur. Garmezy and colleagues (1984) and Murphy and Moriarty (1976), as cited in Grizenko and Fisher (1992); and IOM (1994), present a protective model that assumes that protective factors buffer stressors. Protective factors may help improve the child's coping mechanisms and adaptation to his or her environment (IOM,1994). This research suggests that to enhance a positive outcome, community interventions should reduce risk factors and promote protective factors.

The degree to which the lives of children and their families are influenced by these factors depends on the developmental level of the child; the interactions among risk and protective factors; the number of risk factors experienced simultaneously; their intensity and duration; and interactions between risk and protective factors experienced within families and within the larger environment. Children are affected by the dynamics and interactions of the families in which they live; families in turn are influenced by the surrounding community (Bronfenbrenner, 1979; Szapocznik & Kurtines, 1993).

The complex role that risk and protective factors play in affecting certain outcomes presents a challenge to designing effective community prevention/early intervention strategies. Early intervention planners and researchers can glean three important points from the literature on risk and protective factors. First, the enhancement of protective factors and the amelioration of risks can be effective in the promotion of positive outcomes. Second, an intervention that targets many risk factors is likely to be more successful than one that targets only one or two. Third, interventions must comprehensively address strengths and vulnerabilities at the individual, family, and community levels. An individual is affected not only by his or her own genetic and biological make-up, but also by the environment in which he or she lives.

Risk and Protective Factors Embedded in Community Characteristics

Risk and protective factors reside in community mores, values, culture, and structures. In their article "What Makes Early Intervention Programs Work?," Berlin, O'Neal, and Brooks-Gunn (1998) argue that community characteristics play an integral role in the effectiveness of early interventions. These characteristics can include aspects of the environment that increase families' stress and vulnerability, such as neighborhood poverty and violence, and aspects of the environment that influence the extent to which program participants can access services.

In recent years, policymakers, program staff, and researchers have focused on the concept of the community as a target for decreasing risk for children and families, increasing protective factors, and assessing the impact of organizational structures on negative outcomes such as alcohol and other drug abuse. Community-based risk factors for alcohol and other drug abuse include the following: community disorganization; lack of community bonding; lack of cultural pride; lack of cultural competence; community attitudes favorable to risk-related behaviors such as drinking and illegal drug use; ready availability of alcohol, tobacco, and other drugs; inadequate youth services; and lack of opportunities for pro-social behaviors (Gardner, Green, & Marcus, 1994). While these community risk factors were delineated for prevention of substance abuse, many are relevant for the prevention of emotional, behavioral, and mental disorders in young children and their families and help identify where intervention can be targeted to bolster protective factors.

The community also has many protective factors that can enhance a family's capacity to care for their youngest children. Included in the protective factors of a community is ready access to information, adequate childcare, safe neighborhoods (supportive community policing as well as neighborhood watch programs), employment opportunities, recreational opportunities, good health, mental health, and substance abuse services, and crisis services. Over the past ten years, there has been a significant interest in community-based early childhood programs. Some of these programs focus on young children with disabilities eligible for services under the Individuals with Disabilities Education Act (IDEA). Other programs, such as Head Start and, more recently, Early Head Start, which serves birth to three-year olds, as well as public and private preschool and educational programs arose from the War on Poverty. In addition, many states are now funding programs for "at-risk" preschool age children.

Over the past several years, the federal government and community agencies have been increasingly interested in evaluating the effect of prevention strategies using the community itself as a measure of analysis. In an article on the evaluation of the Community Partnership Program (CPP), which was conducted for the Center for Substance Abuse Prevention (CSAP) in the Substance Abuse and Mental Health Administration (SAMHSA), U.S. Department of Health and Human Services (USDHHS), the authors state that CPP is not a "prevention program" but a macro-strategy for preventing substance abuse. It is based on the belief that effective prevention of substance abuse requires a coordinated, community-wide strategy, involving a broad range of organizations and institutions, encompassing many prevention activities that are sustained over the long term (Cook, Roehl, Oros, & Trudeau, 1994). Activities for these community-wide endeavors include the following: (a) public education, (b) prevention programs, (c) therapeutic recreation programs, (d) community organizing and empowerment, (e) advocacy for policy change, and (f) other community activities. The evaluation sought to assess the effectiveness of these activities and strategies on alcohol, tobacco, and drug use in communities that had received funding for these activities.

The rationale for developing this type of complex community evaluation study, whereby the unit of analysis is the community itself, is that effective interventions require a comprehensive community approach. This same type of comprehensive community approach is now required to focus on children from birth through 8 years of age in order to prevent not only substance abuse but emotional and behavioral disorders as well. The Comprehensive Services Initiative funded by the Center for Mental Health Services, Substance Abuse and Mental Health Services Administration, has initiatives in over 30 communities across the country that provide systems of care for children with severe emotional disabilities and their families. Some of the creative efforts spawned through this and other federal funding are included in the section highlighting promising practices.

Continuum of Children's Mental Health Services and Supports

The physical, mental and emotional health of the very young child provides the foundation for all further development. In infants and toddlers, emotional growth, patterns of attachment and increasing competency in the ability to form relationships, and the emergence of self-confidence are as crucial to overall development as are physical growth, cognitive or motor skills.

Children who are at risk for mental disorders, those with other health or developmental disabilities and those exhibiting emotional and mental disorders need a range of multiple, diverse, formal and informal services and supports that recognize child and family strengths and address individual needs.

Communities can respond to this continuum of mental health risk factors and disorders by taking a developmental perspective toward intervention. By starting with the provision of universal interventions (mental health promotion) for all children and families, communities have the advantage of avoiding misdiagnosis, promoting positive interactions, and being economically wise. As the pathway continues from promotion to prevention and early intervention, the community as a whole benefit from the services and supports provided.

Promotion activities target all young children and their families. Communities that provide home-visits to all, newborn parent training, education focusing on social and emotional development, and universal screening are investing in smart beginnings.

Preventive measures are usually geared to specific populations considered to be at risk because of biological or environmental factors. Preventive services are available before there are diagnosable symptoms. Examples of preventive approaches include intensive home visiting programs for mothers of low birthweight, premature babies born into families impacted by substance abuse. Organized, ongoing training and consultation by a mental health provider to childcare programs on emotional development and behavior management might be another preventive intervention. The increase in family resource centers as a neighborhood support strategy in communities where families face multiple stresses or isolation illustrates another effective prevention strategy.

Early intervention services and supports for children who have a significant delay or disability in psychosocial development are essential in order to help them achieve their full potential and improve the quality of their relationships. Beginning at birth, some children are already impaired in their daily functioning and relationships. Even though our ability to diagnose mental and emotional disorders has not kept pace with clinical understanding of the development of such problems, some diagnostic categories exist for infants and toddlers including failure to thrive, pervasive developmental disorders, autism, and attachment disorders (Schrag, 1987). In addition, preschoolers and young children can be diagnosed with post-traumatic stress disorder, depression, conduct disorders, and attention disorders. Well-trained clinicians familiar with very young children can use observation, family interviews, and clinical judgement, along with screening and testing to help determine the most appropriate diagnosis and treatment.

Communities that have a mechanism for interagency, interdisciplinary approaches to intervention can best provide the family-centered, strengths-based services and supports needed by young children and their families. Individualized plans that are developed with families allow for a range of interventions that are delivered with the intensity needed for a specific child and family, and across settings. One family with a young child diagnosed with autism spectrum disorder might need intensive services and supports including a trained aid to help with many hours of behavioral intervention, respite services, and sensory integration services, while another may need a community preschool program with specialized staff and a home intervention program. A family impacted by substance abuse or parental mental illness with a baby diagnosed with failure to thrive may require intensive family intervention, home visiting and nutritional services. As needs change from family to family and over time, so must interventions vary. Communities need mechanisms for providing cross-system services, good case management and both formal and informal supports.

Increasingly, research points to the wisdom of communities investing resources "up-front" in the areas of promotion, prevention and early intervention. Meeting the mental health needs of all young children and families through careful planning, integration of services and supports, creative funding and the full participation of families, providers and other community members, makes good economic sense and helps assure good outcomes.

OUR MOST VULNERABLE CHILDREN AND COMMUNITIES

An honest and informed discussion of risk and protective factors within the community is essential to the development of policies and activities based on the capacities, skills and assets of neighborhoods and communities. Community members interested in building the necessary supports for young children and their families, while focusing primarily on the strengths their neighborhoods have to offer, must also be very aware of the vulnerabilities demonstrated by some children and embedded within the community.

Fortunately, most young children explore their worlds in physical safety and emotional security, but for a sizeable minority the experience is quite different. The separation of child and community can stem from the all too real barriers of danger and fear. With increasing frequency, children are being denied access to neighborhoods due to a variety of hazards. Young children may lack independent play skills that encourage creativity and autonomy because in many communities it is unsafe for children to explore their neighborhoods.

For this vulnerable group, there is a widespread perception that they are entering a wide range of early childhood settings "...with fewer intellectual, social and emotional school readiness skills [and that they] have a precocious knowledge of life issues, that they lack the emotional and cognitive ability to understand and integrate (Edelfsen & Baird, 1994, p. 567, as cited in Knitzer, in press). Instead of security and growth, these children face the "double jeopardy" (Kaplan-Sanoff, Parker, & Zuckerman, 1991, as cited in Knitzer, in press) of poverty compounded by exposure to environmental and biological risks, either alone or in combination.

U.S. and international studies of children raised in adverse environments show that these children develop substantial cognitive deficits by the time they are 18 months old (Infant Health and Development Program, 1990; Ramey et al., 1992). Other important research indicates that a stressful social environment can activate hormones that actually hastens the elimination of neurons and adversely affect a child's brain functioning, providing a scientific basis for the observation that children who experience extreme stress in their early years are at greater risk for developing a variety of cognitive, behavioral and emotional difficulties. These difficulties can manifest themselves in a number of ways, including impaired school performance, the inability to manager anger, disproportionate use of special education, and other negative outcomes (Knitzer, in press).

The rationale for an increased focus on prevention and early intervention activities with young children stems from research data and experience across the fields of health, mental health, child welfare, education, substance abuse, and juvenile justice. Early disruptions in emotional development and caregiving relationships can have long term negative consequences. Many of the problems evident in older children and adolescents are believed to originate in early childhood. Serious emotional, behavioral, and mental disorders in older children and adolescents are often manifested in chronic delinquency and antisocial behavior; school failure; depression; suicide; and alcohol, tobacco, and other drug abuse. The Institute of Medicine (IOM) estimates that at least 12 percent of children and adolescents in the United States (about 7.5 million) suffer from one or more mental disorders, including autism, attention deficit hyperactivity disorder, severe conduct disorder, depression, and alcohol and psychoactive substance abuse and dependence (IOM, 1994, p. 4). The prevention and early intervention of these problems in early childhood may avoid significant personal and social costs in later childhood and adolescence.

Second, reports from early childhood program staff indicate that children are entering programs with more serious and challenging behaviors and emotional needs than in the past. While no epidemiological data are yet available to confirm this observation, violence and other stressors are increasingly becoming a part of the early childhood experience. Research on a sample of children under age 6 seen in a Boston City Hospital indicated that 10 percent had witnessed a knifing or shooting (Groves, Zuckerman, Marans, & Cohen, 1993). Community violence, a serious consequence of community disorganization and lack of bonding, is a major issue today for young children and their families and a significant risk for the healthy social and emotional development of young children and the ongoing support of their families.

In a recent article, "Growing Up in a Violent World: The Impact of Family and Community Violence on Young Children and Their Families," Groves (1996) reviewed a number of studies that examined the impact of three kinds of violence on young children: media violence, family violence, and community violence. In addition to listing implications for practice and further research, the author recommends that any effort to address the problems of violence and its effects on young children and families must involve comprehensive and multidimensional strategies:

> A single-focused intervention will fall short of its goals...No single institution can take on the task alone. Schools must unite with health, mental health and law enforcement agencies to provide services and support to families. Social institutions, such as churches and civic groups, must join the effort as well. (pp. 47-48)

A study conducted in Alaska showed that 46 percent of children served were "at risk" because of emotional and developmental delays, chronic health problems, physical or sexual abuse, or alcohol and other drug abuse by parents (Mead, Stewart, Cordes, & Clarson, 1993, as cited in The American Orthopsychiatric Association, 1994). In a national survey, Head Start program staff reported child abuse and substance abuse in families to be of increasing concern (Office of Inspector General, 1989).

Head Start staff also report increased concern about the mental health of their children, families and staff (Yoshikawa & Knitzer, 1997, as cited in Knitzer, in press). Most typically, complaints focus on the levels of provocative, inappropriate, and challenging behavior of the children. Family needs too, in some programs, overwhelm the staff and challenge the very core of Head Start's commitment to strong parental involvement. High levels of parental depression are not uncommon. In a study of one Head Start program, 47 percent of the parents reported poverty-related sadness, demoralization and other indices of despair (Lamb Parker, Piotrkowski, Horn, & Green, 1995, as cited in Knitzer, 1997), a pattern repeated in other non-Head Start samples as well (Johnson & Walker, October 1991, as cited in Knitzer, in press). In some programs, high levels of parental involvement in substance abuse, and familial or community violence also pose enormous challenges to the staff.

Similar reports are emerging from the childcare community. For example, although there are no systematic data, childcare providers in communities across the country report that more and more young children are being "expelled" from programs. A recent call to a childcare technical assistance center illustrated a troubling trend. Instead of a request for help managing the difficult behavior of a child, this childcare director asked for help in developing a "discharge plan" for expelling children who act out. Unlike the situation for older children, no review or referral to either mental health or special education agencies is required (Knitzer, in press). Teacher reports on children entering kindergarten suggest that increasing numbers of children are less prepared to cope with the demands of that environment. A national survey of 7,000 kindergarten teachers reported that 35 percent of their students were not ready for school, with 42 percent of the teachers reporting a worsening of the situation during the past five years (Boyer, 1991, as cited by Knitzer, in press).

As communities begin to build and implement the necessary mental health systems for young children and their families, special attention must be paid to those with or at risk for mental health problems.

Over the last ten years, the child mental health field has created a strong framework for developing community-based programs and services, particularly for children and adolescents with, or at risk for, serious emotional disturbances and their families. Stroul and Friedman (1986) initially articulated this framework in *A System of Care for Children and Youth with Severe Emotional Disturbances*, pointing out three core values for systems development: a system of care must be child-centered and family-focused; programs and services should be community-based; and the system should be culturally competent, with agencies, programs, and services responding to the cultural, racial and ethnic differences of the population (pp. 4-5). The essential building blocks for an early childhood mental health system proposed earlier in this chapter reflect the learnings of the system of care movement.

One caution shared by several communities who have tried to extend their system of care initiative for severely disturbed adolescents downward (to serve infants, toddlers, and preschoolers) is that a system of care for the youngest children and families looks very different from that for older children. The players are different, the needs differ and the settings also vary.

To be successful, an early childhood mental health system of care must be provided in natural settings such as family homes, childcare centers, primary health care clinics, and schools. It must address the needs of the child in the context of the family and promote the well-being of the whole family. Mental health service providers should be trained in typical and atypical child development, family systems and classroom consultation. They must work respectfully with families, childcare providers, health care providers, and substance abuse providers. In addition, families, childcare providers and community members must recognize the value and skills that mental health professionals have to offer. The stigma of mental health will lessen as new relationships are formed.

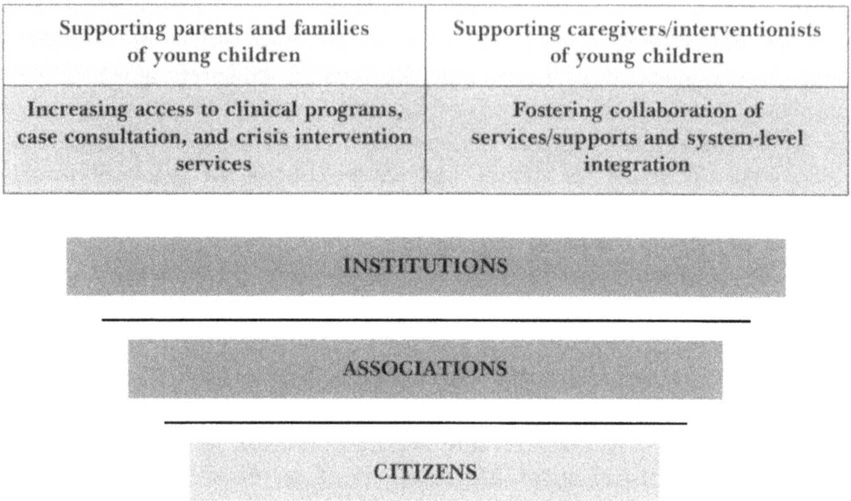

FIGURE 6.2. The differing roles individuals, associations, and institutions can play in the reinforcement of essential components.

COMMUNITY STRATEGIES AND APPROACHES

Each community has a unique combination of assets upon which to build it's future in relation to promoting and supporting children's mental health. These strengths manifest themselves in citizens, associations and institutions, with each asset category having something to contribute to the secure placement of the four building blocks for a community-based early childhood mental health system (Kretzmann & McKnight, 1993). As the building blocks are discussed in further detail, it is important for readers to keep in mind the differing roles that individuals, associations, and institutions can play in the reinforcement of these essential components (see Figure 6.2).

Supporting Parents and Families of Young Children

At some point, all parents of young children need support during the course of childrearing. The provision of constant nurturing and the building of caring relationships are learned skills that require reinforcement by family, friends and the community at large. Families of children with or at risk for emotional or behavioral problems are often faced with challenges that go beyond the everyday challenges of family life. This includes disruptions in patterns of daily living, frustrated communication patterns, an undermining of familial roles, a sense of loss, and isolation from family and friends. These parents can benefit from more intensive behavior and stress management skills. Families faced with multiple challenges require competent intervention programs that meet their complex and changing needs.

Community-based services and programs that are truly supportive of parents and families are often times delivered in natural settings, such as family homes; respect developmental processes, and are flexible and individualized to meet the needs of both children and parents; and are sensitive to the cultural and ethnic values of the families. Family support programs provide a variety of services that "empower and strengthen adults in their roles as parents, nurturers and providers" (Weissbourd & Kagan, 1989, p. 21).

Increasingly, family resource centers and other family support programs are recognizing the need to partner with other agencies, organizations or providers to expand the repertoire of interventions provided in order to meet the needs of families with complex challenges such as mental illness, physical illness and substance abuse. The Federation of Families for Children's Mental Health (1992) defines family support as formal and informal services and supports including tangible goods as defined by families. In essence, family support is whatever it takes to care for or live with a child who has an emotional, mental or behavioral disorder. Regarding the role of family support programs in prevention and early intervention services, Weissbourd (1991) stated that "What they can do is enhance the competency of parents and enable participants to build skills, utilize resources, and develop the confidence necessary to advocate on their own behalf" (p. 70).

Since each family has its own structure, racial and ethnic identity, roles, values, beliefs, and coping styles, respect for and acceptance of this diversity is a cornerstone of family-centered early intervention. Respecting and accepting family diversity means acknowledging that there are strengths and resources present in *all* families. Therefore, professionals must learn to recognize and build on these positive attributes as part of their work with families. This approach holds equally true for all families, regardless of their ethnicity, cultural background, or socioeconomic circumstances and forms the foundation for services that are culturally and developmentally competent.

In their review of the literature on the sociocultural influences on infant development, Coll and Meyer (1993) found support for the importance of integrating family culture into service delivery approaches. The authors highlight the success of culturally relevant interventions such as *Cuento* or folktale therapy that conveys the knowledge, values and skills inherent in Puerto Rican heritage, thereby fostering pride and reinforcing adaptive behavior. Other practices include

Does your community:

- ✔ Have family support groups for parents of young children with emotional/behavioral disorders?
- ✔ Have courses for parents on emotional development?
- ✔ Have family resource centers?
- ✔ Have information on emotional/behavioral disabilities available in a variety of languages and formats?
- ✔ Have parent-to-parent networks?
- ✔ Have respite programs?

FIGURE 6.3. A checklist for building family support.

enlisting the support of cultural folk healers, elders or religious leaders who often provide families with advice and strategies for solving problems with their young children. Also, since many African-American families have complex extended family households or closely knit networks of friends and family, it is often a serious therapeutic error to focus treatment on the mother and child only, ignoring the positive impact of significant family and surrogate family members (Tatem, Mosely, Boyd-Franklin, & Herzog, 1995). The Kauai, Hawaii, study found that the support of alternative caregivers, such as grandparents or siblings, is a protective factor, thereby reinforcing the importance of including the extended family in treatment planning and intervention (Werner & Smith, 1992).

Family Support: Promising Practices

Avance is a family support and education program that began in Texas in 1973 and serves Mexican-American families. Each year Avance serves 2,000 families with young children in Houston, San Antonio, and the Rio Grande Valley. Avance operates in public housing, in elementary schools, and through its family-service centers. Its Parent-Child Education Program provides home visits by trained staff members (many of them former participants), weekly classes on child growth and development, and information about community services, English classes, and high school and employment preparation courses.

Avance also stresses a two-generation program approach. The program provides free childcare so that mothers can attend classes. Often, when their children are older, mothers serve as volunteer aides at the childcare center, thus learning more about child development. Avance staff members, most of whom have some college education in relevant disciplines, emphasize individual attention to the child and support for the mother. Avance also supports fathers—staff encourage fathers through job training assistance, parenting education, and social support networks.

Evaluations show that Avance programs have improved families' ability to provide an emotionally stimulating and nurturing environment for their young children, positively influenced mothers' childrearing attitudes and knowledge, and expanded mothers' use of community resources (Carnegie Task Force, 1994).

The *Teen Parents and Babies Program* (TPBP) of Syracuse, New York, provides weekly home-based visits to low-income teen parents who are, due to factors such as substance, physical, or sexual abuse, deemed at high risk for poor parenting of their infants. It is a comprehensive program with several goals, one of which is prevention of child abuse and neglect. Services primarily begin prior to birth and continue through the second year of the child's life. A home visitor demonstrates for parents developmentally appropriate physical, emotional and cognitive stimulation of the infant. The program provides sensitive support to help young parents become attuned to their infant's needs and basic parenting education on subjects such as childbirth and breast-feeding. Infants with suspected developmental delays are referred by program staff for a more thorough evaluation.

The program is two-generational because the genuine, focused attention provided by the home visitor nurtures the teen parent's self-esteem and improves her sensitivity to and competence with the baby. Family issues such as physical violence or substance abuse are dealt with as they arise. Therefore, the content and intensity of the visits vary. In all cases, the home visitor tries to build a trusting relationship with the family and introduces the family to community resources. In addition, the staff encourage teen parents to find ways to continue their education and develop strong support networks.

Healthy Families America (HFA), whose roots are in the prevention of child abuse and neglect, is a community-based home visiting family support model. HFA programs are intensive, comprehensive, integrated with other community services, and flexible in responding to families' unique needs. Presently over 250 cities in 38 states have HFA programs. Building on the work of HFA is Project Before, a program component of Kan Focus located in Parsons City, Kansas. This initiative, funded by the Center for Mental Health Services, aims to create a system of care for children and adolescents with serious emotional disturbance.

A community needs assessment process determined that a priority need was intensive support for families with young children, high risk factors, and a parent with mental health or substance abuse challenges. The resource assessment showed that although Healthy Families America was effective with overburdened families, the program was much less effective with families who had substance abuse and mental health problems. This became the group of families served by Project Before. Services were provided through intensive case management, pulling together the diverse programs and providers working with each family. Services such as substance abuse and mental health treatment were provided primarily to the adults in the family. Their goal was to break the constant state of crisis that had become the norm for many of the families served. Helping them to identify and build informal social supports to address their isolation became an important part of the home visits.

The work is intense and demanding for the home visitors. The home visitors that were most successful in working with this population and who remained with the program for the longest often were those who had experienced problems similar to those of their clients, in their own families. The program found that the most effective orientation process for new home visitors involved shadowing an experienced home visitor. In addition to the standard training provided by Healthy Families America, priority training topics for Project Before home visitors included family-centered service delivery, substance abuse, maternal depression, child development, infant mental health, collaboration, strength based assessment, and the whole-family wraparound process.

Critical to the success of Project Before interventions is ongoing training, supervision and mental health consultation to the home visitors. Early findings have exceeded expectations about impacts on children and families. At intake, 55 percent of the children were receiving medical care and 35 percent had been immunized. With respect to the mothers, at intake, only 60 percent of the mothers were receiving maternal health care and less than 25 percent of the pregnant women receiving prenatal care. Within a three-month time period, this increased to 85 percent. Utilization of therapy and substance abuse services by the parents also increased, with some parents returning to treatment and others entering for the first time. Within three months, 75 percent of these mothers, considered the most difficult to serve, had gone to work. Project Before has been a catalyst for the development of an early childhood system of care that has rallied key community leaders and agencies. Head Start and Early Head Start, Part C, business members, police, health, mental health, and social services work together to plan and integrate services.

Supporting Caregivers of Young Children

The need for quality childcare and after-school activities is a daily concern for millions of working parents. Every day, three out of five preschoolers are in childcare and millions of older children are in after-school activities while their parents work. Childcare and after-school activities help to shape the way children think, learn and behave for the rest of their lives, but too little attention is paid to the quality of those experiences (Children's Defense Fund, 1998).

Caregivers need a great deal of ongoing support in their efforts to nurture and build caring relationships with young children. Communities can provide a wide variety of services to childcare providers including training opportunities for both professionals and paraprofessionals; space for providers to share information, achievements and problems; and lending libraries for books, toys and essential safety equipment.

For some families who have a difficult relationship with their infant, childcare is seen as a respite. Professionals also may look upon Head Start and childcare as an intervention for troubled children. An assumption is

Does your community:

- ✔ Have a childcare resource and referral agency that understands the needs of children with emotional/behavioral disabilities?
- ✔ Provide an early childhood association that offers ongoing training in social-emotional development, mental health screening, and behavior management?
- ✔ Provide safe escort for home visitors?
- ✔ Train home visitors, childcare providers and teachers in understanding family systems?
- ✔ Have a childcare director's support network?
- ✔ Have a mental health consultation program for childcare providers and teachers to access?
- ✔ Have lending libraries that include books on children's mental health, early childhood mental health curricula, and toys?
- ✔ Have recreational and stress reduction programs for child care staff?
- ✔ Have a mechanism to assess and maintain high quality child care?

FIGURE 6.4. A checklist for building caregiver support.

made that through interaction with the childcare provider, new patterns of relating will be learned and the child will "be cured." This assumption is inadequate. Childcare providers who work effectively with groups of challenging, but typical children, are often untrained to meet the special needs of those children with extraordinary needs or behaviors.

For this very reason, it is essential that caregivers (as well as family support workers) working in programs for infants, toddlers and preschoolers, have access to mental health consultation, case consultation, and back-up support to address issues of burnout, cultural and workplace conflicts, and other staff issues. Furthermore, caregivers who express concern with a child's emotional/behavioral development should have access to multidisciplinary assessment and therapeutic services when necessary. Because of the demands of their work, these services need to be provided on-site and at flexible times.

Caregiver Support: Promising Practices

The Day Care Consultants Program located in San Francisco, California is a collaborative effort between three of the cities' most experienced mental health organizations: Jewish Family and Children's Services, the Infant-Parent Program at UCSF, and the Child, Youth and Family Section of the Division of Mental Health. These organizations, with financial support from the Miriam and Peter Haas Fund, have created the Early Childhood Mental Health Services project. This model program, targeted to serve San Francisco's low income children aged two to five, trains early childhood mental health consultants to work directly with the city's public and nonprofit childcare centers and the children's families. The Day Care Consultants Program provides consultation to center administrators and staff, parent education and support to families, and clinical intervention for at-risk children and families.

Mental health consultation, whether it focuses on a particularly difficult child or on an equally distressing but more general program issue, is centered on and conducted through relationships. The relationships involved in the consultation process are those between consultant and consultee and between caregivers and children. The consultant's impact on the caregiver is reflected in the caregiver's impact on the children for whom she provides care. The consultant understands not only the concerns about a particular child or program issue but also the feelings that these situations create in the caregiver.

Through the relationship with the consultant, the caregiver comes to feel that her experiences with children are valued and understood, and she in turn becomes better able to understand, value and empathize with the experiences of the children for whom she cares. Ultimately, it is this increased awareness and understanding of the child's experience at which consultation is aimed.

The relationship between consultant and caregivers is developed over time through meeting regularly, usually weekly, with the staff at each childcare site. Through these weekly discussions, in conjunction with periodic program observations, the consultant becomes intimately familiar with the setting. The familiarity and trust that develops permits the consultant's participation in all aspects of program planning.

In addition to program consultation, case consultation is provided to caregivers who are concerned about a particular child in their program who may be very upset when separated from a parent; very upset with transition; unable to play; unusually quiet and withdrawn; likely to hurt himself or others; unable to form relationships; particularly fussy or hard to comfort; phobic; or having difficulty controlling behavior. Case consultation includes on site observation, meetings with staff, helping caregivers work with families, direct work with families, and referral for additional developmental and social services.

When case consultation proves insufficient, therapeutic groups are provided. Currently, two groups are conducted in childcare centers for children with pervasive mental health problems. In addition to the child therapeutic groups, consultation is provided to staff to help them address the children's individual needs and to the parents of the children.

The Ounce of Prevention Fund's (OPF) Developmental Training and Support Program (DTSP), located in Chicago, Illinois, grew out of the need of community-based direct service staff with whom OPF worked to develop more effective strategies for working with teen parents and their children within the context of their relationships, environment and culture.

The DTSP is based on the belief that change and growth in people occur through strong, positive relationships. Training activities, therefore, are all designed to strengthen relationships. Through ongoing training, over the course of at least two years, home visiting, supervisory and executive staff of the program develop new insights into the parent-child relationships they encounter and learn new ways of working that bolster relationships within the families they serve and within the program itself.

The OPF Developmental Training and Support Program helps programs to redirect their services from a parent-centered approach focusing on parents' crises to a parent-child relationship approach that builds on family strengths to enhance the successful development of children, parents, and families. By adopting this method, programs implement a crucial sequence of support—where supervisor and staff, staff and parent, and parent and child all learn from and respond to one another's relationships. The DTSP calls this "a chance of enablement."

The most critical content of each monthly training session is distilled from discussions of the work that staff members are doing with their families, why it might be happening, and the staff member's contribution to the success they are seeing. When successful, the final result of the DTSP is to inspire and empower programs to incorporate the methods and values of the training into their community-based organization's service delivery system.

As part of the DTSP, supervisors meet with staff on a frequent and consistent basis. Caseloads are kept small enough so that staff can establish meaningful and productive relationships with parents. Supervisors are trained to support these relationships through regular, reflective supervision. Parent Child Observation Guides (PCOGs), videos and the Denver Developmental Screening Test are used not only to enhance discussions and planning for families, but to identify home visitors' strengths and the skills they need to improve their work with families.

Increasing Access to Clinical Programs Case Consultation and Crisis Services

As we noted earlier in the chapter, children's mental health can be viewed along a continuum. Communities must have in place programs and supports for those young children and families most in need, starting with children with serious emotional disturbance. For children exhibiting symptoms of mental illness a range of services and supports must be available. Many of these young children should be eligible for services through existing programs such as Part C and Section 619 of IDEA, although in many communities this is not happening in a systematic way. Unfortunately the expertise of many early intervention screeners and evaluators does not include knowledge of infant mental health, parent-child interaction, or functional assessment of emotional and behavioral disabilities. Early childhood mental health professionals can train other providers, join community child-find efforts, and be available for consultation. Services should be flexible, family- and child-centered, and provided in homes, childcare, and other community settings.

Local interagency coordinating councils and community mental health collaboratives can combine efforts in order to provide comprehensive mental health services and supports to those children and families most in need. The wraparound model used for older children with serious emotional disturbance can be effectively used with families of very young children in order to provide intensive in-home and community-based services, informal community supports, and to meet concrete needs.

Does your community:

- ✔ Have mental health providers trained in early intervention?
- ✔ Have behaviorally-based programs available in a variety of settings?
- ✔ Have on-site mental health consultation readily available to home visitors, childcare providers, and teachers?
- ✔ Have in-home mental health services and supports?
- ✔ Have wraparound services targeted to young children and their families?
- ✔ Have crisis teams available in case of emergencies such as family or community violence?
- ✔ Have therapeutic intervention programs available (ideally in existing Head Start, child care settings or schools)?
- ✔ Have a hot line available for families and caregivers who need immediate help?
- ✔ Have substance abuse services available that includes a focus on the relationship between parent and child?

FIGURE 6.5. A checklist for increasing access to clinical services, case consultation, and crisis services.

Vulnerable young children and their families in emergency shelters, involved with courts, and in other high-risk settings, should be the focus of community outreach efforts and should have adequate access to the early childhood mental health system of care. In addition, young children, families and child-serving programs experiencing crises related to violence, community disasters or family-specific experiences should have *immediate* access to crisis intervention (Stroul, 1996).

Access to Clinical Services, Case Consultation and Crisis Services: Promising Practices

The Early Intervention Center (EIC) of the Positive Education Program (PEP) represents an early intervention program specifically designed for young children with serious emotional and behavioral problems. EIC is a parent-driven early intervention program located in Cleveland, Ohio. The program focuses on the use of parents as the primary change agents for young seriously troubled children through a combination of individualized learning for parents, behavioral intervention, group support, the offering of formal courses in child development, and group experiences for the children staffed by parents and staff. Parents learn first by rehearsing and role playing in the observation room with the help of coaches and then testing out what they have learned in real settings. The coaches are often parents themselves who have successfully completed the program, with resource consultants who are either childhood educators or mental health professionals providing support.

In an effort to accommodate working families, the program provides services on weekends and evenings. Special efforts are made to engage fathers in the care of their children. Coaches or resource consultants help shape interventions that really work by accompanying parents to the mall, grocery store or by observing meal times and bed time routines. Individual plans are developed for each child, implemented in the center and at home, and evaluated for effectiveness by the parents and staff. Transition to a less restrictive environment, such as regular education or special education, is an ongoing goal.

The Families and Schools Together Track Program (FAST Track) involves children attending kindergarten in selected schools in four communities of the United States. (Durham, NC; Nashville, TN; Seattle, WA; and rural central Pennsylvania). The FAST Track program is a developmental and clinical model for the treatment of youth conduct disorder through the strategy of preventive intervention for families with children showing early aggression and peer difficulty. This program integrates five intervention components designed to promote competence in the family, child, and school, in order to prevent conduct problems, poor social relations, and school failure. The components are (a) parent training; (b) home visiting/case management; (c) social skills training; (d) academic tutoring; and (e) teacher-based, classroom intervention.

FAST Track participants include families with children exhibiting aggression and peer difficulties. The program takes a multi-systemic focus that not only attempts to build appropriate skills, attitudes, and expectancies among families, schools, and peers, but also focuses on building positive relationships among these systems. The FAST Track program treats parents and other family members as collaborative partners in the process of helping their child succeed (Conduct Problems Prevention Research Group, 1992).

The East Baltimore Mental Health Partnership is a project housed within Johns Hopkins Hospital that is building a collaborative system of care for children with serious emotional disturbance and their families. Funding comes from a variety of state, federal and local sources. Primary financial support for the early childhood effort comes from the Substance Abuse and Mental Health Services Administration. Presently program staff provide on-site mental health services to several Head Start programs in Baltimore, Maryland. These services focus on children, staff and families, and are designed to provide support to and build on the existing strengths of individuals, families and organizations.

The mental health services at the various Head Start Centers differ depending on program needs. Although grounded in a common core, services are flexible, responsive, and individualized. All efforts emphasize staff development and relationship building with the staff at the center.

Training has focused on emotional development, behavioral strategies, grief and loss, and myths about mental health. Use of videotaping is frequently used to illustrate behaviors, interactions and relationships.

Services to individual children are provided in a variety of ways, including in-class interventions, small groups (socialization, loss, and so forth), and family therapy. Groups for caregivers include parenting, self-esteem, and kinship caregiver support.

Since the program is impacted by community and family violence, including shootings, child abuse and substance abuse, clinicians are multi-trained, interdisciplinary, but all have a primary focus on early childhood. In response to frequent crises, a community crisis team is available to center staff and families. The children in the program who are often witness to violence also receive intensive support in dealing with trauma. Recently a shooting of a staff member occurred right outside a Head Start center. A number of children and their parents watched this tragedy unfold. The clinical consultants as well as other staff from the mental health center provided immediate and ongoing counseling and support.

The East Baltimore Mental Health Partnership has recently joined members of the clergy and other citizens and organizations in a community-wide effort to reduce youth homicide. Clergy and clinicians talk about community violence and behavioral health at victim's funerals and other community events.

Fostering Collaboration of Services and Supports and System-level Integration

Families with young children living in communities are not typically dealing with single issues or accessing services from only one organization. This is especially true for families with young children with, or at-risk of developing, emotional and behavioral problems—substance abuse coexists with violence; behavioral and emotional disorders in young children coexist with speech and language problems (Knitzer, in press). A thriving community infrastructure rich with interagency linkages, service coordination and collaboration between various service

Does your community:

- ✔ Have an interagency effort that addresses the mental health needs of young children and their families?
- ✔ Provide cross agency service providers?
- ✔ Train case managers to work across systems?
- ✔ Have a community mapping project that identifies community needs and resources?
- ✔ Provide supervision to providers that work collaboratively across mental health, child care and education, and substance abuse?
- ✔ Have a philosophical and financial investment in early childhood mental health?
- ✔ Encourage a Part C and special education system that addresses the broad needs of the child, family and community through collaboration with mental health, substance abuse, social services and other agencies?
- ✔ Have a commitment to developing an early childhood system of care that supports the mental, physical and developmental needs of young children and their families?

FIGURE 6.6. A checklist for fostering collaboration and services integration.

entities is better equipped to meet the diversity of needs represented by all young children and families.

In order to foster collaboration at the community level, open lines of communication between clubs, organizations and associations must be established. Agency representatives must have the opportunity to communicate with their counterparts, gain an understanding of the abilities and constraints of other programs, and see the roles of their own agency with a perspective that includes the roles of others (Swan & Morgan, 1993). This dialogue, and the resulting appreciation of other's efforts, can lead to the development of trust between agencies and organizations. Trust is a critical element in the honest analysis of the overall community system available to young children and their families. The community service delivery system can undergo rapid change as roles and responsibilities are realigned in an effort to reduce duplication of services and to fill in gaps.

Many communities across the country have demonstrated innovative approaches to the establishment of interagency linkages, service coordination and collaboration. Through initial funding from the federal Center for Mental Health Services, Vermont has seeded a state and regional initiative to develop a comprehensive system of care for children from birth through age 6 and their families. Key agencies and family members have joined with community leaders, university faculty and others to plan, implement and evaluate this effort. The Community Wraparound Initiative in Chicago, Illinois has developed a strong interagency planning and delivery system by tapping into existing Local Interagency Coordinating Councils and Local Area Networks originally established by the Special Education and Mental Health systems. Services and supports are developed according to a wraparound model that provides both formal and informal help to families with young children impacted by mental health or substance abuse problems. Services are provided in family homes, Head Start locations, as well as substance abuse and community mental health clinics.

Fostering Cross-System Collaboration and Services Integration: Promising Practices

In Stark County, Ohio, the Head Start Community Action Agency has joined forces with a local child and adolescent mental health agency to provide an on-site team of paraprofessional early interventionists and a mental health supervisor to Head Start staff, children and families. The early intervention team has access to the full range of flexible, wraparound, diagnostic, and treatment resources of the mental health center, which gives it the capacity to continue even the most troubled children in the Head Start program. In addition to helping with more traditional Head Start mental health activities, the early intervention team makes home visits and offers a variety of wraparound support to families, including in-home behavioral aids and respite care.

The Village Early Intervention Project (VEIP) on John's Island, South Carolina, is the first systematic blending of mental health and substance abuse services for families with very young children in the state. The initiative, funded in 1995 for three years by the Substance Abuse and Mental Health Services Administration, is so successful that it will continue providing services and supports through fees-for-services and with state and community funds.

When the project started, there were no mental health or substance abuse services on the Island although there were many families in need of services. Over time, strong involvement of community leaders, especially clergy, helped foster acceptance of the program. A new community center provides therapeutic childcare, mental health and substance abuse services, and a place for families to meet. In addition, home visits are provided to all families. A natural helper hired by the program provides an ongoing link to the community, and is responsible for most of the growing referrals. Additional staff include mental health counselors, a substance abuse counselor, childcare providers, and a consulting psychiatrist. All staff are trained in Multisystemic Therapy, Multi-Component Behavioral Treatment, infant and child development, and cultural competence.

Individualized wraparound plans are developed for all families, with the intensity and scope of services and supports differing depending upon need. The family and therapist identify and prioritize child and family strengths and needs, build a support team, and locate informal and formal services and supports. In addition to treatment needs, families often identify tangible needs for food, housing, transportation, babysitting, and so forth. Services are available around the clock, including a response to crisis situations such as domestic violence, attempted suicide, child abuse, and behavioral intervention for children whose behavior is out of control.

The Family Health Promotion Program (FHPP)/Servicios de Integracion Familiar (ICFS), sponsored by CODAC Behavioral Health Services, is a culturally appropriate community development program serving families of children from birth to age 7 in the Connie Chambers Public Housing Development and the Drachman Elementary School area in Tucson, Arizona. CODAC is a private, nonprofit agency providing a full continuum of drug, alcohol, and mental health services for children, youth and adults in residential and outpatient settings.

The FHPP/ICFS program features an on-site family resource center, parent education on children's health and development through regular home visits, an early childhood development center, and other services. In order to achieve integrated service delivery, a family services team is convened for each family participating in the program; this team is responsible for the development and implementation of a coordinated family services plan. Although the primary purpose of the FHHP is to reduce risk and bolster resiliency, the coordinated services plan expands services to include more intensive, coordinated services such as child or family therapy and substance abuse services.

Several initiatives stand out among the diverse array of services and supports available to program participants. Since 1993, the Connie Chambers Early Childhood Center has provided full day, full year early preschool programming for children 3 to 5 years of age living in and around the housing project. For the past three years the center has received state block grant funds to serve four-year-old at-risk children, and is accredited by the National Association for the Education of

Young Children (NAEYC). This is one of the few NAEYC-accredited programs located in public housing.

A Head Start program is also located in the housing project and there is collaboration between the two centers, such as home education, afternoon placements for the Head Start children in Connie Chambers, and shared resources for serving children with disabilities, including an art therapist. A prevention/promotion philosophy is pervasive in the childcare program through the development and use of the Building Me Curriculum, a risk and resiliency framework. The needs of children with severe mental health challenges are addressed through the coordinated services plan and consultation with a mental health professional.

The Neighborhood Services Center (NSC) enhances the coordination and availability of family centered services. NSC offers childcare, a learning center, recreation facilities, and family self-sufficiency programs to greater Santa Rosa residents. Services related to housing, employment training, job opportunities, education, wellness, recreation, public assistance, and other essential information is available. In addition, a primary health care clinic has been established. It is staffed with family medicine residents from Arizona State University and is open one day per week providing regular health care to children and families.

Funding for these integrated initiatives come from federal grants, state funds, Medicaid, and foundations. Strong partnerships have been formed with many community organizations including parks and recreation, public schools, community mental health, public health, libraries, police department, Planned Parenthood, Head Start, Pima Youth Partnership, city of Tucson water department, Part H, and others.

CONCLUSION

> Community residents are demonstrating the will to take control of their own destiny. They want a better life for their family ...and a better future for their children. [They] realize that healthy families go hand in hand with healthy communities. (Family Resource Coalition, 1995, p. vi)

The outcomes for children and families are increasingly linked to the communities in which they live. Every family with young children depends on a wide range of formal and informal supports in order to meet the increasing demands of society. Research, anecdote and experience point out the need for communities to focus on the total development of young children and their families. Whether by virtue of environment or biology, increasing numbers of infants, toddlers, and preschool children experience or are at risk for mental illness. When families have a child with a mental illness, they require a variety of individualized, respectful services provided by skilled personnel. When children are at risk for mental illness because of multiple factors, early intervention can help prevent or lessen poor outcomes.

Communities across the country are beginning to address the complex mental health needs of young children. Increasingly, programs are being targeted to children impacted by family or community violence, substance abuse and other risk factors. Enlightened communities provide universal screening and family education. Less frequently provided is the secondary support needed to maintain children with mental health problems in their natural settings such as childcare or preschool.

Comprehensive, integrated service systems that pull together all child and family serving agencies and programs including child development, mental health, health, and substance abuse are almost nonexistent in communities. The lessons learned through initiatives such as Part C of IDEA and the Comprehensive Mental Health Services Sites can serve as a catalyst for community development. They guide the way to an integrated approach to services—both informal and formal—and provide opportunities for infrastructure development and community collaboration.

It is hoped that this chapter will be useful as a challenge for action, ensuring that the mental health needs of our youngest citizens and their families are recognized and met in the community. Assessing need, evaluating existing capacity and creating community support for focusing on early childhood mental health will help strengthen the fabric of our communities.

REFERENCES

American Orthopsychiatric Association, Report of the Task Force on Head Start and Mental Health. (1994, April). *Strengthening mental health in Head Start: Pathways to quality improvement*. New York: Author.

Arst, J. (1996). *Working toward a good start in life: Mental health approaches in early childhood settings*. San Francisco: Miriam and Peter Haas Fund.

Berlin, L. J., O'Neal, C. R., Brooks-Gunn, J. (1998, February/March). What Makes Early Intervention Programs Work? *Bulletin of Zero to Three: National Center for Infants, Toddlers, and Families, 18*(4), 4-15.

Bronfenbrenner, U. (1979). *The ecology of human development*. Cambridge, MA: Harvard University Press.

Carnegie Task Force on Meeting the Needs of Young Children. (1994, April). *Starting points: Meeting the needs of our youngest children*. New York: Carnegie Corporation.

Chamberlin, R. (1996). Primary prevention and the family support movement. In G. Singer, L. Powers, & A. Olson (Eds.), *Redefining family support: Innovations in public-private partnerships* (pp. 115-133). Baltimore, MD: Brookes.

The Children's Defense Fund [Online]. (1998). Available: www.childrensdefense.org/ccmenu.html

Cochran, M., Larner, M., Riley, D., Gunnarson, L. & Henderson, C. R. (1990). *Extending families: The social networks of parents and their children*. New York: Cambridge University Press.

Coll, C. T. G., & Meyer, E. C. (1993). The sociocultural context of infant development. In C. H. Zeanah, Jr. (Ed.), *Handbook of infant mental health* (pp. 56-70). New York: Guilford.

Conduct Problems Prevention Research Group. (1992). A developmental and clinical model for the prevention of conduct disorder: The FAST Track Program. *Development and Psychopathology, 4*, 509-527.

Cook, R., Roehl, J., Oros, C., & Trudeau, J. (1994). Conceptual and methodological issues in the evaluation of community-based substance abuse prevention coalitions: Lessons learned from the national evaluation of the community partnerships program [Special Issue]. *Journal of Community Psychology*, 155-169.

Dunst, C. J. (1993). Implications of risk and opportunity factors for assessment and intervention practices. *Topics in Early Childhood Special Education, 13*(2), 147.

Family Resource Coalition. (1995). *Know your community: A step-by-step guide to community needs and resources assessment*. Chicago: Family Resource Coalition

Federation of Families for Children's Mental Health, Family Support Committee. (1992). *Membership brochure*. Alexandria, VA: Author.

Gardner, S., Green, P., & Marcus, C. (Eds.). (1994). *Signs of effectiveness II. Preventing alcohol, tobacco and other drug use: A risk factor/resiliency-based approach*. Rockville, MD: Substance Abuse and Mental Health Services Administration.

Grizenko, N., & Fisher, C. (1992, December). Review of studies of risk and protective factors for psychopathology in children. *Canadian Journal of Psychiatry, 37*, 711-721.

Groves, B. (1996). Growing up in a violent world: The impact of family and community violence on young children and their families. In E. J. Erwin (Ed.), *Putting children first* (pp. 31-52). Baltimore, MD: Brookes.

Groves, B., Zuckerman, B., Marans, S., & Cohen, D. (1993). Silent victims: Children who witness violence. *Journal of the American Medical Association, 269, 262-264.*

Henderson, P. (Ed.). (1995). *Children and communities*. London: Community Development Foundation.

Infant Health and Development Program. (1990). Enhancing the outcomes of low birthweight premature infants. *Journal of the American Medical Association, 263*, 3035-3042.

Institute of Medicine. (1994). *Reducing risks for mental disorders: Frontiers for preventive intervention research*. Washington, DC: National Academy of Sciences.

Knitzer, J. (1997). Early childhood mental health services through a policy and systems development perspective. In S. J. Meisels & J. P. Shonkoff (Eds.), *Handbook of early childhood intervention* (2nd ed.). New York: Cambridge University Press.

Kretzmann, J. P. & McKnight, J. L. (1993). *Building Communities from the Inside Out: A Path Toward Finding and Mobilizing A Community's Assets*. Chicago, IL: ACTA.

Office of Inspector General, Office of Analysis and Inspections. (1989, November). *Dysfunctional families in the Head Start program: Meeting the challenge* (DHHS Publication No. OAI-09-89-01000). Washington, DC: U.S. Government Printing Office.

Ramey, C., Bryant, D., Wasik, B., Sparling, J., Fendt, K., & LaVange, L. (1992). The Infant Health and Development Program for low birthweight, premature infants: Program elements, family participation, and child intelligence. *Pediatrics, 89*, 454-465.

Schorr, L. B. (1997). *Common purpose: Strengthening families and neighborhoods to rebuild America*. New York: Doubleday.

Schrag, E. (1987). *Sensitivities, Skills and Services: Mental Health Roles in the Implementation of Part H of PL 99-457, The Education of the Handicapped Act Amendments of 1986*. Washington DC: Child and Adolescent Service System Program, National Institute of Mental Health.

Stroul, B. A. (Ed.). (1996). *Children's mental health: Creating systems of care in a changing society*. Baltimore, MD: Brookes.

Stroul, B. A., & Friedman, R. M. (1986). *A system of care for children and youth with severe emotional disturbances* (rev. ed.). Washington, DC: Georgetown University Child Development Center, National Assistance Center for Children's Mental Health.

Swan, W. W., & Morgan, J. L. (1993). *Collaborating for Comprehensive Services for Young Children and Their Families; The Local Interagency Coordinating Council*. Baltimore, MD: Brookes.

Szapocznik, J., & Kurtines, W. M. (1993). Family psychology and cultural diversity: Opportunities for theory, research, and application. *American Psychologist, 48*, 400-407.

Tatem, J., Mosely, S., Boyd-Franklin, N., & Herzog, E. (1995). A home-based, family systems approach to the treatment of African-American teenage parents and their families. *Zero to Three, 15*(4), 18-25.

Weissbourd, B. (1991). Family resource and family support programs: Changes and challenges in human services. In D. G. Unger & D. R. Powell (Eds.), *Families as nurturing systems: Support across the lifespan* (pp. 69-85). New York: Hawthorne.

Weissbourd, B., & Kagan, S. L. (1989). Family support programs: Catalysts for change. *American Journal of Orthopsychiatry, 59*(1), 20-31.

Werner, E. E., & Smith, R. S. (1992). *Overcoming the odds: High risk children from birth to adulthood*. New York: Cornell University Press.

chapter 7

State-Level Supports for Community-Based Services

Gary J. De Carolis
Department of Health and Human Services, Rockville, Maryland

INTRODUCTION

True leaders know that honesty, dedication, creative thinking, political and business savvy, and undying respect for the power of a community of individuals to influence radical change are among the most critical characteristics of people who succeed in their efforts to make this world a better place. To these ends, Vice President Gore has spearheaded a continuous process of reinventing government in which system reform is achieved through unprecedented collaborative efforts and significant reductions in bureaucratic red tape. First Lady Hillary Rodham Clinton (1996) has uplifted and empowered the community and "village" as the overseers of care for its members, especially its children and families. Gandhi and Mandela stood prepared, as have many others, to die for the greater good of their community.

As the chief of the Child, Adolescent, and Family Branch of the Center for Mental Health Services of the Substance Abuse and Mental Health Services Administration of the United States Department of Health and Human Services, I currently have the privilege of overseeing system reform efforts in more than 30 states by administering the Federal Comprehensive Community Mental Health Services for Children and Their Families Program. While this grant program financially supports reforms in selected communities, the Branch is also responsible for ensuring that the mental health needs of all children in America are given priority, let alone parity, in our health care delivery system. To this end, I have made every attempt to support the development of outreach and technical assistance materials and services that are intended to empower families and communities everywhere to initiate local reform efforts with or without the incentive of a federal grant. One of those materials is a guidebook titled *Making It Happen*. Because I firmly believe that this book well describes the essential stages of system development and enhancement, I have elected to borrow from its text to validate the sequence of events I will describe as inherent to successful system reforms. In this chapter I attempt to share with you my knowledge of those key factors and my specific operational experience as a leader of a statewide effort in Vermont. I will use Vermont as a case study to illustrate the process of system reform as well as the critical roles of the leader, stakeholders and communities in achieving the desired outcomes.

This chapter will also describe the central role of leaders in mobilizing the communities to carry the reform processes from concept to implementation. Critical discussions will include the following: defining your vision, institutionalizing core values, building stakeholder support, using needs-assessments effectively, and ensuring interagency collaboration. There are also brief discussions about developing core services, establishing operational strategies, implementing training and technical assistance, and making continuous quality improvement.

It is important to note that my goal, as a public entrepreneur, then and now, is the same: to find better ways to engage stakeholders in a collaborative venture toward the realization of a comprehensive, coordinated, community-based, culturally responsive system of care for all children and their families. With this in mind, I invite you to join me in an exploration of my lessons learned about system reform at the community level.

Like every other state in 1985, Vermont lacked a *cohesive* system addressing the mental health needs of children within home- and community-based systems. Stakeholders in childcare had been crying for a more effective way to deliver services to children and families with serious emotional disturbances. The agencies responsible (mental health, education, juvenile justice, substance abuse, child welfare, etc.) had until then existed and operated as discrete, insular entities, creating a loose patchwork of care fraught with inefficient gaps and overlaps. In the last 14 years, the state of Vermont has reinvented its system of care for children with serious emotional disturbances by limiting bureaucratic inefficiencies and allowing the communities to assume a central role in system reform, design and operation.

In 1985, the Department of Mental Health and Developmental Disabilities secured a five-year strategic planning grant called the Child Adolescent Service System Program Grant. The purpose of the grant was to develop an integrated, cohesive system of care for children with serious emotional disturbance and their families.

BUILDING A SYSTEM OF CARE

In developing a system of care for children with serious emotional disturbances and their families, leaders must provide all stakeholders with a vision and sense of purpose. It is the leader's job to elucidate core values and principles upon which the reform effort is founded, and to engage all those involved in the movement to adopt those principles. Once a leader has engendered broad-based agreement on values, it is then possible for the leader to join key stakeholders in the processes of operationalizing those principles and restructuring the system. Critical steps in this redesign process include conducting and using needs-assessments and developing family- and community-driven infrastructures with extensive interagency collaboration.

System Reform Leaders must be able to gain support for the goals, values, and mission of the new system. As Covey (1992) explains, "principle-centered power elicits a willingness to risk doing the right things, because they are valued, they are modeled by the leader, and they are sanctioned by the vision clarified by the leader." Principle-centered power occurs "when the cause or purpose or goal is believed in as deeply by the followers as by the leaders" (pp. 104-105).

For these and many other reasons, in both my roles as Branch Chief and system leader in Vermont, I was careful to express a clear vision of the method and goals involved in constructing a system of care for children with serious emotional disturbances. That vision was and is centered upon five principles that I believe shape the entire process of reform: (a) family involvement as partners in all aspects of the undertaking; (b) an interagency approach to address the needs of the children; (c) a focus upon strengths rather than pathologies in building individualized service and family centered treatment plans; (d) cultural competence in constructing systems that are responsive to the unique needs of all people in a community; and (e) the central notion of a "home-in-community" underlying system design.

Establishing Infrastructure and Support from Key Stakeholders: Community Involvement and The Vermont System of Care Steering Committee

In an effort to extend my principle-centered vision to all those involved by developing a broad based agreement on values, I first created a steering committee consisting of families, providers, and administrators across the child service systems of juvenile justice, education, mental health, substance abuse, and child welfare. This committee incorporated the state and local legislatures with the inclusion of two House members and two Senate members in the steering committee. Two of the most critical features of this steering committee were the active involvement of family members and the commitment of representatives of every significant child and family-serving agency in Vermont. I used the principles of the Federation of Families for Children's Mental Health to guide my thinking about instituting and operating a truly family-driven system of care. I took heed of Vice President Gore's call for the development and improvement of interagency coordination (Gore, 1993) to reduce inefficiencies, duplication, and overlap of tasks and regulations in shaping my thinking about interagency collaboration.

Schoenberg (1995) explains that once the leader has crystallized and extended his/her vision of core values and principles to the people, s/he must then create a groundswell of support among key stakeholders such as child-serving agencies, schools, families, and community members. From the inception of the steering committee, we realized the importance of including the community in an open forum with committee members to share information and garner their support through involvement in the system design process.

Kouzes (1987) notes that "by consulting with others and getting them to share information, leaders make certain that people feel involved in making decisions that affect them" and that "by seeking diverse inputs, leaders...provide a more open forum for competing viewpoints to be aired...enabl[ing] the leader to incorporate aspects of people's viewpoints into a project and demonstrate to others how their ideas have been heard and included" (p. 161). In an effort to open a public forum of information exchange with the communities, I had the steering committee meet around the state in 12 catchment areas of Vermont, which have essentially become the twelve community systems in Vermont. We would meet every other month as a body of the whole, meeting in the off-month in subcommittees, and thus taking over two years to complete the tour of the state of Vermont. It was necessary that as the leader, I not only have vision but also the foresight and "patience with the process" to "maintain a long-term perspective" (Covey, 1992, p.107) through those first two years.

Schoenberg (1995) suggests having "family members...share their stories" through "parent presentations" and public forums in order to gain community support. The steering committee meetings always began with a public forum so that the families and community representatives could elucidate their needs and comment on the strengths and weaknesses of the community. It also allowed us to convey our intentions and educate communities about the goals of our work. In some cases we also enlisted some community members to become part of the central steering committee. After the public forum, community members could stay and listen throughout the official meetings in which we addressed issues such as arriving at a common definition of "serious emotional disturbance," drafting legislation to institutionalize the reform movement, and creating interagency agreements or blended funding mechanisms.

Families First

From the start, we placed immense importance on involving families and communities in developing policies. Schoenberg (1995) states that "active participation in all aspects of program development, service delivery and evaluation is essential to ensure that services respond to the real needs and concerns of children and families" (p. 1). When I first met with community mental health center children's directors, I expressed the idea of including families as equal players in designing services. The response was less than enthusiastic, as many of them, in their clinical training, had been led to believe that families were the problem for any child who walked into a clinician's door. In order to legitimize the role of families, I began to bring families from other states into meetings with children's directors of mental health, child welfare, district directors, and others. Schoenberg remarks upon the importance of "find[ing] family members who are willing to share their stories. Personalizing the impact that a failed system has on families can help the community better appreciate the need for a new and different system of care" (p. 20). The first families that became members of the steering committee were those I had met in the public forums. They were those who were coming to speak about their children who were in out-of-state placements, were about to be sent out of state, or were thrown out of school, or entering into custody in order to get services. Many of the parents I met in this manner eventually became a core group of family members in the development of the Federation of Families for Children's Mental Health in Vermont. As a leader, I had made it a principle to have families represented at the table regardless of the type of meeting.

Small Incentives Go A Long Way

In his best-selling novel, *All I Really Need to Know I Learned in Kindergarten* (1993), Robert Fulgrum reminds us that the rules of life are at once simple and complex. Acknowledging the contributions of others seems to be a matter of human decency and yet few leaders take the time to do so. Realizing that small incentives can influence loyalty and foster competence and trust, leaders should find creative ways to maximize their resources so that those resources touch every person involved with the system.

For example, in Vermont, the Child Adolescent Service System Program grant made it possible to buy dinner for the steering committee whose members would come to a meeting from all across the state, and to have meetings at bed-and-breakfasts so that the people could enjoy some rest and relaxation while working until late in the evening. Another example was the allocation of resources to the Federation of Families for Children's Mental Health and all its neighborhood based programs. This decision sent a clear message that the services families wanted most would be attended to first and that they would be led by family representatives. The level of commitment and participation was strong throughout the whole effort, as the committee members volunteered their time to work often until midnight or one o'clock, or staying over to go to work early the next day, sometimes a few hours away from their office. Family members rallied and supported one another throughout the state and donated countless hours of their time to ensure the success of the reform movement. People worked tirelessly with little reward because they were invested in a common vision.

Finding and Communicating Common Ground

Schoenberg (1995) refers to the importance of the leader's vision in maintaining a clarity and commitment to the mission of a new system, as well as in "facilitat[ing] the learning of key stakeholders, remov[ing] the barriers to their commitment, and creat[ing] the initiative to get the service underway" (pp.17-18). As leader of this effort, I used this forum for information exchange with the communities to generate local publicity and support for our work, as well as to involve the public in this statewide effort. From my experience as an elected official in Burlington, I knew that the success of an idea within a community depended on that idea being heard, changed, massaged, and ultimately owned by the community itself. Holding the meetings in the 12 local communities rather than in Waterbury, where the state government human services bureaucracy is located, provided an opportunity for the steering committee to listen and hear; to minimize personal nuances and maximize public wants; and to develop their ideas in the real world rather than in their own prejudices and perceptions of how a system should function. One of the most important tasks at hand in the initial stages of system reform is the identification of common ground.

Common Language Leads To Radical Change

Because there were many diverse stakeholders who participated in the system design, there was a need to develop a common language to align the array of issues and parties and to foster a broad-based agreement on values. First we focused on development of a common definition of serious emotional disturbance. The seven or eight definitions of "serious emotional disturbance" extant in Vermont and throughout the United States at the time reflected the absence of a common language, and contributed to an inefficient patchwork of service in which children received service in one system while simultaneously being denied service in another system.

The first step in building a common language was the agreement upon a common definition of "serious emotional disturbance." A subcommittee of the larger steering committee worked for two years to formulate a precise definition across agencies that would be used as an operating standard. The committee parried and conciliated with a host of related considerations and positions challenging their attempt to arrive at a common definition. For instance, federal laws impacting the operation of state departments, as well as the particular definitions of different state departments, hindered any easy resolution. The private and public sectors also had differing definitions. The complicating effect of money, evidenced by the use of broad definitions by well-funded departments and more restrictive definitions used by less-funded departments, further added to the difficulties. Overcoming these challenges, we did arrive at a common definition and proceeded to have each department sign an agreement to use that definition in determining eligibility for service.

There were significant changes in many systems in Vermont as a result of this effort. For example, the Department of Education, which had used the federal definition of serious emotional disturbance in selecting children eligible for services in special education, now implemented our broader definition to expand service to children with emotional disturbances who had previously been denied service. As a result, education, regular education, and special education now began to work together.

Listen to the Community: The Village that Will Raise These Children

When communities heard about a planning grant, they were not enthusiastic about spending money on planning. People seemed more interested in immediate fixes such as an extra therapist or program. Their complaints of lack of service and three month waiting lists that led to out of state placements would not be alleviated by the addition of a few therapists or programs, but could only be effectively addressed by rethinking and restructuring the entire system. As the leader of this effort, I had to gain the trust of the communities in the notion that formulating a plan to change the entire method of supporting children and families in communities would make the greatest difference down the road, more so than merely adding therapists or programs. Kouzes (1987) explains that "leaders who build trusting relationships within their team are willing to consider alternative viewpoints and to make use of other people's expertise and abilities" (p.165). As a leader, I went about building trust by performing a needs-assessment that involved and included families and parents, as well as professionals. I also attempted to gain the people's trust over the long term by providing for some short term needs.

Assessing Community Needs

> The overall purpose of a needs-assessment is to determine the service needs of a target population. This information is then used to decide what services will be put into place in the community. Needs-assessments also bring stakeholders together to create a shared vision...; invest stakeholders in the service system...; define action steps based on identification of community needs...; provide data that can be useful to obtain funding for system and individual program development. (Schoenberg, 1995, p.18)

The needs-assessment conducted early on out of our office proved immensely useful. Schoenberg has noted that there are many kinds of needs-assessments, from determining the shape of a completely new service delivery system (long run) to establishing the rationale for providing a particular service in a community (short run). She also suggests that children and families should be included as experts on the services they need. Our needs-assessment went out to hundreds of professionals from all fields and all agencies across the state, as well as to parents and families throughout the state. We then ranked the needs, and submitted the top one or two needs in a report to the legislature. Our needs-assessment revealed that families' greatest unmet need was respite care. Prior to that needs-assessment, consultation of families for determining needed services had been all but nonexistent. The accepted method had been to consult a professional or clinician working with the family to determine what service was most needed. Based upon the need for respite care expressed by the families themselves, I pursued and obtained a respite care grant at the federal level to give communities a short-term visible product, while at the same time we moved on a five-year planning scheme that would ultimately end in system change. Our ability to provide for some early needs of community mental health centers built trust and hope that change was occurring and enabled the effort to keep moving forward. Thus, in order to engender trust over the long term, we pursued grants to implement some services in the short run.

The needs-assessment also provided an information base that helped direct our efforts over time. Over the long term, the legislature would address the number one need in one year, and move on to the next need the following year. For instance, therapeutic intensive home-based services was the number one need in one year, and when that had been addressed and satisfied, we moved on to the next need which was therapeutic foster care. Schoenberg (1995) has noted the value of phasing in system development and incremental change, given the difficulty of implementing major changes all at once. By prioritizing our change management plan, we never overwhelmed the legislature by submitting dozens of proposals simultaneously.

CORE SERVICES

Ideally, findings from needs-assessments and the good guidance of family-driven interagency teams are used by leaders to set an agenda for the development or enhancement of core services. Katz-Levy, Lourie, Stroul, and Zeigler-Dendy (1992) have enumerated seven core services that provide optimum care for children with serious emotional disturbances: crisis services, home-based services, case management, respite care, therapeutic foster care, transition services, and school-based services.

As noted above, our needs-assessment identified respite care as the most urgent and we therefore made it the identified core service we would pursue first. The grant for respite care, which I mentioned above, was given to the Federation of Families for Children's Mental Health to manage and implement through community mental health centers. The family member heading the grant was Judy Sturtevant, who was responsible for distributing the respite care dollars to community mental health centers across the state. In order to get all the communities involved, the money was sprinkled across every part of the state. Although each community could only serve a few families at a time, this distributional spread of the money enlisted support from families and neighborhoods all around the state.

Another core service was made possible through the acquisition of a suicide prevention grant. Vermont had a very high suicide rate. The suicide prevention grant trained natural supporters for children so they could better identify children who were at risk of suicide. This was a very powerful grant because it helped Vermonters express their feelings with others.

We also discovered a need to develop wraparound care, intensive family-based services, and therapeutic foster care. To test the efficacy of these services I worked with one of the twelve catchment areas to build a model program of core services. We quickly realized that in order to bring up these services properly we would have to simultaneously invest in training and technical assistance that would infuse the kind of cultural change and new thinking required to implement these services in a meaningful way. For example, previously, in community mental health centers, the clinicians did not visit the families' homes, but in intensive family-based services, clinicians would need to go into the homes. This represented a significant practice change for these workers. Therefore, they required substantial retraining and support to take on their new roles. This model program proliferated and the program managers of Intensive Family-based Services became their own support group developing standards for their work, as well as forming a training cadre that developed a curriculum for themselves. This same program of support developed for the providers of therapeutic foster care and respite care. They would hold conferences for their peers in therapeutic foster care or respite care on an ongoing basis, and ultimately they created practice standards that were used across the state.

As a leader, my task was to facilitate the spread of the model program to other communities, which we accomplished through funding the conferences and other technical assistance for the replication of variations of the model program. Thus, as a leader it was necessary for me to find ways to use my limited pool of funds wisely. Investments in activities such as training the trainers or leaders of programs that increased that impact exponentially were viewed in a positive light. In addition, as in the case of the development of the respite program, whenever it seemed sensible, I used the grant funds to pay for staff who pursued other funds to support the services-development activities. Once we opened the doors of the new system, children and families were there and interested in accessing the new services. The role of the leader at that time was to balance the system development responsibilities against the program implementation requirements. Next we will discuss the realities of daily operations of a system of care through the lens of community based leaders.

EFFECTIVE STRATEGIES FOR PROGRAM IMPLEMENTATION

Good leaders are visionaries who can also see the trees and the forest. They are people who either possess the skills or who know how to delegate the responsibility to people who posses the skills required to hit the ground running during the initial phases of program implementation. Program implementation experts are inordinately talented at continuously improving and monitoring the balanced operation of the system. Schoenberg (1995) notes that the following steps of program implementation are essential for insuring financial, administrative, and clinical viability of program services: (a) Selecting a Program Design, (b) Considerations in Budget Development, (c) Implementing Services that are Marketable, (d) Finding and Keeping Staff, and (e) Maintaining Momentum. In moving on to the next stage of state-wide system reform efforts in Vermont, I will briefly discuss a few aspects of program design and focus on momentum issues involving the media and legislation and the role of political will in keeping it together. In Vermont, I spent most of my time on these aspects of implementation and delegated the others to my trusted colleagues and co-workers. The work of these other individuals created a groundswell of leadership-building that I believed would be necessary to maintain momentum for the services-delivery system.

Selecting a Program Design

Earlier we discussed the critical roles of defining, communicating, and inculcating the values and principles that are intended to drive the system reform effort in your community. As a firm believer in principled leadership tactics, I went about the business of building a program design that mirrored the values I wished to impart in Vermont: striving to achieve the existence and continuous improvement of family-driven, community-based, culturally responsive, coordinated and comprehensive care. As I have already noted we went through all the necessary steps of program design: developing a philosophy of care, defining goals and desired outcomes, describing our population and identifying a means of managing the challenges and strengths of the system so that it could maintain its momentum. We also worked with community leaders to establish the logistics of the program structure. The structure included services site locations, hours of operation, hiring and training staff, defining and setting standards for new services, and establishing clinical and case management guidelines for describing pathways for children and families who would flow through the services system. The key to our success was the initiation of local interagency teams that drove the implementation in communities throughout Vermont.

In Vermont Interagency Teams Influenced System-Wide Changes

> In Vermont, interagency collaboration at the state and local levels was codified into law in 1988. Local interagency teams meet regularly and are composed of the directors of the local child-serving agencies [e.g. child welfare, education, community mental health, substance abuse, juvenile justice, and other community providers] and a parent(s) of a child(ren) with an emotional disturbance. Their objectives are to (1) develop coordinated services plans for children whose needs cannot be met by their individual treatment teams, (2) design new services in their region, and (3) bring unresolved problems regarding systems and individual treatment issues to the attention of the state interagency team. The State Interagency Team is composed of similar representatives from the state level offices as well as family members. This team addresses individual problems and suggests solutions. This hands-on case review allows state officials insight into needed reforms in the system. Teams at both levels work together to plan, implement, and more recently, govern new service delivery. (Schoenberg, 1995, p. 22)

As a leader, I used my knowledge of state-of-the-art technologies to develop local interagency teams that worked together to find creative ways to help children and families get the resources they needed. We spent a great deal of time traveling around the state (outside the steering committee capacity) to bring people together. We would, for instance, give $3,000 to a community mental health center to forge their leadership role in the community, to bring people to the table, pay the parents to attend, have coffee and cookies, and enlist community support. These interagency teams worked on individual cases as well as on larger scale system reform and strategic planning. Initially, I requested people to bring a difficult case to the table, in theory, not in practice, that they were unable to resolve, and attempt to try to meet that child's needs as a group. Eventually, they started to bring real cases to the table, and without our prompting, began to try to solve those problems among themselves. It was in this very kind of loose exercise that the local interagency teams were created.

They learned that individuals in different departments were uninformed about each other's limitations imposed by law, and about the resources available to each department. As Heifetz states in a chapter entitled "On a Razor's Edge" (1994), a leader "disorients people so that new role relationships develop; rather than quelling conflict, one generates it...challenging people...and raising conflict about direction" (p.

126). Similarly, I knew that the interagency teams would provide an opportunity for conflict to generate understanding. Typical conflicts included: child welfare workers criticizing mental health workers for not being present to meet children in their crises and merely engaging in an hour of therapy that ends once the child leaves the office; mental health workers attacking child welfare workers for being unwilling to engage a child unless he or she were in their custody; and other departments accusing the education department of restricting their definition of "serious emotional disturbance," in order to deny access to services to youngsters who did not fit the criteria of a child in need of services. However, as the individuals from different departments began to collaborate on cases, they gained a better understanding of the limitations and responsibilities of other departments. For instance, the mental health worker realized that the child welfare worker was prevented by law from interacting and spending money on a child before he or she was in their custody. The child welfare worker also realized that the mental health department, through Medicaid, was able to provide a broader range of services than the child welfare department, but that given the child welfare law, had chosen not to deal with children in custody. The mental health department also had limitations to the community mental health center by the contract they had with the state department of mental health. Over time, a mutual understanding of the responsibilities and limitations of departments produced more collaboration and better coordination of services and benefits on every case, as Kouzes (1987) explains that "leaders must help to break down barriers between people by encouraging interactions across disciplines and between departments" to produce collaboration which will ultimately improve performance" (p. 158).

System reform leaders bear significant responsibility in ensuring the public trust. Those spearheading interagency teams are particularly challenged by a multitude of issues and regulations that drive and govern the day-to-day work of the interagency partners. Generally, interagency work should result in increased access to a broader array of services delivered in a consumer-friendly manner. As a leader, the task of creating interagency teams to institute change required that I define specific goals and construct a path to achieving those goals.

One such goal was to increase access to services through the implementation of interagency teams. In the first year of the grant, the education department had identified some 400 children as having a serious emotional disturbance. After modifying their definition of serious emotional disturbance, by the fourth or fifth year of the grant, the figure increased to between 800-900 children. The education department was willing to make this commitment because they felt that the cost of increasing access to services would be offset by the resources beyond those of the education department that could be provided for children. Another significant effect was the shift in perspective. Children were no longer locked into one department or another; they were no longer seen as mental health children or child welfare children or education children, but as "our" children, allowing the departments to share resources more effectively.

Another goal I had was to ensure privacy and confidentiality while simultaneously continuing information sharing between interagency teams. As a leader, I had to convince major departments to allow us to relinquish information on a particular child and family to other participants in these teams. The departments agreed to this shift in policy provided that the parent would agree, and that the information would be available to only those involved in formulating a treatment plan or some other systematic program for that individual child or family.

The efforts of the state interagency teams resulted in a process of reform at the state level triggered by the needs of individual children at the local level.

Another goal that I defined as leader of this effort was to increase customer satisfaction of the services by integrating and streamlining the system through interagency collaboration. Vice President Al Gore (1993) has called for leaders to "redesign the organizational chart...to melt the rigid boundaries between organizations...[to] organize needs according to customers' needs and not bureaucratic turf" (p. 48). Eighty-seven percent of the children passing through this interagency process had their needs addressed at the local level. The remaining 13 percent did go to the state level for resolution. The problems confronting the state interagency team effort concerned policy glitches, program gaps, and lack of money. For instance, by law, a child in state custody would be assigned to a child-welfare case worker; but if the child's problem was a mental health issue rather than a state custody issue, a mental health case worker would obviously be more effective in addressing the real needs of the child. As a result, an effort was made to reach an interagency agreement at the state level to change policy so that the system could function more effectively in sharing responsibility to satisfy the true needs of the child.

Financial Management

While it is the job of system administrators to create and manage a budget for the services in their purview, it is even more critical that the leaders possess the skills and talents necessary to maximize all resources that could be brought to bear on the successful operation of a seamless system of care. In addition, in this age of managed care and new ways of paying for and delivering services, leaders are faced with choices about setting rates for services that are accompanied by substantial risks. The consequences, pros and cons of choices such as case rates, capitation, and risk sharing solutions must be studied carefully by leaders along with stakeholders to protect the public trust and ensure that appropriate services are available for all children and families in need. Furthermore poor choices in this regard can lead to the devolution of the provider infrastructure and hence the service system itself. In my role as Branch Chief, I have worked hard to ensure that system leaders receive adequate training on these matters so that our systems remain intact and are able to thrive in a managed care environment.

I also believe that true leaders are looking for dollars to sustain their systems the day they start-up, not toward the end of the grant allocation. Creative leaders who operate on system of care principles and who regularly listen to key stakeholders will find that the system will take care of itself by providing stories of unmet need and cost. Clinically effective interventions designed to meet that need will compel legislatures and other funders to support the continuous improvement of the system.

An outgrowth of the interagency method was the collaboration between the three commissioners of education, child welfare, and mental health. The three commissioners as well as the Secretary of Human Services were very faithful in coming to the biannual retreats to discuss the issues of the mental and emotional needs of children. As a result of this sharing of information, the commissioners responded to the need for intensive family-based services, and collaborated to form a legislative budget proposal to fund the service across the state within three years. In the first year, the child welfare department received much of the money, due to the commissioner's relationships with the governor and house and senate members, as well as his articulate and compassionate efforts. Eventually, the mental health department began to receive money due to their use of Medicaid. However, the significance of these events is that rather than competing with each other for funding, the three commissioners were collaborating and uniting on issues, thereby sending a powerful message to the members of the legislature, who were then more willing to commit new resources due to the concurrence of the three commissioners. It really did not matter which department received the services money since all three departments were working so closely together.

We also found that our interagency teams produced case studies that influenced budget allocations across departments. For example, one of these teams presented a case of a twelve-year-old who had been sexually abused in her natural home, then repeatedly abused in a foster care place. This young woman became suicidal while in a residential treatment placement with nine boys, gouging her eyes and cutting her arms. The local level response to her situation was to send her case to the State Interagency Team recommending an out-of-state placement. The state team was unwilling to send her to another facility after she had already been rejected by family and community. The state team approached the Secretary of Human Services with a proposal to develop a treatment plan separate from the nine boys that would stabilize her and then move her into a small intensive therapeutic group home with two or three other children that was unique to her needs. The secretary provided the team with money to give to the local community to develop an intensive, 24-hour treatment plan, seven days a week, which included medications and a very close intensive case manager, a school program, and other components.

We systematically collected and compiled information from cases like these, and the state interagency team would give the results of the cases to the commissioners of child welfare, mental health, education, and the Secretary of Human Services at the biannual meetings. The compiled information would assist the commissioners in developing budgets based on real world experiences, triggering state level reform based upon cases at the local level.

A critical issue in financial management is developing and implementing a plan for sustaining the system. Next we will explore the role of the media and communications in ensuring the fiscal viability of system reform efforts.

The Role of Communications in Maintaining Momentum and Sustaining the System

In system reform, the leader is responsible for engaging the media to inform the public as well as in garnering support and maintaining momentum for the new system. In addition to enlightening the communities about the mental health needs of children, the media also conveyed the inadequacies of the local system to the people. Leaders need to be prepared to manage media inqueries and strategically seek media coverage of milestones in their movements histories.

For example, the public forums I had spoken of earlier were preceded by press releases describing the agenda and inviting the public to attend. Radio stations would often invite us for an interview before the meetings, and other times the stations would come to the public forums and broadcast the meetings on television. Community and regional newspapers were very often also at the meetings.

As a state leader, my job was to convey information from the state and federal level to local communities and vice versa. We would have talk shows, TV, radio and newspapers to circulate information about programs. We had a press conference in the city hall of Burlington when the three commissioners signed an interagency agreement to develop a state interagency team. The media helped legitimize the system reform that was beginning to take place by reporting such events. This extra layer of support provided by the media usually caught the attention of politicians who pay close attention to the newspapers, TV, and radio. As a result, politicians would be well informed when approached with proposals. Press releases were also used to inform administrators and legislators about the results and progress of programs.

Schoenberg (1995) states that is the responsibility of the leader to create incentives for staff to change to the new system by providing recognition and rewards for staff who are able to move beyond their traditional roles in order to facilitate positive outcomes for children and families. Toward this end, we developed a newsletter in Vermont for the professional and parent community to share information about new technologies, as well as to recognize good work. Every issue highlighted an individual who was making a positive contribution in these developing systems of care. This type of public recognition served to validate and motivate team players in the new system of care. It was also an extremely effective vehicle for mentoring and role-modeling clinical leadership skills. The newsletter, which still exists today, is also well known as a forum for debate and discussion of controversial issues.

Finally, in this era of managed care it is essential that families and communities learn to articulate the values, principles and success of the reforms they have crafted so that they are part of the good that will result from local managed care efforts rather than victims of the potential perils. A key to success here is learning to describe your reform movement in a manner that is marketable to multiple stakeholders, especially those in the business community. Communications consultants can be inordinately supportive in helping analyze outcome and cost data and generating reports and print and broadcast media materials to further your cause in this situation. The waves of rapid and unpredictable change that have accompanied the managed care movement in this country are only further evidence of the need to find ways to institutionalize those reforms that have been successful before the right to do so is lost to privatization and individuals who have no sense of this history. Next we will discuss one strategy for institutionalizing a reform: the development of legislation.

Culminating Momentum: Institutionalizing System Reform through Legislation

It is all too common that system reform efforts and movements die shortly after the grant dollars that sparked their inception disappear. It is the responsibility of leaders and communities to ensure that effective system reforms remain viable. One way to accomplish this is to develop support from advocates who through educational efforts may be inspired to create regulatory support for maintaining the new system. Those who receive funds from federal sources are restricted from lobbying legislatures in any way. Leaders of federally supported movements must learn how to enlist the support of advocates who will implement this part of the work if and when they feel the new system is worthy of their efforts. This kind of support is not usually hard to garner if leaders have taken the time to be inclusive of families and community leaders at all phases of the program design, implementation and evaluation. Additionally, leaders may fund conferences and other educational forums to educate stakeholders on system accomplishments as well as advocacy skill building.

In Vermont, the momentum of community desire and information gathered from the state/national level coalesced and culminated in Act 264, which codified the body of system changes. A subcommittee of the advisory board steering committee was created to develop public policy, and they decided to draft legislation to codify much of what we had developed through this grant program such as local and state interagency teams and family involvement. A number of families were on this committee and they added a section discussing the involvement of families in designing and implementing individualized treatment plans. The professionals would not have considered this idea, nor the idea that the plan be developed after the child came in for a screening, had it not been for the involvement of the families.

In contrast to other laws that function as an overlay on a community's inaction, this law emerged and culminated from the momentum of changes and events that were already occurring. Because the reforms were already in progress, that momentum gave legitimacy to the law and kept the state moving forward to approve the law. The legislators who missed many of the steering committee meetings early on were actually very effective in passing the law and overseeing future appropriations. The legislators were able to collaborate and pass the proposed statute with minimal language modifications. Another factor facilitating passage was the absence of entitlements in the legislation, except for the entitlement to an individualized treatment plan. It was determined that the cost of entitling services to all children in Vermont with serious emotional disturbances would have been too much for any state legislature to deem acceptable. We believed we could progress year to year with the mechanisms we already had in place, thereby instituting a "de facto" entitlement, rather than a "de jure" entitlement.

Keeping It Together: Maintaining Political Will

In contrast to the nature of momentum which provides support for leadership and impetus for change, conflict and controversy may undermine reform efforts unless they are judiciously handled by the leader. It is important for a leader to endure and persevere through conflict that will inevitably arise with change. If a leader cannot withstand the challenging, questioning, and attacking by his or her opponents, the leader will not succeed in bringing his or her idea to fruition. I have seen ideas foreign to politicians in one year being espoused by the very opponents of that idea the next year. People require time to allow the idea to sift through their minds before they begin to understand and appreciate it. In his article "On a Razor's Edge," Heifetz (1994) refers to this type of phenomenon as a "ripening" in which conflict and confrontation are necessary for the development of an idea. System change is founded upon confrontation and the ability to handle confrontation. Confrontation clarifies the vision. Unless a leader confronts and challenges the status quo, change is impossible.

As Heifetz (1994) has stated, "exercising leadership from a position of authority in adaptive situations means going against the grain." He explains that "leadership is a razor's edge because one has to oversee a sustained period of social disequilibrium during which people confront the contradictions in their...communities." The leader must "raise conflict about direction" (pp. 126-127). Along a similar vein, my job was to act as a lightning rod, to speak to the direction Vermont was heading at the state and local levels. At times when I would speak to the issues, direction, and mission, confrontations would emerge around individuals who were unwilling to change along with the reform. In one such situation, a community mental health center encouraged the individual to retire and in another situation reorganized itself and placed the individual in a position that was less directly involved in the collaborative work. In many cases of hiring or promotion, we would pass over someone who, by experience, would appear to be the logical person to hire, and select an individual whose philosophical leanings were congruent with the collaborative system. As a leader, I feel that we must not avoid confrontation (as many systems are apt to do, thereby becoming stagnant without momentum or leadership) but must follow through with actions that may be perceived as painful or hurtful, ultimately with the best interests of the community in mind.

STAFF DEVELOPMENT

Considerations in Hiring

As the momentum behind the interagency system developed, many staff members were unwilling to collaborate in the new culture. These individuals would either reform or leave, and in most cases, staff members would leave. The new breed of person was one who saw their mission linked to the missions of individuals in other systems, an individual who viewed families as part of the solution and not part of the problem, one who perceived his or her role as a clinician being involved beyond the office, in the school, home, and community. The work environment was no longer limited to the office, but included the entire community itself.

Leading a system reform often requires a changing of the guard. It is critical for leaders to possess the ability to assess the strengths and potential of old staff, the fortitude to release those who need to move on, and the foresight to recognize and hire the right mix of new and successful team players. Because we redefined roles and goals of the system, we sought out staff with a skill and mind set different from those who worked in the old system. We would define the role, create standards for it, hire new people, and meet with them monthly. One example of nurturing service reform was when we created new positions called therapeutic case managers. We hired a child psychiatrist to be their clinical supervisor. The therapeutic case manager would be dealing with children who had in the past been sent out of state, and now were in their community. To work with these children, the therapeutic case managers needed the clinical knowledge and support, as well as a proper understanding of their new roles, to effectively care for the therapeutic needs of these children. Providing the monthly forums for open discussion between and among the therapeutic case managers was critical to the ultimate success of this new clinical service.

The Provision of Training and Technical Assistance

As noted earlier, it is the responsibility of a leader to facilitate the spread of the model program among local staff and other communities. In Vermont we accomplished this by funding conferences and other forms of technical assistance. An example of individualized technical assistance in Vermont was peer to peer matching. This allowed us to take what had been learned in a particular geographic region by a professional, parent, program, or team and bring that learning to another geographic region that could benefit from that particular piece of knowledge. Investments in activities like train the trainers or leaders programs increased the likelihood of reaching a maximum number of people throughout the area. I also am a firm believer in finding ways to influence and foster creative thinking. Therefore I believe it is critical to give people a chance to leave their communities and attend national or regional meetings where they learn about new ideas that have been generated in other places as well as nationally accepted standards of practices. I have also found that bringing in national and regional experts to consult with sites not only provides needed guidance but creates incentive for local stakeholders because they tend to view this consultation as a gift. Training and technical assistance only works if it occurs on a regular basis, is reinforced through supervision and strong leadership and if it is informed by hard evidence of techniques that work. Next we will explore the crucial role of managing, teaching and leading with good data.

MAKING EVALUATION HAPPEN

Performance based contracting and report cards for service delivery performance have become mandates of federal, state and local government entities throughout this country. Thanks to technological advances, businesses thrive on information such as productivity reports they receive on a daily and hourly basis. Responsible leaders in this day and age must carefully select the methods by which they will measure the effectiveness of their efforts at both the management level and the clinical level. It is equally important to know whether or not the reform movement made the community stronger and whether or not it influenced services providers to deliver services that actually helped children and families find ways to function more productively and in a developmentally appropriate manner.

Leaders now know that their constituents will demand that they cycle back information and data about system performance to the community and that this is a critical aspect of maintaining support and enthusiasm for their efforts. Data also serves to assist program officials in deciding upon the future path and next steps of the system.

In Vermont, we established a relationship with the local university to work collaboratively on studies they already had underway as well as to commission outcome studies we would require in order to provide the community with the feedback it anticipated receiving. From the onset, we expressed a value for evaluation by conducting extensive needs-assessments and validated those assessments by funding new services in the order of the community demands we discovered thorough the process.

Later when we acquired a Robert Woods Johnson Foundation grant, which was a systems of care service implementation initiative, we performed studies on the cost of implementing an individualized treatment plan for children which was a part of the therapeutic case management wraparound system. Many services that were called for in the plan were, in the end, not needed, and after three months actual costs began to go down as the children improved. We also performed studies analyzing the cost of sending a child to an out-of-state placement, which was shown to be more expensive than the cost of wraparound programs. Thus, these cost studies demonstrated that in wrapping services around a child in their home community, we could get good results for less cost.

Our data analyses also showed that our individualized care system, if offered to all children who needed that level of support, would require substantial up-front investments, but that the ultimate cost per child would be lower. For instance, a child in foster care with unaddressed mental health needs would require more money to address those needs. At the same time, money would be saved in the out-of-state placement, as these children who were being over-served or served in inappropriate, high-end, expensive, out-of-state placements would be incorporated into the wraparound system within their own communities. In addition, our data showed that the outcomes for these children being served in their communities were much better than if they were being served in a distant out-of-state placement where the clinical gains could not be transferred to the home and family.

As I mentioned earlier, we also had a close relationship with Dr. John Burchard at the University of Vermont. Burchard was performing studies of children in residential treatment and children in community, analyzing success indicators for children such as school attendance, grades, crime rates, and other such factors that would increase for children in communities when they returned from residential treatment, but would then taper down. We studied the contrast between children who returned from the isolated residential treatment to the open community, and children who had treatment services wrapped around them in their communities. The differences between the two were significant.

As the Branch Chief and person responsible for overseeing the Community Mental Health Services for Children and Their Families Program, I have worked closely with evaluators who have orchestrated that largest comparative outcome study in the history of child mental health service delivery. There have been many lessons learned from this effort and many incredible success stories. Among the most critical lessons for me as a leader has been how important it is to build relationships with both researchers and communications experts who can help you share stories about the data in ways that are palatable, powerful and honest for your diverse constituencies. Equally important has been the involvement of multiple evaluators and stakeholders in the evaluation design, implementation, and evaluation of the findings and the process of evaluation itself. Multiple perspectives have enriched the evaluation and shed new light on the findings. Allowing time for this level of inclusion is not always easy but it pays back in dividends when all parties have confidence that the data are truly representative of the outcomes and useful for informing the next phase of developing your system.

CONCLUSION: RETROSPECTIVE VIEW OF SYSTEM REFORM AND IMPLEMENTATION

My discussion has progressed through the stages of system development as delineated by Schoenberg (1995). The first step in starting system reform requires that the leader elucidate the core principles of the reform effort. The leader must then garner support from key stakeholders, perform needs-assessments, and perhaps most importantly, provide the infrastructure for interagency collaboration. Next was to discuss a few of the core services we provided in Vermont including respite care, therapeutic foster care, intensive family-based services, therapeutic case management, and wraparound care. The third stage involved strategies for program operations such as selecting program design, considerations in budget development, implementing marketable services, finding and keeping staff, maintaining momentum, and hints for keeping it together. I focused upon the role of the media in maintaining momentum by providing public support and information dissemination, as well as upon the political will of the leader that is necessary for keeping the reform effort together. The next stage involved considerations in training and technical assistance, in which the new breed of person viewed his or her mission linked to that of other individuals in other systems and considered families as part of the solution and not part of the problem. Among the many issues involved in the final stage of system evaluation, I chose to focus upon the role of data analyses and management in cycling back information to the officials and the community, thereby maintaining public support and providing new directions for the future.

Ultimately, the responsibility of the state and leader is to support communities in building a system of care for children with disabilities and their families. One hundred years ago, the state's solution for people with special needs was to create a community outside natural communities. In the end, they found that they were unable to create community outside community; they found that what people truly need is the neighbor, the sense of belonging to a community, the sense that they can contribute to a child regardless of the extent of his/her disability. That fabric of community is very powerful, and costs not a penny, while also being priceless in its relationship to children with special needs. The responsibility lies not only with the community, which is a subdivision of the state, but also with the state. The state must give communities the policies, services, and supports necessary to provide an effective system of care. This is the beginning and the end of the state's responsibility to the community. States err when they, for political reasons, refuse to support innovative ideas at the policy level that communities have formulated themselves. A state's refusal to consider ideas formulated by communities prevents the communities from flourishing. The ideal situation is when the community enlightens the state while the state ensures support for ideas and systems most helpful to the people. It is important for the state to realize that the solutions to many problems are actually present and embedded within the communities themselves. If the state's officials go beyond their offices into the communities, they will find the answer to almost every problem.

If one looks at America today, one will see isolated community pockets of excellent public policy, services, and support to children with disabilities and their families. The challenge as we move into the 21st century is how to knit these pockets together, strongly and deeply enough so that all of America's children with special needs and their families can grow and flourish.

REFERENCES

Covey, S. (1992). *Principle-centered leadership.* New York: Simon & Schuster.

Clinton, H. R. (1996). *It takes a village and other lessons children teach us.* New York: Simon & Schuster.

Fulgrum, R. (1993). *All I Really Need to Know I Learned in Kindergarten.* New York: Ivy Books.

Gore, A. (1993). *The Gore report on reinventing government*. Washington, DC: National Performance Review.

Heifetz, R. A. (1994). *Leadership without easy answers.* Cambridge, MA: Harvard University Press.

Katz-Levy, J. W., Lourie, I. S., Stroul, B. A., & Zeigler-Dendy, C. (1992). *Individualized services in a system of care* (monograph). Washington, DC: CASSP Technical Assistance Center, Georgetown University.

Kouzes, J. M. (1987). *The leadership challenge: How to get extraordinary things done in organizations.* San Francisco: Jossey-Bass.

Schoenberg, S. (1995). *Making it happen: A guide to program development for services for children and adolescents who are experiencing a severe emotional disturbance and their families*. Child, Adolescent, and Family Branch of the Center for Mental Health Services, Substance Abuse and Mental Health Services Administration.

section IV

Examples of Community Support in Action

The five exemplary chapters in this section begin with a parent's perspective of how services and supports should be organized in a way that family well-being is enhanced, without adding more undue stress caused by the system of care. Speaking as the director of a national family and parent support and advocacy group, Family Voices, Polly Arango, in Chapter 8, articulates both the needs of families and the necessity for family involvement at each level in the system in order for programs to be effective. Each of the chapters that follow provide unique perspectives on this theme. In Chapter 9, Peter Evans describes projects in international settings and suggests that there are many lessons to be learned from the international arena. From the perspective of Part C Early Intervention Programs, Adrienne Akers and Diane Behl, in Chapter 10, tackle the uneven distribution of services within community settings and the need to coordinate and integrate existing efforts so that they make sense to families who use them. Similar themes are found in the last two chapters—Chapter 11, by Glenna Boyce, Diane Behl, and Therese Johnson, and Chapter 12, by Sharon Carnahan, Carnot Nelson, and Thomas Gordon—which use examples of environmental risk and child abuse and neglect programs.

chapter 8

Supporting Families with Young Children in the Community: A Parent's Perspective

Polly Arango
Family Voices

Each person is born into a family and, throughout life, continues to be connected in some way to a family. This history and experience as a son, daughter, aunt, uncle, mother, father, brother, sister, grandparent plays a significant role in how that individual understands the word *family*. No matter the years of course work and professional experiences, every person who touches a child and a family brings to that relationship perspectives and biases that reach way back into their own childhood in a family, and their later pursuit of family as an adult.

In this chapter, I will first describe what I learned about the complex nature of family through a series of shared conversations with child and family advocates living in New Mexico. These conversations followed a mandate from the New Mexico State Legislature to analyze the status of the state's children, and to make legislative and policy recommendations for improvements. This group, appointed by the governor and the legislature, represented the ethnic and cultural diversity of the state, bringing a broad range of life experiences and ideas about family to their deliberations. As a consequence, the group's collective ideas about what it means to be a child, parent or a family sometimes hindered or even halted consensus-building. Several advocates from different backgrounds and perspectives decided to look for an acceptable definition of family. Finding no acceptable definition that encompassed the views of the group, this smaller group wrote, critiqued, brought their ideas back to the larger group, and decided that a *broad description*, rather than a *strict definition* of family would be more helpful and was achievable.

The following description captured, to the satisfaction of the advocates, what *family in New Mexico* means. Several years of policy recommendations, legislative triumphs, and progress for children and families in New Mexico have flowed from the description below. Take a moment to read the description, and then reflect upon the diversity and strength within every family, including your own.

A DESCRIPTION OF FAMILY

We all come from families. Families are big, small, extended, nuclear, and multigenerational, with one parent, two parents, and grandparents. We live under one roof or many. A family can be as temporary as a few weeks, as permanent as forever. We become part of a family by birth, adoption, marriage, or from a desire for mutual support. As family members, we nurture, protect, and influence one another. Families are dynamic and are cultures unto themselves, with different values and unique ways of realizing dreams. Together, our families become the source of our rich cultural heritage and spiritual diversity. Each family has strengths and qualities that flow from individual members and from the family as a unit. Our families create neighborhoods, communities, states, and nations (developed and adopted by New Mexico's Children's Continuum/House Memorial 5 and New Mexico Advocates for Children and Families, 1990).

Some Families

The following stories of nine families represent a composite of many families I have met and talked with over the years. With their own unique compositions, geographic locations, economic and social situations, and racial and ethnic backgrounds, each family's story illustrates what families expect and need from, and contribute, to their communities.

The Curtis family of Texas

I have three children, with the oldest now almost ready for college. I have been divorced from my husband, a military officer, for several years. During our marriage, we lived all over the country, and sometimes it was hard making friends, changing schools, finding good housing, and working with the military's health system, especially for our oldest daughter who has diabetes. My ex-husband and I both now live near Houston where we both claim family roots that go back many years in the African-American community. I work at our state health department where I assist families when they come into health clinics. My children live with me in a suburb of Houston, but we all commute into the city so that they can attend Catholic schools there; my youngest daughter is in kindergarten, my son is in fifth grade, and my oldest daughter is now a senior in high school. The kids see their dad fairly often (Diana Curtis).

The Hayden family of Wisconsin

My family and I live on a dairy farm that has been in my family for four generations. I farm and also drive a school bus during the year, and my wife works as a cook at school. This way we have good health insurance and a steady income, no matter what might happen to milk prices. Our three children are now in high school, middle school, and preschool. We like living on the farm, even though it is seven miles from town. Most of our social life revolves around our church and 4-H. I hope one of our children will choose to farm like I did. I like being my own boss, working hard, and looking up at the stars at night (Mike Hayden).

The Sturgis family of Iowa

Believe it or not, Janet and I have five kids! Both of us are registered nurses. I work in an emergency room, while Janet takes care of the kids. She's home-schooling two of them right now while she stays home with the baby. We grew up in a big city, but decided after college to raise our children in a smaller community. We like living in our town because of the organized sports for the kids, a university for all of us when we are ready, and special services for our oldest daughter who has cerebral palsy. I coach Little League, take our daughter to therapy and Special Olympics, and like being around my kids (David Sturgis).

The Martinez family of Arizona

I am a single mother with four children. My youngest is two, and the oldest is eight. My first husband and I divorced, and my second husband died. I knew I couldn't do it alone, so after his death, I moved back to Arizona from California to be near my family. The five of us live in a mobile home community where my mom and dad also live. But I hope to own a real home in a nicer part of town some day. I was on welfare for a while, since my ex-husband never paid child support for the two oldest kids. Now I am working, taking care of an older gentleman who needs help with everything; a friend next door takes care of my little one while I work. My three older children go to an after school program which helps a lot. I worry about them getting into the wrong crowd. Even though I was able to get off welfare, Medicaid still covers my kids' health insurance. Things are beginning to look up (Trish Martinez).

The Alonso family of New York

My husband, son, and I live in Brooklyn. Bob is a musician and I manage a restaurant. Max is four and has autism. This is a good place for us to live, because New York has many programs and experts for Max. He goes to a special preschool that also provides child care for him if my husband can't take care of him while I am at work. We take turns taking Max to specialized speech therapy sessions across town. We want him to go to public school, but we worry about whether the school in our neighborhood will accept Max. We're checking into it now with neighbors in our building who have a child with cerebral palsy. They say it can be done, but you have to be persistent (Cheri Alonso)!

The Williams family of California

Here in Los Angeles, it's hard to raise your kids right. My ex-wife and I try to do a good job with our two boys, and both of us are there for them. Both of us live in the same neighborhood we lived in before the divorce. This means our kids can go to the same school and keep their friends. I work two jobs, but I'm off weekends so that's when I have the kids. My ex-wife has more flexible hours and takes our oldest to gymnastics and our youngest to a reading program at the library. Still, it's a constant juggle with phone calls, keys, and lost clothes. At least we don't have to travel across town to stay connected (Sid Williams).

The Woodward family of Michigan

I live in a medium-sized city with my son who is five. My ex-husband lives nearby. We were married for almost 10 years when he left. My son has many health problems related to a serious illness he had shortly after birth, so he continues to need in-home nursing care. It's nice that his dad still lives close by. Although I travel in my job, the nurses help take care of my son when I am gone. But, I still need to ask my ex-husband or my parents who also live nearby to help out when I will be out of town. The hardest thing for me and for my son has been to try to have a normal life when we also have medicines, doctor appointments, emergency room visits, and medical equipment taking up so much of our lives—and our space. David doesn't participate in sports, but he is learning to play the piano. He is taking free lessons from a friend and he loves it (Marianne Woodward)!

The Johnson family of South Dakota

I am a single mother and live on an Indian reservation where I grew up. I drive to work in town and I'm trying to raise my two kids by myself. If I did not have such a huge and wonderful family, I doubt I could manage alone. My sisters and brothers all live nearby, and we have raised our kids together. In our culture, cousins are more like siblings than cousins! And I am more like a mom to my nieces and nephews than their aunt. Because we live on the reservation, we expect that federal Indian programs will keep their promises to us and provide us with good education and health services. But that is not always the case. Because the BIA schools didn't have some special services that my kids needed, I brought them with me to school in town most of the time. We patch together our health care, using my health insurance at work and Indian Health Service (Naomi Johnson).

The DesJardin family of Colorado

My husband, three children, and I live in Denver where we just bought a house last year, a fixer-upper, mainly because of the safe neighborhood and a bus-route around the corner. We spend every spare moment working on our house, it seems. Because my husband is a freelance computer expert who mostly works at home, I work in downtown Denver at a bank so that we can get health insurance. My husband does a lot of our childcare since his work is either at home or at night. When neither of us can be at home, the children go next door where my neighbor provides licensed, in-home childcare (Nancy DesJardin).

COMMUNITIES

Families look to their communities for formal and informal assistance as they raise their children. But is there a way to think about and organize these supports? Having developed a description of *family*, the same group of New Mexico child advocates tackled *community* a few years later. They did so because they concluded that their efforts on behalf of children and families would be more effective if placed in a familiar context—the community. The New Mexico advocates realized that everyone, even state legislators, agency directors, and corporate CEOs, belongs to a family and a community—a suburban neighborhood, a collection of city blocks, a small town or village, an Indian reservation, or an isolated farm or ranch. Therefore, they reasoned, if public and private policymakers could gain a better understanding of the basic needs of families, then perhaps state and local budgets, corporate policies, even school hours and recreation opportunities, would engender community supports to better match family realities and requirements.

What Young Families Need From Their Communities

The ideas generated by the New Mexico advocates resonated with the state legislature, were incorporated by the governor into his new Department of Children, Youth, and Families, and over the years have seeped into discussions and agreements between advocates, policymakers, and the business community. Six domains were identified as necessary connections between families and communities:

1. food;
2. shelter;
3. employment, economic security, and *childcare* (*added by the author*);
4. *lifetime* education for children and adults (*author's change*);
5. health services for all family members; and
6. social supports and recreation.

Food

Given the pace of family life, the dietary requirements of some children, and the sometimes long distances to grocery stores, making or finding affordable and nourishing meals can be a challenge. The Alonso family takes a subway and buses to a grocery store to find the selection of foods they and their son with food allergies can afford. Living on the reservation means Naomi Johnson must shop in town and not forget necessities, "because the trading post in our village is very expensive." For most families, nearby supermarkets make grocery shopping easier, but "finding fresh vegetables and fruits that we can afford makes grocery shopping a chore," notes David Sturgis. Some parents, like Trish Martinez and Nancy DesJardin, devote hours to scanning grocery ads, clipping coupons, and shopping for food sales. They also make sure their children are enrolled in summer and school lunch programs.

When a child has special health needs, nutrition and meal planning become more critical. Fortunately, Diana Curtis has been able to get help in most of the communities where she has lived. She and her daughter currently participate in a diabetes support group that includes field trips to restaurants and grocery shopping. Janet Sturgis learned how to make the right kinds of meals and snacks for her daughter by using her professional connections with a registered dietician. On the other hand, Marianne Woodward admits that she has been frustrated about her son's diet, despite inquiries to his therapists and pediatrician. Families whose children have special dietary needs often find help by talking with other parents, who always seem to have creative ideas and practical solutions.

Almost every family concludes that finding the time in busy schedules to make mealtime pleasant is the biggest challenge of all. For the Hardens, breakfast begins at 6:00 a.m., with everyone at the table, "because this is the only meal when we're all here." For other families, meals are eaten on the run during the week, especially in homes with teenagers like the Curtis' family. But on Sunday nights, everyone pitches in for a family supper filled with conversation and laughter.

Shelter

All families want a place they call home. However, finding affordable housing is a challenge for many families. Although Trish Martinez and her four children live in a small three bedroom mobile home, she dreams of having a "real home someday," perhaps through a low-cost housing program. Meanwhile, Trish often shares her modest trailer with a niece and sometimes with other single parents with no place to go. Families in New York City, like the Alonsos, consider themselves lucky to be in rent-controlled apartments. However, they worry about their neighbors in a third floor flat with no elevator: "I don't know how that mother can carry her daughter with CP up three flights of stairs at least once a day," notes Cheri. The Hardens live in a house on the family farm where three generations have raised their children, while the Johnsons recently moved from cramped quarters into a new home built by their tribe. After Marianne Woodward's divorce, she and her son gave up their dream home and moved into a condominium where she set up an office in a spare bedroom. The Hayden, DesJardin, and Sturgis families have achieved the American dream in different ways: inheriting a family farm; or buying and renovating an old house.

Employment, economic security, and childcare

Parents need jobs in their community that pay enough to support a family. It is also important that workplaces acknowledge family obligations, including time for school and doctor appointments, flexible work hours that acknowledge family schedules, and family-friendly benefits, such as health insurance, disability, and retirement plans. A community's informal and formal supports for families are illustrated daily throughout the country as millions of young families struggle to find childcare that is loving, safe, and with an appropriate developmental environment. Some families find it most comfortable and cost-effective to rely on neighbors, family, and exchanges among other parents for childcare. Only a few families can afford live-in nannies or caregivers.

Fitting together a job and childcare is a constant challenge, whether families have one or two parents, draw down professional salaries, or work for minimum-wage. All families have the potential to become adept at juggling jobs, nurturing and enjoying their children, keeping the house clean, and trying to spend some time together with spouses and other adults. Today, many two-parent families find that both mothers and fathers must find employment in order to pay expenses generated by their households. Other families, like the Sturgis', have made a conscious decision for one parent to stay home to care for the children and to try to live on one salary. When possible, families like the Williams' work flexible hours around family schedules.

For single-parent families, it is often a struggle to arrange child care while the parent works. On the days her ex-husband takes care of the children, Diana Curtis works late in exchange for being able to leave work early when she must pick up her children at school and take them to sports and other activities. Trish Martinez recently moved off welfare into paid employment. She not only takes care of her elderly client during the day, but also baby-sits a niece overnight, cleans several houses, and bartends most weekends. Because Marianne Woodward must travel in her job, she moved to be near her own family so she could be sure to have dependable childcare.

With increasing numbers of single-parents and dual-wage couples, more communities now offer a variety of safe and affordable licensed childcare: a nonprofit community-run facility, childcare at a job site, a family daycare home, or a private childcare facility. Before a mother goes back to work after maternity leave, as Nancy DesJardin recently did, she will typically expend hours of anxious telephone calls and interviews exploring the availability of a secure and loving place for her baby. Families with the most persistent childcare problems are those who, like Cheri Alonso, have a youngster with special needs. Childcare providers with the skills for working with children with special needs are frequently more expensive and harder to find than typical providers.

Two other issues, transportation and summertime/holidays, add to the complexities of employment and parenting. Transportation to work can be complicated: an aging minivan that refuses one morning to make the trip across town to a job; keeping two cars running to get to two places of employment; a lack of emergency or daily transportation in most rural and suburban areas; skimpy bus schedules, even in large urban areas. Summer and school holidays always present challenges to employed parents, because few communities offer adequate and affordable summer recreation and childcare programs that address the developmental, social, and physical aspects of youngsters of all ages. Fortunately, community-supported programs, such as Boys and Girls Clubs, continue to expand their year-round programs and activities to meet the needs of children and families in communities.

Education for their children and themselves

From preschools through the public education system and on to technical schools and college, community members have a right to expect lifelong learning opportunities that are accessible and affordable. Nancy DesJardin and Diana Curtis remember their early parenting classes, often linked to childbirth or home visiting programs, as the place where they found answers to their unspoken questions, friendships with other young families, and validation of their own expectations and ideas about child rearing. Sid Williams and Cheri Alonso had positive experiences with preschools and childcare centers for similar reasons. In families where a child with a special need arrives, early intervention programs, whether home- or center-based, are critical. David Sturgis praises the therapeutic preschool where his daughter with cerebral palsy started classes and therapies within months of her diagnosis. "That set us on a path for her development and for us with friendships, peer support and links to other resources that we never would have found for ourselves," he says.

As children enter kindergarten, the traditional educational process begins. All families expect their neighborhood schools to provide an education that prepares their youngsters for a happy and productive adulthood. When families have children with special needs, things can sometimes get complicated. One of the Williams children has an exceptionally high IQ; Mike Hayden's son has attention deficit/hyperactivity disorder; the Sturgis's daughter has cerebral palsy with speech and mobility complications. But these families indicate that, armed with good information and persistence, they have been able to keep their youngsters in their neighborhood schools where they learn alongside their peers.

Some parents, like Sid Williams, seek higher education for themselves. "My night classes at the community college took me off my sales route and gave me a job with higher pay and more flexible hours," he notes. Nancy and Steve DesJardin take turns attending classes on parenting and home renovation. Trish Martinez obtained a GED in a class held in a neighborhood school before she ventured into the job market. Janet Sturgis updates her nursing certification by attending conferences and short courses. "This brings me into contact with other adults–and helps me maintain my mental health!", observes Janet.

Health services for their children and parents

Access to adequate health care for children has begun to receive the policy and media attention it deserves. The rapid growth and development that occur during childhood and adolescence require different health services and coverage than those designed for adults. Infants and children should visit their health providers for well child checkups more frequently than adults. Families can follow health guidelines from the American Academy of Pediatrics and a document called Bright Futures (now available in a version for families through the federal Maternal and Child Health Bureau). Unlike adults, children depend on someone else, usually a parent, to oversee and guide their health care, so a third person enters the discussion between patient and provider.

Swift and complex changes in health care systems in the United States have thrown families, employers, and health providers alike into a sea of unknown and untested configurations. In fact, finding affordable health care today is now more challenging than ever. Some families, like the Hardens, DesJardins, and Woodwards, have had to keep jobs they might have otherwise left, solely because of the employee health benefits offered. When Trish Martinez went off welfare and began to work, the state continued her children's health coverage, but she lost hers, so she hopes and prays she doesn't get sick or injured. Sid Williams and his ex-wife, like the Curtis' family, have patched together their health coverage. Sid admits, "It's a pretty bare-bones plan."

In families where there is a child with special health care needs, access to affordable health insurance and broad benefits coverage takes on heightened urgency. As a nurse in a large hospital, David Sturgis has good health benefits for his family, which is especially important for his daughter with cerebral palsy, who needs specialized equipment, therapies, and medicines. On the other hand, the Alonsos have not been able to convince their insurance carrier that their son's autism requires access to specialists. Finding consistent pediatric care, now referred to as a *medical home* by the American Academy of Pediatrics, has been a challenge for Mike Hayden and his family, "The school district's health plan keeps changing, so we are always getting different doctors who never get to know my kids or me." Naomi Johnson has a similar complaint. Although Indian Health Services has a clinic on the reservation, "The doctors come and go, and we're constantly having to tell our stories to the new ones. It's also difficult to get a referral for a specialist because of funding problems."

If a family seeks health services beyond visits to a family practitioner or pediatrician, they must understand the coverage available in their benefits' package. For example, many plans do not cover dental or mental health services. Diana Curtis and her family have sought counseling, especially during the divorce and again as her daughter was a teenager learning to deal with diabetes. But even under the military's plan, "We had to fight hard and almost make things sound worse than they were in order to get a few sessions with a psychologist." Dental care is an even greater problem. Many insurance plans do not cover dental care, or in the case of Medicaid, many dentists do not accept patients who are on Medicaid.

Communities can assess how healthy they are by acknowledging that health extends beyond hospitals and doctors' offices, and includes services such as counseling centers; immunization and anti-tobacco campaigns; the inclusion of parenting, sex education, and drug information classes in school curricula; and citizen involvement in health policymaking boards. The need for clean water and a safe place to dispose of household garbage is another community health issue that is sometimes ignored. "One reason we moved to our town is that I knew it was clean. Our state and community have made healthy water and a healthy environment a priority," says David Sturgis.

Social supports and recreation

As parents enter the world of raising children, they begin to look to members of their community for guidance, friendships and validation. They wonder if what they are doing is right for their babies—who soon will be preschoolers, kindergartners, and adolescents. An unspoken bond seems to exist between pregnant women as they catch each other's eye in a crowd, among young parents as they walk their babies in strollers, or as they watch toddlers at play in a park. Not only do young families seek out one another, but they also find that talking with other parents, joining playgroups, and spending time with their relatives eases the challenges of parenthood.

"As a single mother, I couldn't live in a place where I didn't have my family to lean on and the after-school and summer recreation programs for my kids," declares Trish Martinez. Sid Williams frequents the local community center on the grounds of the elementary school, where after-school programs, sports activities, dances for teens, and parenting classes take place.

The military often provides opportunities for personnel to socialize and offers activities for children and families, but Diana has had to hunt for similar supports in her suburb and in Houston itself. "Actually, the Catholic school seems to understand that families need extra help these days. They have weekend and evening programs for single parents, for younger children, and especially for teenagers. We have to pay for them, but it's worth it." The DesJardins would like to have a community center in their town. "Why can't our schools be used for this? They're empty at night, on weekends, and in the summer, and they are so close to where we live" says Nancy. Naomi Johnson describes a range of activities on her reservation, from parenting programs and Head Start, sports for boys and girls, and an exercise class she attends two nights a week.

David and Janet Sturgis helped to start a swimming program for youngsters with cerebral palsy. This turned into a summer camping program which later linked their daughter with a local Girl Scout troop. When Marianne Woodward noticed that her son loved music, she joined a program at the local library that introduces youngsters to music through a visiting musician program and trips to free performances. Cheri Alonso found a community respite program that gives her and her husband a night off every month while a trained special provider cares for their son.

Families as partners in planning and implementing community services

As community citizens, families have responsibilities to participate in planning public and private services that effect families. In the workplace and as members of civic and education organizations, families can provide their insights, perspectives, and expectations. However, public and private institutions that seek input from families must also make allowances for childcare, work schedules, and cultural diversity. The participation of energetic, realistic, and committed families will assure the development of healthier communities.

For example, Mike Hayden spends at least one night per month as a member of his county zoning commission where his priorities are the protection of agricultural land, controlled development, and a healthy environment—legacies for his children and grandchildren. Trish Martinez joined a fraternal lodge that offers recreation for her children, with an opportunity to chair the committee that brings other single parents together. Naomi Johnson dreams of serving on her Tribal Council, but until then, she coaches a soccer team and volunteers at the reservation library. Marianne Woodward says that, "I complained so much about the children's hospital visiting hours and clinic practices that they put me on the hospital board!" Sid Williams volunteers as the representative from his apartment complex on his town's youth commission: "Not that I know much about how government works, but I do know what kids need." Although Cheri Alonso's husband has little time to spare, he serves on his neighborhood library's advisory board, with a dual focus of developing a tape and CD lending program and on including more youngsters with special needs in the library's programs. Mike and Janet Sturgis share a position on the United Way board because, "We think this is a place that has the resources to make things happen for a lot of families."

Every community has its unique and endearing characteristics. Families who know their community cares about them will be more likely to contribute to their neighborhoods. If a community's message and actions acknowledge the importance of families and provide them with the supports to they need to raise their children, families will thrive. Every family, no matter what their configuration and economic circumstances, can benefit from support as they struggle to deal with the realities of parenthood—a cranky infant, a sudden job transfer, home repairs, access to child care, or adequate transportation. A healthy community is a place where families live in safety and security, where they contribute to their neighborhoods, where their children are loved, and where the future for everyone holds promise.

chapter 9

International Perspectives in Community-based Services

Peter Evans
Organization for Economic Cooperation and Development Centre for Educational Research and Innovation (OECD/CERI)

BACKGROUND

While predicting the future remains a hazardous occupation, there is, nevertheless, one issue that remains a key concern for all countries and which has implications for the successful education and early experiences of young children. The world's globalized economy demands its citizens become better educated if they wish to participate in the labor market and avoid the possibility of social exclusion associated with poverty and the denial of rights. In response to globalization, in many countries of the world, educational systems are undergoing reforms that seek to improve their effectiveness and the standards obtained by the children whom they serve. In addition, concerns about equity of provision are raised which includes the move to the full inclusion of children with disabilities into mainstream schools.

A further and very forceful pressure for change comes from the emergence of the so called knowledge economy which is set to replace the current industrialized economies of many countries in the next millennium. Here, knowledge and learning are becoming indispensable assets, not only to the individual but also to companies and are replacing manual skills in importance. Knowledge and an openness to lifelong learning give enterprises flexibility and afford a greater opportunity to adapt to changing market opportunities. Thus, the knowledge economy stresses, in particular, the importance of high level literacy and numerical skills along with problem solving skills, the ability to work flexibly and in teams.

For many governments, the response to these trends and pressures has been to decentralize decision-making and planning, since this is viewed as a way to reduce central government costs, to promote local flexibility and increase allocational efficiency (Klugman, 1997). In addition, the recognition that client need can be better met through more responsive local service structures that can involve the community in its entirety, and that this is more important than agency bureaucratization, is now widely held to be a preferred model of service delivery (OECD, 1996). While this model is certainly desirable, the need to maintain an effective link between national policymaking and local delivery is strengthened by globalization and by international agreements, which can impact on individual citizens or groups. This chapter will describe some examples of local services delivered in the context of national policy frameworks outside of the United States. But before turning to these developments, two other important factors are pressing for reforms to be made. They are changing demographics and the growing emphasis on human rights including children's rights.

Changing Demographics

It is now well known that the balance between the old and the young is changing. The birth rate in most Organization for Economic Cooperation and Development (OECD) countries[1] has now fallen below the replacement rate (Halsey, 1993), which means that our populations are decreasing in size and are only likely to be maintained through immigration. This fact, allied to the increasing numbers of retired citizens, means that all people of working age need to work and contribute to the economy simply to maintain the tax base to support our current standards of living and to maintain retirement pensions. Having a student population who are not learning the skills necessary for survival in the new labor market is simply not acceptable, since not only do they not contribute to the tax base but they also, in many countries, draw long-term benefits from it. Furthermore, the poverty that almost inevitably ensues is associated with a decline in mental and physical health adding yet more strain to public health and social services (Whelan & Whelan, 1995).

Human Rights

Democracies do not stand still and the protection of human rights is emerging as yet another powerful force on education systems. The ratification of the Convention on the Rights of the Child by the United Nations in 1989 is a considerable step forward but there remains growing concerns for issues of equity in education especially with regard to gender, ethnic minority status, and regional disparities. Furthermore, the right for disabled students to be educated in mainstream schools, alongside their peers, is an ever growing policy objective (OECD, 1997).

Taken together these factors indicate the need for substantial reform in the ways in which all children and families are supported and educated and it is perhaps not surprising that in this environment research work that stresses prevention has resonated with policymakers. It presents the dream scenario. Fewer child and family problems, less costs, higher standards, and labor market compatibility. At least these are some of the aspirations.

This chapter will introduce the reader to some of the ways in which various countries outside of the United States are developing community-based services for children who are disadvantaged and disabled. It will begin with a brief description of the OECD and will then provide illustrations of good practice selected from a number of different countries in North America, Europe and Australia, which have been studied as part of on-going work by the Center for Educational Research and Innovation (CERI) of the OECD. It will conclude with a discussion of the Agenda for Action, which provides an informal statement, agreed by a number of countries, of action needed to achieve the full participation of children and families in an inclusive society.

THE OECD STUDIES OF COMMUNITY BASED SERVICES IN MEMBER COUNTRIES

The OECD consists of 29 democratic countries, which are essentially the wealthiest in the world where mandatory universal education has been operating for many years. Children who are failing in school, whether because of disability or disadvantage, are a great cause for concern in all OECD countries, although comparative prevalence estimates are not easy to obtain. The proportion of children said to be at risk of school failure varies between about 15 and 30 percent (OECD, 1995a) and this estimate is generally understood not to include children with disabilities whose prevalence estimates also vary substantially between approximately 1 and 10 percent of the school age population (OECD, 1995b). These figures must be interpreted with caution since they are not based on any true scientific classification procedure but reflect instead a complex interaction of epidemiological factors, educational policy and practice (OECD, 1995b).

Nevertheless, these figures reveal the extent to which the current normative conceptualization of education systems, including schools and other support services, are maladapted to the needs of their present clientele and how far they require substantial additional support if all needs are to be met. In the past failure has been tolerated since the labor market was able to absorb those students with little interest in school learning and with lower academic attainments. However, this attitude is now unacceptable, and the failure of these students can no longer be viewed as the necessary by-product of an inefficient industrial process, but as a challenge to be met by the system which must play a much greater part in helping to produce citizens who are fully included and able to take full part in society.

However, to change complex systems where there are intricate links between policy and practice is not easy. International organizations like the OECD, inter alia, provide a forum whereby reform can be promoted and discussed away from the hurly-burly of national decision-making. When different nations with their different histories and cultures share their experiences and exchange information and research data, similar problems and goals are often identified. This very process is important in helping the key players to move along their thinking, policymaking, and practices in their own countries and to identify possible solutions. Examples of innovations responding to these challenges studied by CERI are described.

The examples given here are drawn from case studies described in full in the OECD, 1996 and 1998 reports. Involving communities and coordinating services to support disabled and disadvantaged children and families has roots which can be traced back at least to the turn of the century (e.g., Webb & Webb, 1963). The key idea of partnership can be identified in a number of different countries in their approaches to policy about care. In Germany for example, the current philosophy of social care is based on earlier determined principles of an obligation to work and subsidiarity—whereby help and care are first seen as the responsibility of the family, relatives, and the neighborhood, then of voluntary and statutory agencies and finally of national organizations. More recent developments have stressed service cooperation and coordination in planning preventive services for children and youth that meet their needs across the age range. In the Netherlands, cooperation between education, primary health care, youth welfare work, manpower services, justice, the police, and social services has been stressed in an effort to develop a preventive youth care policy, and the link between education and labor market entry has recently been given special emphasis (Rauwenhoff Committee, 1990). This chapter, however, is mainly concerned with young children and the remainder focuses on this age group whose politico-economic importance is growing since the link between this period and later educational success and job market entry is becoming more and more appreciated.

Preschool Programs

While preschool programs feature strongly in some OECD countries, across the OECD as a whole there remains a lack of general provision for children in this age range. Perhaps it is partly because the statutory responsibility for children of this age cuts across many government departments or ministries, that this period provides interesting examples of the widest collaboration to develop support for families and children. Three examples will be described more fully, from New Brunswick in Canada, from Germany, and the Netherlands.

Canada (New Brunswick)—healthy children and families ready to learn

The Province of New Brunswick is on the eastern seaboard of Canada bordering on Nova Scotia, Quebec, and the state of Maine in the United States. Community based support services for families and children have been being developed there since the mid- to late-1980s. Services for young children and their families are developed in the context of the early childhood initiatives (ECI). The ECI bring together the collaborative efforts of the public health and medical services division and the family and community services division of the government of New Brunswick. They have been developed within a general framework of service integration throughout the province, which was stimulated by the recognition that parents, teachers and administrators need a better access to support from other professions to help to improve all children's level of education. The ECI are planned to bring young children to school who are as healthy and ready as possible to achieve their potential. There are seven major components. These provide:

1. Enhanced prenatal screening and intervention in order to increase healthy pregnancy outcomes;
2. Improved postnatal screening and intervention in order to enhance factors and conditions known to foster healthy growth and development;

3. The retargeting of preschool clinics to 5.5 years of age in order to support the healthy growth and development of preschool children;
4. Home-based early intervention services aimed at improving childhood outcomes and enhancing family self-sufficiency;
5. Integrated day care services with goals to achieve full participation of the high priority child in developmentally appropriate childcare services, and improved childhood outcomes among high priority children;
6. Social work prevention services whose goal is the secondary prevention of the abuse and neglect of children, through the strengthened parenting competencies of high priority parents; and
7. Home economics services whose goal is to have priority families develop skills in the areas of resource management and family development with the intention of stimulating greater self-reliance.

The services are coordinated across the entire province via a single entry point system through the public health nurse. Regional public health coordinators register priority families, conduct an assessment and refer the families to a range of existing government and community based services including the school districts. At 3.5 years, a student health profile form is completed on each child and is passed on to the school before entry into kindergarten.

Germany—supporting the community to avoid stigmatization and marginalization

Bremen is the smallest state in Germany. It is a Free city with a strong tradition of autonomy and pride in the city among its inhabitants. Bremen has developed an inclusive organizational structure for supporting families and young children who are disabled and disadvantaged that is planned to take responsibility for a population regardless of whether or not any particular individual has a problem. This is an approach intended to serve the whole community and not to marginalize certain groups as problematic. An orientation to the citizen as a consumer and receiver of services is a key requirement.

At the center of this organization of social services are two principles. First, the idea that the needs of clients must be identified in the context of the stage of life in which they are, and that help must be holistic. The second is that the diagnosis of need must be made in a neighborhood context. This principle also implies that regionally located agencies of social services should be working together to reintegrate clients into regional structures and living space (Dolls & Hammetter, 1988) and in this way an attempt is made to create a community.

From the point of view of service delivery, the first principle is operationalized through the division of Bremen into four regions, each of which has a service with subgroupings of professionals (Bezirkssozialdienste) that focus on demographic groups (e.g., children and their families, youth and their families). There is also a complementary service that focuses on specific issues that are dependent on demographic factors but which require a specific professional knowledge (e.g., in counseling for children or sociopsychiatric care).

The second principle is operationalized through the regional division of social services with professional groupings organized to meet the needs of neighborhoods of some 5,000 to 10,000 people.

The particular example to be described more fully here is that of Huchting, which is a disadvantaged area of Bremen with some 25 percent of its population receiving welfare benefits. Several different committees coordinate the different local organizations and institutions. An area committee and its director coordinate the various Bezirkssozialdienste. At the local level there is a committee consisting of social pedagogues (from the welfare office) who are responsible for the district, and one expert from each welfare organization in the district (i.e., from kindergartens, youth clubs and institutions, playgrounds, the City Farm, the local council, the social center, school psychological services, nonprofit organizations and health services).

The committee has a very important role in bringing all service providers together for discussion and cooperation. It also serves to link the community with the remaining hierarchy bringing emerging issues to the attention of management; a task achieved by a local coordinator.

A range of services is provided in Huchting. These include a Mothers Center, which is run by and for women and their families. The center provides a social forum for women to meet, share and support each other with the philosophy that a mother's well-being is essential for the child's well-being. The center collaborates closely with all of the other associations in Huchtings Social Services Center, and health guidance and advice on child rearing and on disabled children is provided.

The regional department of social services provides a support service for children and their families, which offers counseling and broad practical advice (e.g., on education and budgeting to families in need in their homes). The goal is to help families develop improved management and coping skills. In addition, they run a Family House, which has an educational focus with social workers and educators making up the staff with a main goal of developing self-help skills and the building of strong family relationships. In addition to these services, child guidance and health services are provided that work within the two guiding principles already described. The City Farm provides space for children to go to help them to develop social structures and learn to take responsibility.

The city, churches, and other voluntary organizations run daycare centers. They focus on 3- to 6-year-olds. The Dietrich Bonhoefer Center, for example, is part of the Protestant church and pioneered integrated preschool education for disabled and nondisabled children. The state-run kindergarten emphasizes the teaching of social skills and play and provides speech and psychomotor therapy. Both organizations cooperate more widely with schools, child guidance and so forth and the other facilities noted above.

These various facilities are supported and funded in many different ways—from the European Unions social fund, federal and state budgets, the Church, the lottery, and a whole range of sponsorship activities.

These provisions in Huchting emanated from both policymakers and professionals working at ground level. The system has short lines of communication between the key players at different levels of the system and this is seen as a major strength. Cooperation between the various agencies was stimulated through a workshop that brought together different professionals from nurseries, pediatrics, child guidance, social welfare and school psychology. It identified the gaps in the service provision based on available data. The directors of these services continued to meet informally and monitor progress. The work is facilitated by the one-stop-shop principle and the sharing of knowledge and information by professionals. Nevertheless, problems remain, such as the duplication of services and the negative competition that arises, and the different expectations of different professionals in terms of identifying solutions to problems. Social workers, for example, do not always agree with the approach taken by the Mothers Center and want to focus only on the child and not the synergic relationship of mother and child.

Despite the time over which this coordinated work has been taking place, there is still much to be done. It is recognized that success cannot be achieved without cooperating with other services. This benefits not only the clients but also the professionals who can operate holistically. Furthermore, it expands knowledge of practice and takes away the stress of dealing with poverty from any one particular service.

The approach taken in Bremen has produced many positive experiences and some of these have been described in the previous paragraphs. There still remains the problem of short-term funding for good cooperative projects, which are just beginning to take off. At the regional level, the Huchting committee has been instrumental in bringing about an integrated approach. It perceives itself as a powerful pressure group for improving service delivery in the area according to the principles of targeting demographic groups and through the neighborhood approach. The efficiency in solving problems is also emphasized. Cooperative social work at the local level is seen as a powerful force for staff development, as well as a means to achieve more effective provision for clients. The effectiveness of the Committee is believed to be enhanced by the coordinator, who keeps open channels of communication between local services, and between the local services and the strategic level. At this level there are difficulties in developing links between different government departments, nevertheless, informal arrangements exist and the importance of cooperation is recognized.

There will always be some overlap in the programs offered by different agencies—no single program can be expected to meet all the needs that will exist in any community—and so maintaining cooperation is important in providing comprehensive coverage for clients and providing choice.

Holland—providing home-based support to strengthen preschool provision

In Holland, welfare and health care policies were decentralized some years ago; in recent years, there has been a move to decentralize aspects of education policy with the goal of creating a more coherent response to the problems of deprivation. Within this general policy framework that covers all children and youth, preschool-age children have not been excluded.

Home-based support is an important element of preschool provision for disadvantaged families and for those who have children with disabilities. In Holland, a project called MOVE, developed in Emmen, is a good example of how this can work. The development of community based services that will sustain themselves is complex and the determinants need to be right as the following example shows.

Emmen is situated in the northeast of Holland. It is a community of some 54,000 people, with the greatest industrial concentration in the north of Holland and an unemployment rate in 1994 of 15.5 percent—about twice the national average. Holland has used the principle of the educational priority area (EPA) in order to target funds to disadvantaged families. Because of its background Emmen has been engaged for over 20 years in national projects intended to help it overcome its traditionally low level of education. For example at the end of the 1980s Emmen participated in an experiment on integrated municipal youth policy which encouraged the development of neighborhood networks for youth care services. One outcome of this work was the identification of high numbers of delayed children of preschool age and the need for preventive services which would expand the possibilities for toddlers and the involvement of parents.

The EPA in Emmen comprises a network of services for children at risk—especially of primary-school age as well as developed preschool playgroups. The latter caters for some 9 percent of the 0-4 age group, which while being indicative, almost certainly underestimates the size of the at risk group, which in primary schools covers those with low socio-economic status accounting for about 25 percent of the population.

Perhaps as a result of this long-term engagement with services for the disadvantaged, Emmen also has available a large number of services for children and families, which are publicly advertised on posters, and which parents can use to help obtain advice or support and so on. From these posters it is clear that more than 11 institutions deal with the pre-school period and that in many cases more than one institution covers the same area. For example seven different bodies deal with nourishment and support with upbringing.

It was in the context of this ongoing collaboration at the community level and following further attempts to coordinate or integrate services concerned with compensatory policy, under the general rubric of a Foundation for Educational Priority, that project MOVE was born in Emmen. MOVE was the implementation plan that followed a working party report that formulated the following policy goals intended to make services supply more attuned to customer demand. The central objective, the realization of an integrated set of measures, offering optimal chances of development for children aged 0 to 6 carried three sub-objectives:

1. stimulating and improving the development possibilities for young children by offering family-oriented activities;
2. backing up and strengthening appropriate child rearing methods and neighborhood services; and
3. preventing and/or decreasing problems in the development and upbringing of young children.

MOVE also responded to the need to coordinate the growing number of programs that were being offered for 0- to 6-year-olds. These were seen as:

1. being fragmented and lacking continuity;
2. often operating in isolation and not coordinated with other programs to benefit the recipients;
3. too linked to the possibility of external funding sources;
4. not fully thought through;
5. driven by particular civil servants or institutions; and

6. providing a dislocation between supply and demand, whereby the supply was either determined independently of client need, or with no evident means to get the service to the client, or where the methods used to identify clients were viewed as stigmatizing and for this reason self-defeating.

The project's name, MOVE, was deliberately chosen to reflect both the Dutch abbreviation of the project and the English verb to move—indicating the intended movement towards integration of services in other communities. It is recognized that the problems caused by educational deprivation call for a broad range of solutions. To increase their chances of success, children and their parents need to be positively encouraged and supported through cooperation between education and welfare including health care, help services, welfare work, and child care. This cooperation must result in a clear and well tuned supply of facilities for parents and children. On the one hand, family-oriented programs are needed; on the other hand, an accessible infrastructure of services, which calls on parents to play an active role in the stimulation and guidance of the development of their children.

The project plan was devised to support the ongoing work based on the objectives of education priority policy (i.e., to improve educational opportunities for the disadvantaged). Particular goals were to have by 1997:

1. seventy-five percent of children in the priority programs participating in the preschool program;
2. all preschool playgroups and schools affiliated to the priority program collect information on the course of development of priority children; and
3. seventy-five percent of priority parents with a child between 3 and 12 years participate annually in events which help them make an active contribution to the learning and development of their children.

The main innovative element in MOVE is the figure of the go-between mother. She may well be a member of the appropriate ethnic minority and works on building up a relationship with the family in the home and links their demands to the existing supply. In other words, an investment in relations and trust is the basis for change, which forms around meeting family needs. The go-between mother develops made-to measure approaches in linking supply and demand. For example by:

1. specific approaches to link the family with the facility;
2. activities to stimulate the development of young children;

3. made-to measure activities to support the childs upbringing; and
4. methods to signal problems and develop preventive strategies.

Introducing a new approach such as MOVE requires a coordinated effort across many levels of the system, which, in the example cited, was certainly helped by earlier national policy and the involvement of Emmen in the practice emanating from it. Furthermore, needed additional funding was secured through collaboration between the management and field level workers and a local foundation provided support in developing the methodology and training of staff. The team leader was a key appointment and after training carried out preliminary developmental work on the implementation of the project by making contacts locally and assembling a basic package of facilities. The management team supports the go-between mothers in identifying appropriate services and in their work with the families.

Comment

These three examples from Canada, Germany, and Holland show in different ways how services have been brought together to support families and children of preschool age. They have developed in a context of more general reforms to service provision that have involved their own forms of central government in decision-making and over a very substantial period of time. Although the realization of the work is very different between the countries, and this to some extent reflects the more multicultural base of the European examples, they are similar in that educational success is a common goal around which a wide range of services are united in supporting families and children.

School-Age Children

The examples described above that concentrate on preschool children have focused on coordinating services in the context of community support with parental involvement being given a priority in promoting preventive approaches. As children become older parental involvement in the education of their children remains imperative, but can change form.

The examples to be featured in looking at community support during the school age period come from Portugal, Finland, Canada, and Australia. They reflect responses to very different problems in urban and rural environments. In Portugal the issue is street children—children with little or no parenting; in Finland, on supporting families and especially coordinating social services and health. In Canada, the problems of organizing community services in a rural region is highlighted and in Australia an approach to involving Aboriginal communities is reviewed.

Both Portugal and Finland have been in the throws of rapid economic change, but in different directions. Portugal has been expanding fast in order to integrate itself fully into the European Union whilst on the other hand Finland has been experiencing uncharacteristically high levels of unemployment following the collapse of the Soviet Union. Both countries have looked to involving communities more fully in finding solutions to help children in difficulties.

Portugal—taking services to children living on the streets

Portugal has a high level of poverty (Vasconcelos, 1993) allied to insufficiently developed social support. In Lisbon, for example, the capitol city, Ramirez (1988) reported that less than 40 percent of children in the city between the ages of 3 and 6 were attending public childcare services even though the proportion of working women was very high. Many, even very young, children are simply locked out on the streets or left to the care of others or the extended family. It is only since 1984 that Portugal has begun to develop a network of state child and family protection services in cooperation with other public and private organizations. Private initiatives in this area are currently favored in Portugal and childcare centers are now managed by private social solidarity institutions (IPSS). Such an organization, the Institute for the Support of Children (IAC) was set up in 1983 to contribute to the integrated development of children and to the protection and promotion of their rights. There was an insistence that there should be close cooperation with the community in order to create the dynamism and coordination needed to meet the needs of children and their families. Its focus since 1989 has been on the problem of street children.

The aim of IAC in regard to young street children is to help them to continue their education and to establish appropriate parenting with natural parents or relatives or in some other suitable caring arrangement. The program has four steps. The first is to gain children's trust and to make friends with them. Contact with their families is not made until the children are ready and desire it. The second step is a period of transition whereby the relationship between the social worker and the child is strengthened and other professionals such as educators and nurses are introduced. At weekends, for instance, an attempt is made to encourage them to live in a group and to develop a normal lifestyle.

The third step is to reintegrate them into some form of family life either with parents or relatives or community provision. The fourth and last step is to develop participation in home and at school as appropriate.

These arrangements provide for great flexibility and this is encouraged. For example through personal contact between a social worker and the local zoo, the zoo agreed to take on some of the children and to help in giving them educational and socializing experiences.

Official support for this work comes from a number of sources including the ministry of education who provides teachers to work on the street with the children via the street school. The ministries of health, employment and social security, justice and youth, and institutions that cover education and health are also involved, as are other local authorities such as the town hall.

This work has developed against a background of some difficulty in dealing with local bureaucracies. Despite this, groups such as the press, the police, and shopkeepers report a reduction in the numbers of children on the streets of Lisbon. Changes have come about and there has been a growth in the development of preventive strategies. This includes the planning of activities in schools and local communities, promoting parent associations, and improving cooperation between parents and teachers—improvements that have started following the realization that the needs of children and families have to be met more effectively if progress is to happen.

Finland—decentralization and the local coordination of school-based and daycare services

In Finland the position is quite different. Here there has been a strong tradition of social welfare for many years and education, health, and social services are free although taxation is high. The recent downturn in the economy has led to a reconsideration of the structure and function of some of these top-down services along with a search for greater economies.

Services organized in this way are inevitably highly regulated, and following the recognition that a rationalization was required, laws and policies were adopted to help to make the services more responsive to local needs. Especially significant in these changes was the adoption of a policy of Local Population Responsibility (LPR). According to this principle, a multiprofessional team of social welfare and health professionals is given responsibility for a small geographically defined area containing 2,000 to 4,000 people. The aim is to improve the coordination, functioning, and accessibility of services to better meet the needs of service users. Important focuses of this policy are family-centered approaches, community care, and prevention.

Along with this policy came changes in the law which adjusted the nature of the funding process, allowed for flexibility in the place of provision and facilitated the sharing of client information. Taken together these reforms gave substantially increased freedoms to municipalities to spend monies and organize services with more versatility and more relevance to meet local demands. Mäkelä, Winter-Heikkila, Astrom, and Rokka (1993) argue that LPR holds possibilities for fostering creative local experiments involving multiprofessional and nonhierarchical teams provided that inherent difficulties between status and pay for the professionals involved and their practice ethics can be overcome.

In the town of Jyväskylä, there is an elementary school and daycare center that is unusual in Finland since it provides day care services and elementary school for children aged between 1 and 8 on the same site. It serves a new residential area with a socioeconomically mixed population with a number of families with serious problems. The main purpose of the combined provision is to integrate the educational content of the day care program with the school curriculum. It is also expected that children with problems will be identified earlier and that transition between the two facilities will be easier than if they are separate. In addition, school aged children will be able to benefit from onsite after school care which will be a great deal more convenient for parents. Joint training was provided for staff before the facility was opened in order to familiarize them with each others' working practices and perspectives.

Considerable emphasis is placed on collaboration with parents and the community. They are seen as equal partners and staff get to know them and to ascertain their personal interests and their goals for their children. They are invited to annual assessments of the children and the facility is open for community use outside of school times. It also provides other community services beyond its basic day care educational functions. These include a day care worker for parents of sick children, a nurse and a local social worker to help families in crises, and a meal service for elderly residents. The center also collaborates with local churches on various projects and the local library to provide children with books.

Canada (Ontario)—reaching isolated families in remote rural areas

Ontario is Canada's wealthiest province. It is a large landmass with many families living in remote rural regions. Children and families who live in remote regions are often underserved in terms of professional services and present a challenge to their delivery. The northern part of the Canadian province of Ontario provides an example, where services, which are taken for granted in southern Ontario, did not exist prior to the development of the Integrated Services for Northern Children (ISNC) program. Parents were obliged, for example, to take their child several hundred miles for psychological or speech assessments.

The children (and, of course, their families) most negatively affected by this situation were those with multiple difficulties needing the support of a number of professionals who cross ministry funding divisions and agency mandates. This problem came to be recognized by government reorganization and led to an inter-ministerial protocol and adjustments in the ways ministries functioned vis-à-vis their responsibilities regarding assessment services for children. Further review of the way the services were working led to the establishment, since early 1990, of the ISNC program (Lewko, Shea, Volpe, Lees, & Salhani, 1998).

The ISNC program is intended to improve services access in remote and underserviced areas using a network of satellite workers who are based in the communities and who are linked to urban based resource groups comprised of professionals from different disciplines. These workers are key as they serve as single entry points for all referrals and as case managers for all children and families who are part of the ISNC work.

Three things are unique about ISNC. One is the use of satellite workers who perform outreach, process all service requests, coordinate services, provide follow-up, problem solve, and support involved professionals. Their role as actual community members allows them to be part of both natural and professional support systems. Another feature is the effective use of a management information system for case and program monitoring. This system creates an electronic web that holds a program together. Finally, there is the continuous systematic program evaluation plan. This is integral to the functioning of the project and provides a tangibility to its implementation and development and establishes a firm foundation for its philosophy and goals.

South Australia—services for the children of indigenous peoples embedded in a statewide strategy

Aboriginals and Torres Strait Islanders have a disadvantaged position in Australia. Reports indicate that their mean income is less than two thirds that of the national figure. Retention rates in school are one-third that of other students; unemployment rates are 2.6 times that of other Australians; life expectancy at birth for females is 20 years less; and they are 15 times more likely to find themselves in prison.

The Australian government has, over the past few years, made considerable progress in implementing policies of social justice for all Australians with particular concerns for the plight of the indigenous peoples. Reconciliation, or the bringing together of indigenous and nonindigenous peoples became formal government policy in 1991 following the creation of a Council of Reconciliation.

The Murat Bay District Council in the South Australian community of Ceduna has received national recognition for its work with the Aboriginal community. A local economic plan, jointly negotiated, has been drawn up to address efficient and effective service delivery networks within the local council boundaries to meet the needs of all community residents. This plan essentially coordinates the budgets of a number of different responsible agencies to avoid overlap and waste. The Aboriginal community was not easily engaged in this development and the council needed to take considerable initiative to reach out to engage them.

In addition, the council benefited from the South Australian attorney general's crime prevention initiative. Through discussion with residents five areas were identified that needed to be addressed to fight crime: youth, domestic violence, alcohol and drug abuse, education and skills development to combat unemployment, and community development. Eighteen different program needs emerged (see Collins & Miller, 1992).

1. A homework center away from the school environment to support children who lack the necessary supports at home.
2. A school breakfast program.
3. A local women's shelter/hostel/accommodation center and crisis intervention services for domestic violence and child abuse.
4. A detoxification/rehabilitation center.
5. Literacy programs for youth and adults.
6. A mediation service.
7. More police aides to assist with communication with specific groups.
8. Support services for victims of crime.
9. More cross-cultural information, interaction and integration.
10. More involvement of the elderly and youth to alleviate fears about each other.
11. Family support systems related to child-rearing.
12. More adequate parental supervision of children.
13. Easily accessible information on parental rights and responsibilities.
14. Housing facilities for homeless youth.
15. More employment opportunities for the entire population.
16. Availability of and access to leisure facilities for those under the age of 18.
17. Transportation to cater for the needs of youth.
18. More adequate street lighting and public telephones in the Housing Trust area.

To begin the task of implementing these reforms, committees were set up for each of the five areas. Their function was to determine priority areas for funding, to give advice about implementation, to evaluate the results, and to submit progress reports to the district council.

The education sector is also particularly responsive to the needs of Aboriginal children. An Aboriginal pre-kindergarten has the goal of helping to socialize Aboriginal children in an environment which is sensitive to their culture, helps them with Aboriginal language, and prepares them for regular kindergarten. In the kindergarten, Aboriginal health services are provided as well as dentistry. Since many of the children are transients, whose basic needs have not been met adequately, the staff coordinate with the local child care and family day care centers.

As in other countries, these developments in Ceduna operate within the context of a more general strategy for the development of community-based services.

The complexity is well illustrated in an example from South Australia where a strategy for coordinating services for school children with social and behavioral problems has been outlined by Stratmann (1988) and which incorporates the following:

1. Agreement to be reached at the chief executive level as to the range and extent of services to be provided by each agency at the local level.
2. Interagency networks (school response teams) relating to specific clusters of schools be formally identified and effectively maintained.
3. To facilitate interagency coordination, clusters of schools be identified which are as compatible as possible with the Health and Welfare Sector boundaries, and with the clusters of schools being identified as a base for superintendents within the Education Department.
4. Multidisciplinary, district based student support teams be established in the Education Department. It was suggested that initially these teams would be made up from existing personnel in the Education Department from project teams and support services, guidance officers, social workers, attendance officers, etc. They would offer services to students referred from the same cluster of schools referred to above. The team managers would have a major role in the maintenance of the interagency networks as well as being the points of contact for school based personnel and accepting responsibility for case management plans for individuals.
5. Specific programs enhancing teacher skills in behavior management to be developed.
6. At least one form of withdrawal facility or program be available in each Education Department area, on the basis that it is used also as a vehicle for staff development and as a catalyst for change within the referring schools.

7. More joint welfare and education intensive personal supervision for some students be provided through the Department for Community Welfare Intensive Adolescent Supervision Program, in close cooperation with Education Department personnel.
8. Expansion of specialist Child and Adolescent Mental Health Services and Department for Community Welfare personnel, deployed specifically to support school children with social and behavioral problems.
9. The co-location of community health, education and welfare services be formally adopted as policy in the Department for Community Welfare, Education Department and Health Commission, and every effort be made to identify school premises which could be made available for co-locating services on a permanent or visiting basis. This would provide a service base for clusters of schools and, where possible, might provide the site for a withdrawal facility.

Comment

These examples of community-based services developed to meet the needs of families and young children of school age in a wide range of very different and difficult circumstances reveal how effective such an approach can be. The cases speak for themselves in the levels of complexity and variety that are involved in developing services that respond to the needs of people. Given this evidence it is not surprising that centrally administered delivered services have difficulty in addressing the true needs of the families and children involved.

TOWARDS THE FUTURE

If countries, both within and outside the OECD, are to continue to grow and prosper in the next millennium then all will have to respond rapidly to the economic and social developments that are taking place throughout the world. This means substantial changes in the way education, health, and social services operate. This chapter has given examples of how communities can become part of these reforms. This is accomplished essentially through the implementation of a services integration agenda that puts the needs of families and children at the heart of planning and involves the whole community, including businesses, churches, and the voluntary sector in a constructive elaboration of common social and educational goals in the creation of the new civic society.

Providing community-based services requires substantial coordination and cooperation between a diverse range of actors across a vertical structure running from the community through to government, which usually sets the legal framework and has responsibility for justifying the use of the taxpayers money which in turn supports the developments on the ground. At this level it is important not to forget that community-based services will have, and will need to have, strong support from central government. As we have seen, this must be accompanied by changes in the law as necessary, which may have to cover issues relating to the sharing of budgets across departmental boundaries, the training of professionals and allowing for information on clients to be shared across professional groupings. This last issue is of some concern to civil rights groups.

Creating these changes is neither easy to initiate nor to sustain. They need a great deal of determination and forward vision. The fact they are happening all over the world is important in convincing a country's administrators that other ways can be better. The international work is very important in this regard. No magic formulae are being proposed since the implementation details are too varied from country to country. What is clear though is that reforms are necessary and the community based services solution is one of the few on offer that is consistent with our democratic future.

The OECD is only one of a number of International Organizations who are helping to develop a positive philosophy toward coordinated community-based systems of care. Friedman, Magrab, and McPherson (1997) point out that the Pan American Health Organization (PAHO), the World Health Organization (WHO), UNICEF, and the United Nations Development Program (UNDP) have played a significant role in influencing nations. They have particularly influenced those in Latin America, Central Europe, Africa, and Asia, to move toward serving children in the communities where they live. Important benchmarks in the movement towards community-based services have included: the designation by the United Nations of 1981 as the International Year of the Disabled; the World Programme of Action in Favour of Disabled Persons adopted by the United Nations in 1983; the Convention of the Rights of the Child ratified by the United Nations in 1989; the Standard Rules on the Equalization of Opportunities for Persons with Disabilities adopted by the United Nations in 1983; and the Framework for Action on Special Needs Education sponsored by UNESCO and the Government of Spain in 1994.

An Agenda for Action

The Fourth International Congress on Serving Children with Disabilities in the Community (Friedman, Magrab, & McPherson, 1997) is an example of this process in action. This conference brought together 19 countries to discuss the ways in which communities can grow to support and foster the development of disabled children. At the end of this conference an Agenda for Action was readily agreed between the representatives of the countries who were present to advocate that nations:

1. Ensure the right of full participation of children with differing abilities in all aspects of community life such as schools, childcare programs, health services, recreational activities, and, ultimately, the work place.
2. Provide preventive and life-long supports and services beginning as early as possible in the life cycle of children in order to foster optimal growth and development.
3. Plan and implement a responsive and accessible service delivery system that is respectful of individual, family, and cultural differences and that allows families to choose the services and supports that are most appropriate for their children.
4. Ensure partnerships between family members, professionals, and policy makers in planning and implementing decisions at all levels—legislative, policy, and program—related to providing care and services to children.
5. Ensure that coordinated and comprehensive systems of support exist—including preventive measures, health, education, social supports, and other needed services—and are offered in an integrated fashion to families in the communities where they live.
6. Increase the awareness of the public at large that people of all abilities can make unique and valid contributions to their community and nation.
7. Encourage individuals, families, private organizations, government, and advocacy groups from every part of society to become involved and to cooperate in maximizing the capacities of individuals of all abilities as they participate in everyday life.
8. Cooperate with other nations in implementing this Agenda for Action.

This agenda is a full one and summarizes the nature of the problem that has been discussed above. It implies reform at many levels of the system from laws and policies at central and local levels through to practices on the ground. It invites collaboration between the private and public sectors. It advocates for the involvement of parents and families. It challenges the ways in which educational, health and social services are conceived and delivered and the way they currently function. This is not trivial since for this to take place reforms to the legal frameworks in which services operate and are financed would need to be in place. The Agenda demands changes in the ways in which clients interact with the system and vice-versa and by this token challenges the relevance of the current skills of many administrators and professionals as well as of the training courses which certificate or license them.

The Agenda for Action asks for a refocusing of the power structure from deliverers to users and such changes are never easy and the stakes are high. But the costs of the failure of the current model are also high. Countries need then to be very sure indeed that moving in this direction is the correct decision, and for this they need time to work through the implications. International discussion and analysis plays an important part in maintaining the momentum.

The Agenda for Action summarizes a way of thinking, with roots that can be traced back at least to the turn of the century, about how children and families in difficult circumstances can best be served. It reflects current thinking about best practices with an emphasis on prevention, coordination and community responsibility working together to meet the needs of children, families, the community, and ultimately the state.

This work is one testament to the willingness of countries to work together to improve the lives of disabled and disadvantaged children. The work is still in progress—there is still much to be achieved.

NOTE

[1]The Member countries of the OECD are: Australia, Austria, Belgium, Canada, the Czech Republic, Denmark, Finland, France, Germany, Greece, Hungary, Iceland, Ireland, Italy, Japan, the Republic of Korea, Luxembourg, Mexico, the Netherlands, New Zealand, Norway, Poland, Portugal, Spain, Sweden, Switzerland, Turkey, the United Kingdom and the United States of America.

REFERENCES

Collins, R., & Miller, V. (1992). *Draft two year crime prevention plan for Ceduna, together against crime*. Ceduna, South Australia: District Council of Murat Bay.

Dolls, M., & Hammetter, V. (1988). *Zielgruppen- und stadtteilorientierte soziale arbeit*. Neuorganisation der sozialen dienste in Bremen-Sd. Frankurt am Main.

Friedman, J. E., Magrab, P. R., & McPherson, M. P. (1997). *International perspectives: Building local systems of care for children with disabilities and their families*. Washington, DC: Georgetown University Child Development Center.

Halsey, A. H. (1993). Changes in the family. In G. Pugh (Ed.), *30 years of change for children* (pp. 64-77). London: National Childrens Bureau.

Klugman, J. (1997). Decentralization: A survey from a child welfare perspective. *Innocenti Occasional Papers, Economic and Social Policy Series, EPS 61.* Florence: UNICEF.

Lewko, J. H., Shea, M., Volpe, R., Lees, C., & Salhani, D. (1998a). Children and families at risk. In *New issues in integrating services* (pp. 127-148). Paris: OECD.

Mäkelä, M., Winter-Heikkila, M., Astrom, M., & Rokka, S. (1993). Local population responsibility—old wine in new barrels? *Journal of the National Research and Development Centre for Welfare and Health*, 11-13.

OECD. (1995a). *Our children at risk.* Paris: OECD.

OECD. (1995b). *Integrating students with special needs into mainstream schools.* Paris: OECD.

OECD. (1996). *Successful services for our children and families at risk.* Paris: OECD.

OECD. (1997). *Implementing inclusive education.* Paris: OECD.

OECD. (1998). *Co-ordinating services for children and youth at risk—a world view.* Paris: OECD.

Ramirez, M. E. (1988). *Criana portuguesa: Que acolhimento?*. Lisboa: Rede da Comisso Europeia de acolhimento de crianas/Instituto de Apoio Crisana.

Rauwenhoff Committee. (1990). *Education-labour market: Towards an effective pathway.* The Hague: Alphen aan den Rijn.

Stratmann, P. (1988). *Interagency responses to school children with social and behavioural problems.* Adelaide, Australia: Department of Premier and Cabinet.

United Nations. (1989). *Convention on the rights of the child.* New York: Author.

Vasconcelos, L. (1993). Pobreza em Portugal - variaao e decomposiao de medidas de probeza a partir de oramentos familiares de 1980/81 e 1989/90. *Documentos de Trabalho. CISEP, No 2.*

Webb, S., & Webb, B. (1963). *English poor law policy.* London: Frank Cass.

Whelan, B. J., & Whelan C. T. (1995). In what sense is poverty multidimensional? In G. Room (Ed.), *Beyond the threshold* (pp. 29-48). Bristol, UK: The Policy Press.

chapter 10

Service Integration at the Community Level Within Early Intervention Systems

Adrienne L. Akers
Diane D. Behl
Early Intervention Research Institute

> *After Lisa was born, and we found out about her problems, I felt so overwhelmed...doctors' appointments, therapists, a jillion different agencies. It was as if I was in a huge, wind tunnel, bouncing from side to side as I was being sucked into it. But when we were finally referred to the early intervention program, it was as if someone grabbed me by an ankle and pulled me back to earth.*
> (Mother of a child with visual and physical challenges)

As parents learn that their baby is faced with special challenges, a myriad of unforeseen events begin to take place. How can a community offer the kinds of supports and services that will help families as they begin to adapt to the unexpected alteration of the family system? What steps can a community take to prevent the unnecessary confusion and duplication of services mentioned in the quote above?

This chapter describes how communities can develop early intervention systems that address important priorities for families that support child development and family well being, including accessibility, availability, and coordination in a family-centered, supportive manner. The construct of service integration will be explored on both a conceptual level as well on a more pragmatic level through a description of how two communities developed family-centered, integrated, early intervention systems. So that the reader can better understand how service integration strategies can be knitted together at the community level, family-centered service coordination will be highlighted by describing how community-based early intervention systems can support a free and open exchange of information, enhance funding options, and develop individualized family service plans (IFSPs) that involve all of the stakeholders.

Early intervention for children with special needs refers to the system of care for children ages birth to three years of age mandated by federal legislation. The tremendous growth of human services during the last decade has increased the need for greater coordination of services for young children with disabilities and their families. In seeking early intervention services, many families have diverse needs and receive services from a variety of private and public agencies, across health, mental health, social services, and education administrative affiliations (Roberts & Wasik, 1990). With this increase, the need to coordinate services both at the family and systems levels becomes critical. Individual programs must be integrated into a system of care that is responsive to family needs in order to prevent the family from becoming confused by a fragmented system (Ooms & Owen, 1992).

Plans for the development of early intervention services provided under Part H legislation (P.L. 99-457 now P.L. 105-17 and referred to as Part C) incorporated a strong emphasis on developing integrated interagency systems that would build on existing services at the state and community levels. At the same time, coordination at the family level was assured through the requirement that services for each child and his or her family must be offered through an Individualized Family Service Plan (IFSP). Coordination at the state, community and family levels was encouraged as a mechanism to provide appropriate, non-duplicative services to children and parents in order to enhance child and family outcomes.

The framework of this chapter draws on the results of a large study funded through the Maternal and Child Health Bureau (MCHB) in which the Opening Doors Project (Roberts, Akers, & Behl, 1997) studied eight communities in six states to investigate and document the strategies used to integrate services for families with young children with disabilities. Insights into parent priorities were obtained via focus groups and structured interviews with individual families. Focus groups with direct service providers, interviews with community and state-level administrators, and reviews of policies regulating the early intervention service system were conducted. In keeping with the importance of developing systems of care that meet the needs of families, we begin with an overview of critical issues identified by families who participated in our project.

PRIORITIES FOR FAMILIES OF CHILDREN WITH SPECIAL NEEDS

Accessibility of services and where to go for help is problematic for many families. Most families do not anticipate the need to interact with a wide array of service providers after their child is born. When a family learns of their child's disability or special health care need, they often experience confusion and frustration as they attempt to learn about and begin to navigate their way through a community's service system. One mother told of her experience in the following quote:

> We really had no direction, like "There are lots of services out there for infants. Let me connect you. Wait until you get home and get your feet on the ground." Fortunately, I have a background in special education...and I did kind of quickly pull all those people together. One person would refer us to [the early intervention program] and then they would refer us to the infant development center where we get several services now. But we...did all the foot work ourselves.

This is an example of "*resourceful families get the resources*." In a similar study by Mahoney and Filer (1996), they found this to be characteristic of families they surveyed. They found that those parents who had more limited skills and resources were the least likely to obtain and receive services related to their needs. Families reporting the greatest intensity of services were those who had sufficient time to participate as well as the resources and personal skills to negotiate effectively for the services they desired. Unfortunately, those families most in need of services are frequently the ones who go without due to a lack of information on what is available, a lack of self-confidence needed to initiate contacts with agencies, or a mistrust of bureaucracies based on negative experiences in the past. Some providers overwhelm parents with a great deal of information at the start, when most families are struggling to stay afloat both emotionally and financially. Unfortunately, this information may not be reiterated at a later time when families are better able to assess new needs as they arise. Because family needs change over time, a family may not identify the need for financial assistance or for parent support at first, yet changes in employment status or coping ability require access to services to be a continual issue. One frustrated father described how confusing service coordination was for his family:

> We learned about [the lack of coordination] when each [agency] came in and said, "OK, I'm from...and I'm going to be your case manager." It was like, "Wait a minute, didn't [another agency] say they were our case manager? Didn't...say they were our case manager?" They are all government agencies or private agencies.... Quite honestly, it is the old left hand

> doesn't know what the right hand is doing. Maybe they both have very good intentions and they are both doing good things, but there is no communication for whatever reason...They are supposed to be working together, but for whatever reason, they aren't.

Coordination of services is often lacking, as evidenced by this family's experience. The father speaking in this example has the skills to obtain what his child and family needs. Yet for families dealing with multiple stressors, the system could easily fail them—families who are unable to juggle multiple providers are likely to be overwhelmed and omissions or duplications in services may occur.

Family support is particularly important to families who find themselves faced with unique challenges. Families of children with disabilities or special health care needs often feel alone—their friends and family may be supportive and try to be helpful, but it is not the same as being able to talk with another parent who has faced similar circumstances. Adapting family life to meet the demands of a child's health or disability-related needs can be stressful, requiring the need for specialized supports. Respite care is reported to be a critical support for families, yet this is typically one of the first services to suffer funding cuts. Mental health services may be needed to ensure that the family can support the development of a child with special needs, but often falls outside the umbrella of the early intervention system in many states.

The parents' priorities described above emphasize the importance of developing an early intervention system that is accessible, coordinated, and supportive of families. This requires that programs and agencies do not operate in isolation but must be integrated to meet the needs of children with disabilities and their families. When establishing a system of family-centered services, it is essential to bridge the gap between the priorities voiced by families and the policies that drive the service system. This philosophical evolution has resulted in efforts to reform fragmented early intervention and human service systems in order to develop a more coordinated, integrated system of care that meets the needs of children and families (Kagan, Goffin, Golub, & Pritchard, 1995; Roberts, Rule, & Innocenti, 1998).

DEFINING SERVICE INTEGRATION

Kahn and Kamerman (1992) have defined the concept of *service integration* as the "systematic effort to solve problems of service fragmentation and of the lack of an exact match between...a family with problems and needs and an intervention program or professional speciality" (p. 5). Service integration, then, is the systems-wide effort with the dual goals of simultaneously improving outcomes for families as well as the efficiency and effectiveness of the human service systems (Kagan et al., 1995).

Family-level service integration strategies can be found in the literature, such as service coordination, a focus on the family as the service unit, case conferences, individualized child and family assessments and service plans, outcome monitoring, home visits, and flexible funds or resources at the disposal of front-line staff. As suggested by Kagan and colleagues (1995), service coordination serves the function of bringing together previously uncoordinated services at the family level. Early intervention's federal legislation defines *service coordination* as "the activities carried out by a case manager to assist and enable (an eligible) child...and the child's family to receive the rights, procedural safeguards, and services...authorized under the State's early intervention programs" (Pt. H, P.L. 101-476; 1990).

Kahn and Kamerman (1992) also provided a list of commonly cited *community-level service integration strategies,* such as interagency agreements; interagency councils or committees; co-location of services; a single point for intake and assessment; flexible or pooled funding; co-application procedures; coordination or consolidation of programs, budgeting, planning, and administration; and comprehensive data and management information systems.

More recently, Kagan and colleagues (1995) studied service integration in four states. In each state, service integration across six human service domains was examined: (a) childcare, (b) health, (c) elementary and secondary education, (d) welfare, (e) justice, and (f) employment. Unfortunately, state early intervention systems was not included in this study. However, Kagan and colleagues made a significant contribution to the field in the understanding of the breadth of this topic. They recognized that in the past, service integration had been viewed as either an attempt to increase the efficiency of the service system *or* to improve services for individuals, children and families. Kagan argues that the goal of service integration is to increase of efficiency and effectiveness of human service systems and to positively impact human outcomes, enabling children and families to experience a higher quality of life. In a more pragmatic sense, service integration has four basic functions:

1. To bring together previously unconnected services;
2. To overturn past practice, policy or bureaucracy;
3. To create mechanisms that work to promote and sustain integrative strategies; and
4. To change relationships for and among people and institutions.

As we shall see in the next section, federal legislation acknowledged the importance of service integration in community and state early intervention systems by creating a mandate to help families make sense of the human services being offered to them.

SERVICE INTEGRATION RELATED TO EARLY INTERVENTION

In 1986, it became clear there the was a need to restructure services to better meet the needs of young children with disabilities and their families. One of the initial goals of the federal legislation known as Part H (now known as Part C) of IDEA was to assist states in building more family-centered, coordinated systems of care for young children with disabilities and their families. Many states did not begin the process of implementing the elements of Part C with a blank slate and had been providing some services to eligible infants, toddlers and their families prior to the implementation of the law. Many of these services were based on a child-focused, deficit-based model as opposed to a family-centered, strength-based model. It would be natural for agencies to resist change in situations where the existing system did not seem to be "broken" and where families appeared satisfied with the services provided. Part C was designed to create a more unified system consistent with state options and to enhance the overall outcomes for eligible families and children through a more unified model of services.

Part C served as a stimulus for the field of early intervention to broaden its emphasis from a child focus to a stronger family orientation. In principle, parents are viewed as partners in the intervention process, and their concerns, priorities, and resources guide the development of the IFSP, the key to the provision of services. The early intervention system builds upon family strengths while addressing family needs (increasing resources, coping, and support) in order to enhance the development of the child. Parent and family partnerships with Part C are encouraged at each level of service delivery, policy development, and implementation (Roberts, Rule, & Innocenti, 1998; Trohanis, 1998).

A family-centered system is one that provides families with a voice, ownership, and options for services (NEC*TAS, 1995). This means that families are in control of the services they receive. Their input drives program policies and they are represented in system development. In establishing family-centered early intervention it is essential to bridge gaps between priorities voiced by families and the state and local policies that drive service delivery.

As a community attempts to integrate its services in a family-centered manner, the construct of well-being, as described by Gallimore and colleagues (1993) and Weisner (1984), provides a helpful way to view the needs of families from a broader, ecological perspective. Well-being is defined as an individual's ability to participate meaningfully and successfully in the daily routines of his or her culture. In their longitudinal study of 100 families who had a child with a developmental delay, Weisner and Bernheimer found that the most important concern (i.e., what supports family well-being) for families who have children with developmental delays is the child's ability to participate meaningfully and successfully in the daily routine of the family. This construct of ensuring that children with disabilities can participate in the family's natural routine is supported in the new Part C legislation that emphasizes the provision of services in "natural environments." This latest emphasis is particularly relevant to communities in their efforts to design systems that support the inclusion of all children and families to participate fully in the community.

Researchers have presented evidence that some programs are adopting a family-centered approach to services (Mahoney & Filer, 1996). Roberts, Akers, and Behl (1996) compared studies of parent perceptions conducted in 1988 and in 1992; parents reporting in 1992 felt that programs focused greater efforts on helping families cope with stresses of having a child with special needs. A study of consumer-based services (Able-Boone, Goodwin, Sandall, Gordon, & Martin, 1992) concluded that parents generally gave positive ratings to the early intervention services their child received. However, parents reported that access to services, service coordination, and the IFSP process did not meet their expectations. These recent studies demonstrate that early intervention systems continue to warrant the attention of policymakers in regard to developing integrated systems of care for children and families.

COMMUNITY-BASED SYSTEMS OF CARE IN TWO COMMUNITIES

Community-based systems of care (Center for Study of Social Policy, 1991; Halpern, 1991; Himmelman, 1992; Melaville, Blank, & Asayesh, 1993) have received attention in the literature and subsequently, particular emphasis has been placed on local efforts to integrate services. Community efforts to collaborate with families and across agencies have been a challenge that more communities are beginning to address. These issues of collaboration are the focus of the following description of how two communities that participated in the Opening Doors study (Roberts, Akers, & Behl, 1997) are seeking to develop family-centered, integrated early intervention systems. For each community, we will describe how the issues of accessibility, coordination and support are being addressed, as well as their challenges in building integrated service systems. It is hoped that these two community case studies will provide readers with insights into how these same issues can be approached within their own communities.

Orem, Utah

Orem is a growing community of 80,000, located 40 miles south of Salt Lake City. The local early intervention agency, called Kids on the Move (KOTM), serves approximately 200 children ages birth through two years and their families through a combination of home- and center-based services and service coordination with other services in the community. KOTM is unique in that it was started in 1983 by two mothers of young children with Down's syndrome who were disgruntled by the lack of services available for children under three in their community. This volunteer play group has grown into a private nonprofit agency now housed in a 15,000 square foot building constructed through local fund-raising efforts. This program exemplifies the power of parents in driving the development of early intervention. Currently, KOTM has a staff of 34, including a public health nurse who is responsible for monitoring the health needs of the children served. Other direct services provided include infant and toddlers classes; speech, PT, and OT services; home visits; and parent groups.

KOTM service coordinators help link families with state and local resources not provided by KOTM, such as WIC, mental health services, respite care, specialty clinics, and so on. This is the primary family-level service integration strategy employed. At the systems level, the local interagency coordinating council serves to advise policy makers and administrators on how to best meet the needs of families.

As mentioned earlier, staff of the Opening Doors Project conducted a series of focus groups with parents involved in early intervention programs and with community service providers to gain a greater understanding of how parent priorities are being met within the community's early intervention system. The examples below are based on these focus groups, interviews, and document reviews.

Accessibility

Although KOTM provides each family with a user-friendly parent handbook, which includes a list of local and state resources, families still reported that they need more information on services available. The home visitor/service coordinator plays an integral role by being available on a regular basis to hear or observe child and family changes that may require the identification of new services.

In Utah, Part C has placed a major focus on entry into the system. The Baby Watch public awareness program is quite visible and has strong private-public support. Originally, Baby Watch was jointly funded through KUTV and Health Trust Utah (which owns several major Utah hospitals). Part C and Health Trust Utah have also collaborated to conduct joint screenings at these hospitals. One full-time state Part C staff person is responsible for improving public awareness and increasing referrals into the system. Child find efforts are supported through a state interagency agreement between the Part C and Part B (State Office of Education) programs to coordinate child find efforts at the local level.

Utah's central directory provides a hot-line that gives resource and referral information to families of children with disabilities. The directory, known as ACCESS UTAH, maintains an information resource center responsible for disseminating and updating the directory to include listings of public and private early intervention services, resources and experts; research and demonstration projects in Utah; and professional, service, and support programs. To ease data transmittal and maintain cost effectiveness, the directory information is disseminated electronically with a user-friendly Windows format. Users who do not have access to a computer may call the toll-free number.

Coordination

Once children and families have entered the early intervention system, services from multiple agencies are often needed. Because the state Department of Health serves as the lead agency for Part C in Utah, health-related needs are accessed somewhat more easily. Public health nurses who work with the local Baby Watch programs are able to funnel children and families into many health services, such as WIC, specialty clinics, and immunizations.

Home visiting places a central role in service provision and coordination. Families in the KOTM focus group reported that their service coordinators helped them understand the system, assisted them with filling out paperwork, and most importantly, provided emotional support. Several of the families had children with complicated medical problems; for them, home visits were the only way they could access services for their child. Although most families initially receive home visits to introduce them to the program and to provide emotional support, KOTM also arranges for direct services to be provided in the home when medically necessary (although this is limited by therapists' high caseloads).

Home visitors in the focus group were generally positive about the benefits of home visiting. However, some marked differences in philosophy and attitude toward parents were clearly delineated in the group. When asked about the relationship they had with parents, a home visitor from one agency stated:

> I do think you have to keep a professional atmosphere...because if you don't, a lot of times parents will start taking advantage of you. I have had parents worm their way to get rides places here there and everywhere...So you really have to keep a professional distance...Sometimes it is really difficult because you are entering into their lives when they have just found out that their child might be blind for life...and they are in a grieving mode and you have to work through this with them. They come to depend upon you and yet you have to keep your distance in a way without becoming too upset or emotionally involved. Other times they get to be such good friends that [they] don't follow through on the...goals you give them.

In contrast, a home visitor from another agency commented:

> On the other hand, I don't expect to come in and start "teaching." I try to become their friend first and then tell them some advice. I think they take it better once you become their friend. They don't want to know how much you know until they know how much you care...I'm not saying being a friend is doing everything for them, because being a friend is helping others do by themselves. So I would never do for them, I would help them do it by themselves. Being the advocate for their child, maybe that is the difference. I don't ever try to fix things for them or do it for them...I'm there to help them get out of a problem by themselves.

In discussing how she assists families with service integration, the same home visitor made the following comment::

> Instead of saying, "These are the therapies you can have: I want you to come to baby group, I want you to receive this OT/PT thing," I say, "What is it you think you need?" If they say, "I don't even know what you have," then I tell them..[then I ask] "What do you think he needs?" [This way I know] it is coming from them...I try to let parent take the lead and help them make the direction...There is a lot more follow through. I almost never take toys in, I use what is there and adapt. [I say to the child] "Bring me your toys and let's see what we can do with them."...In doing that I feel like [I'm saying] "Hey, we really value what you have, we value your family and your goals are good and here is how we can add a little more...information when the need arises."

Helping home visitors to understand their own attitudes about their role in the home and their philosophy of family empowerment seems to be a recurring theme at both local, state, and national levels. This also implies the continuing need for developing and conducting inter-disciplinary preservice and inservice training for personnel working with children and families.

At the community level, the local interagency coordinating council (LICC) for Orem serves to bring together representatives from service agencies, private business, community stakeholders, and families. The purpose of the LICC is to foster coordination through information exchange with its members, and advise the development of community and state-level policies. For example, local agencies have also developed policies to deal with information exchange without infringing on family confidentiality. The LICC also can address issues such as inter-agency training.

Need for support

Because of its strong emphasis on family empowerment, KOTM provides an extensive variety of parent education and support opportunities for families, such as a mothers' group, fathers' group, sibling programs, make-and-take workshops, toddler play groups, a parent resource library, couples' night out, and parenting classes held in English and Spanish.

Although service coordinators were highly valued for their support, opportunities to interact with other parents are important. One mother described how she looked forward to bringing her child to the toddler playgroup because it "lets me have time to talk to other parents." Informal opportunities to interact with other parents of children with disabilities provide valuable support for parents. With limited time to attend parent meetings and with respite care so difficult to obtain, linking parents with a "phone buddy" provides additional support with little or no dollar cost to the early intervention system.

The lack of available respite care seems to be a recurring these among families of children with special needs. Even though many families in Orem have extended families living close by, parents still report a high need for respite care. In Utah, the Division of Services for Persons with Disabilities (DSPD) is the main provider of respite services. Receipt of respite care services is complicated by limited funding and a long waiting list of families in need of respite care services. Currently, Utah's Part C system does not provide funding for respite care.

KOTM maintains a fairly high profile in the Orem community for a variety of reasons: it is located on the same campus as the community hospital; it was constructed using funds from a very successful fund-raising campaign; it is designed and offered for multi-use meetings and training for local family agencies and groups; and the director has served as the moderator of the local interagency coordinating council.

KOTM sponsored and co-sponsored workshops and training that created the opportunity for staff from parallel agencies to form the connections and friendships that seem to enhance the integration of services for individual families. KOTM's visibility within the community supports an attitude and opportunity for multi-agency collaboration and integration.

Local challenges that interfere with service integration

Services that are more difficult to access because of limited availability include respite care, mental health services, and physical and occupational therapy services—as indicated by both parents and providers in Orem. Other services are difficult to access because of the lengthy and complicated application process, such as Medicaid and SSI. Although common application procedures have been under discussion for years in Utah, progress has been minimal.

The Orem area providers echoed another common theme related to service integration. Local providers tend to see themselves as being able to *make service coordination work,* but not because agencies consciously support and promote it. As one provider stated:

> I think that whenever interagency coordination happens...it is in spite of, not because of. In spite of the agency, because the rules are all set up and the agencies do their own thing. The actual people that go into the home...they coordinate and cooperate, but that is all...[it] is not mandated or outlined by the agency...it's not that the services are in conflict, it is just they are sometimes not coordinated.

This comment highlights the continuing need for state agencies to explore policies and methods that support service integration at the local level.

Integrating services for families served through the Division of Family Services (DFS; welfare) and Part C is more complicated. Both parents and providers describe limited communication between the two agencies and difficulties in integrating service plans. DFS workers do not generally attend IFSP meetings and Part C service coordinators do not typically attend DFS meetings. It would seem that agencies should strive to integrate services for those families have the most limited resources As described earlier, service coordinators are essential for helping these families "navigate through the system."

The role of state-level policies in supporting communities

Influence on the provision of services goes beyond local variation and has also been related to the states in which the families reside. Services provided to families are most likely the result of state policies and resources as they are filtered through and applied as program-specific practices. Unfortunately, less attention has been directed at a state's role in human services system reform efforts.

Orem's early intervention system is supported by several state-level strategies. An annual statewide early intervention conference is co-sponsored by Part C and Part B with strong parent attendance. Each year parents assist in planning and participating in presentations at the conference. Utah has been at the forefront in being committed to strong parent involvement in planning, training and technical assistance activities.

Part C discretionary dollars were used from 1993 to 1995 to local technical assistance to all local Baby Watch programs to conduct a self-assessment of family-centered practices and to develop local action plans for the purpose of improving family-centeredness. Issues related to parent support were frequently cited as being important at the local level.

The Utah Parent Center (UPC), based in Salt Lake City, offers a variety of services and resources for families of children of all ages with disabilities. Part C is in the process of purchasing a half-time position within the Utah Parent Center to work for Part C (e.g., conduct training, serve on advisory boards, etc.). In regard to Part C's interaction with parent organizations, the Part C coordinator stated that she is a strong supporter of parent-to-parent activities and encourages all local Part C programs to develop parent-to-parent strategies.

Interagency coordinating councils exist at the state level as well. Although Utah's CSHCN director and Part C coordinator are members of the State ICC, the SICC is struggling with how to best support local ICCs. Part C has sponsored a state conference for LICC members to facilitate local development. Likewise, a Part C staff person is responsible for training and technical assistance to the LICC's regarding integration issues.

State-level challenges

Utah does not use a state-wide IFSP form; local EI programs have developed their own IFSP forms. Past efforts to develop joint forms and co-application procedures resulted in forms being too lengthy and cumbersome to the extent that they were not family-friendly and were not deemed acceptable to the agencies involved.

Although the Division of Services for Persons with Disabilities (DSPD) collaborates with Part C by providing respite care for families, respite care is not provided for by Part C funds. DSPD is continually struggling to provide adequate funding for respite care.

Randolph County, Missouri

Randolph County is located in central Missouri, with the community of Moberly as its main population base with 12,000 residents. The nearest city in which to obtain specialty medical and related services is Columbia, located 30 miles away.

Caring for Kids is an agency that provides early intervention services via home visiting for children at risk for abuse/neglect as well as families of children who are Part C-eligible. Caring for Kids is housed in the Randolf County Health Department in Moberly. Caring for Kids serves families of children ages birth to 21 years, offering some prenatal home visits as well. The program employs a social worker, developmental specialists, nurses, as well as speech/language, physical, and occupational therapists. Within the same building, the Randolph County Health Department houses WIC, well-baby clinics, immunization services, and home health services for adults.

The Part C system for Missouri, called First Steps, involves the use of service coordinators who are independent from any of the direct service agencies. Families are connected with a First Steps coordinator from either the Bureau for Special Health Care Needs or with the Department of Mental Retardation/Developmental Disabilities, depending on the child's primary reason for the disability. Randolph County's early intervention system uses a variety of community-based strategies to meet the priorities of families. These are highlighted below.

Accessibility

Given the high percentage of families in Randolph County that qualify for public assistance, the "one-stop" shopping model offered by the county health department is a strong asset for helping families access needed services. Because Caring for Kids also serves children who are at risk for developmental delays or special health care needs, public health nurses can easily connect families to the First Steps program if they suspect a delay. One of the First Steps coordinators is just down the hall, ensuring that the family can easily make contact. General child health services can be accessed at the Health Department, meeting well-child-care needs for all children.

Coordination

First Steps service coordinators are recognized by families as the one who connects them with needed services. The IFSP was recognized by the majority of families in the focus group as the document that contains all the services and agencies paid for by Part C. Families also appreciated the assistance they received from their service coordinator in completing application forms and taking care of billing. These bureaucratic hurdles are a particular hassle for families so strategies to simplify the process are valued by families.

Many families in Randolph County face multiple challenges due to lower income and education levels in addition to having a child with special needs. To better meet the needs of those in the community that face multiple challenges, three key agencies have established "Baby Boost," a coordinated effort between Caring for Kids, Parents as Teachers, and NECAC, which provides assistance with financial and home-making needs. Baby Boost serves all families living in Randolph County who have a newborn baby and it is funded through a Children's Trust Fund Grant and donations from community organizations and businesses. A nurse from Caring for Kids makes the initial visit to explain the program and to begin health care services. A Parents As Teachers educator is then introduced. Together the family, nurse, and educator identify family needs. Other additional services can be initiated if requested by the family. Baby Boost has been working on developing a common application form and a common service plan to facilitate coordination, ease the paperwork burden on families, and decrease provider time in completing needed paperwork.

An interagency coordinating council for Randolph County, called the Care Council, is dedicated to providing a system of comprehensive services to children and youth with special needs ages birth through 21. The Care Council was originally formed to provide the needed coordination and planning for First Steps early intervention system at the local level. However, given the rural nature of the community, council members believed that they could best serve their community by addressing the full age range of persons with disabilities. The Social Security Administration is represented on the Council, potentially assisting with the issue of accessing SSI.

Addressing support

Unlike Utah, Missouri's Part C system does pay for respite care for families. The value of this support was reflected by one parent's comment: "It has really made a difference for me, and Jane (service coordinator) says they will always pay for it. I do have to find a person who can do it, and that's sometimes difficult."

As this comment demonstrates, respite care can still be a challenge if regulations make it difficult for families even when funds are available. One solution is to have families of children with special needs serve as respite care providers for other families. Although this strategy helps connect families with one another, it could also add to parental burnout. Through interagency councils, community stakeholders can consider other resources for recruiting respite care providers (e.g., university students in health, education, or social work; church or civic groups, etc.).

Challenges faced

Families in Moberly receive many services through home visiting. As noted in the literature, home visiting is an important strategy for developing family-centered services (Wasik & Roberts, 1994) However, home visits from providers representing multiple disciplines or agencies can be intrusive to the family's normal routine. One parent expressed frustration with the frequency of home visits, by stating "It's a pain. I can't schedule anything else. I had to set the schedule so that he could get a nap and so I could get him fed." Another said, "They (providers) tried to tell me their schedule, and services were based on what they wanted, but I had to set them straight. Now we have to reschedule again also I can take him swimming." This demonstrates the important role of the service coordinator in checking with the family to ensure that services are not conflicting with the family unit but actually supporting it.

Also, services provided primarily through home visiting result in fewer opportunities for families to connect with other families. Families are particularly vulnerable to isolation in rural communities such as Moberly. One of the needs voiced by parents in the focus group was the need to talk with other parents. Involvement of parents in the planning of early intervention services and supports can ensure that there are opportunities available to families to interact, be it informally via phone calls or play groups or through more formal parent-to-parent organizations.

State-level supports to community

First Steps state liaisons are assigned to regions of Missouri, with the responsibility of supporting communication among state and community levels. These liaisons attend local interagency coordinating council meetings, offering support and technical assistance to communities. The liaisons also can inform the state-level policymakers about the needs of the communities to develop more community-based service system policies.

The state's First Steps system has placed emphasis on interagency training for professionals and paraprofessionals. For example, First Steps coordinators were invited to participate in training conducted by Parents as Teachers, demonstrating a mutual respect and desire to understand one another's roles in serving families.

Related state departments are working toward developing strategies that would improve service integration for families of children with special needs. The state Maternal and Child Health Bureau, which serves a portion of the First Steps families, has set a goal to streamline the application process and information sharing by establishing a common statewide data management system related to health services. Software packages are being designed to facilitate state and local health information collection, analysis, and reporting of information needed for effective case management.

As in many states, Missouri has several entities working toward community building and collaboration for all families, including those with special needs children. For example, the Danforth Foundation is a philanthropic organization providing support to schools in their efforts to work effectively with families and community entities. Caring Communities is a statewide service integration effort to link the services of schools, neighborhoods and public agencies, and lends the necessary state support to communities. Missouri's child protection reform efforts also focus on encouraging communities to engage in collaborative efforts to protect children from abuse or neglect. The Family Investment Trust serves as the umbrella over these efforts, serving to connect and streamline the array of initiatives and committees underway and to reduce the barriers to changing systems.

ADDITIONAL COMMUNITY AND STATE PRACTICES

Although it is evident that communities play a pivotal role in developing systems of care to meet the needs of its citizens, states also play a role in facilitating this process. States can move toward decreasing some categorical restrictions in regard to eligibility requirements and they can create blended funding streams for state-wide programs. State-sponsored initiatives can offer financial incentives for collaborative community efforts, such as the Families Agencies, and Communities Together (FACT) Initiative in Utah described in Chapter 11.

Although the three priorities targeted in this chapter appear to be of central importance, other concerns warrant attention. The *affordability* of health care has risen to the forefront in the national arena. Children with disabilities or special health care needs or both often have inadequate insurance coverage, which places additional financial strains on their families. Adaptive equipment, respite care, home health care, and mental health services are examples of health-related needs that frequently are not covered adequately (New England SERVE, 1997). Families with incomes too high to qualify for Medicaid yet are unable to afford the premiums required by private insurance companies are particularly vulnerable. The new federally-supported State Children's Health Insurance Program (SCHIP) is helping to fill this gap for uninsured and underinsured children, yet this program does not provide health coverage for their parents. The Division of Serices for Children with Special Health Care Needs of the Maternal and Child Health Bureau lists health insurance as a key indicator of a system of care for children, which highlights the importance of this issue (McPherson & Roberts, 1997). Service integration efforts can help by encouraging parallel agencies and programs to blend their funds to cover unmet health care costs, ensuring consumer representation on interagency councils, and promoting consumer advocacy within managed care organizations.

A system of care should be *comprehensive* in the services it makes available to families. A comprehensive, quality system of care fosters mental health as well as physical health and development. Children with special needs often require psychological services to address emotional/behavioral problems. Infant mental health has been gaining recognition as a concept. However, those with expertise in this model are still relatively rare and thus not typically found in early intervention systems. Meeting the needs of a child with disabilities can be stressful for parents and siblings, ultimately affecting the parent-child relationship, growth, and development of the child (Kysela, McDonald, Reddon, & Gobeil-Dwyer, 1988). Although family counseling is one of 14 required services listed in the Part C legislation (sec. 632, P.L. 105-17) it is one of the least likely to be included on an IFSP and is rarely paid for with Part C funds. Communities need to ensure that mental health providers are included in service integration efforts, such as including them as participants on local interagency coordinating councils. In addition to mental health representation on state interagency coordinating councils, states can ensure that community-level providers are aware of the inclusion of mental health as an early intervention service and facilitate interagency agreements to cover these services when needed.

Coordination of early intervention with physicians is often reported by both parents and providers as a weak link. In many communities, broad-based physician awareness of early intervention programs is lacking. As reported by families and early intervention providers, many children are not screened by their health care providers to detect potential delays (Behl, Akers, & Roberts, 1997). Through the promotion of the medical/health home concept (American Academy of Pediatrics [AAP], 1995), pediatricians are being called upon to play an integral role in monitoring the overall development and to ensure that coordinated, comprehensive care occurs for children, especially those with special health care needs and disabilities. Another AAP-supported effort is Community Access to Child Health (CATCH), which is funded by Wyeth-Lederle Vaccines and the AAP Friends of Children Fund. This project exemplifies community-based efforts to build collaborative partnerships among pediatricians and communities to increase children's access to medical homes and to specific health services not otherwise available. Likewise, early intervention systems must learn how to involve and inform medical personnel in a more collaborative manner, developing strategies to insure physician involvement in meeting the needs of the child and family. Indiana's Part C program, for example, pays physicians to attend IFSP meetings. Many states, such as Florida, have medical residency training components that focus on serving children with disabilities. Such efforts often include parents of children with disabilities as trainers, providing a truly family-centered intervention perspective.

A fundamental component in the development of family-centered, coordinated, community-based care is consumer involvement (i.e., the inclusion of parents of children with special needs as active decision makers in all levels of the early intervention system). At the family level, the strengths, concerns, and priorities of the family should drive intervention plans. Parental input is valued in parallel with other team members in regard to the child's needs. The ecology of the family and family strengths should guide the development of the intervention plan. At community and state systems levels, families must be represented strongly on local interagency councils and advisory boards. As mentioned earlier, parents hired as staff are now being seen as an untapped resource, particularly in the training of service providers and other families.

EVALUATION EFFORTS

As stated earlier, service integration efforts should result not only in a more efficient system but also result in improved outcomes for children and families. The current imperative for coordinated early intervention service systems has far surpassed the methodology for understanding the effects of such efforts, particularly in terms of enhancing the development of the child and family well-being. Although several states are currently conducting evaluations of their early intervention systems (Roberts, Innocenti, & Goetze, 1999), these evaluations have fallen short of defining outcomes beyond child development indices or general family satisfaction. Based on attempts to measure outcomes in terms of standardized test scores for children with disabilities, we now know that such indicators are not sensitive enough to changes in child growth and development; these types of scores are not likely to show change among those with permanent disabilities. Early intervention, therefore, should not be defined in terms of "curing" children with disabilities, but rather, it should be defined in terms of enhancing the development and well-being of children, particularly in terms of enhancing the capacity of families to enjoy their children and to meet their needs. Although evaluations have included family satisfaction with services as an outcome, the methodologies generally have not been sensitive to nuances in interventions (McWilliam, Tocci, & Harbin, 1995; White, 1990). Current research efforts are looking at family well-being in terms of the family's ability to use formal and informal resources and supports, to effectively participate in determining intervention plans, and by their successful adaptation of their every day tasks needed to function successfully as a family. This is the current challenge early intervention systems face—to translate service integration efforts into improved outcomes in terms of child and family well-being. As communities work toward evaluating these outcomes, it will be essential to include families not only as the subjects of the evaluations but as the developers of the measures and methods.

SUMMARY

This chapter focused on three priorities voiced by parents of children with special needs: (a) improved access to services, (b) improved coordination, and (c) improved support for family well-being. Community case studies described how two communities attempted to integrate their services in a manner that reflects a family-centered, community-based approach. By no means do these scenarios represent an exhaustive list of successful strategies. Rather, they serve to demonstrate the ways communities can support the development of family-centered early intervention systems.

Communities and states must value the voices of families and recognize their importance in guiding the development of integrated early intervention systems. Service coordination, community-based care, and a seamless system support integrated services are important, but the key is a partnership that maximizes family involvement and participation in making decisions critical to their children's lives (Roberts, Rule, & Innocenti,1998). Early intervention as a system of care has this foundation in its legislation; it is now the responsibility of communities and states administering this legislation to develop the policies and practices to carry out its mission, supporting child and family well being.

REFERENCES

Able-Boone, H., Goodwin, L. D., Sandall, S. R., Gordon, N., Martin, D. G. (1992). Consumer based early intervention services. *Journal of Early Intervention,16*, 201-209.

American Academy of Pediatrics (1995). *The medical home and early intervention*. Elk Grove, IL: The Medical Home Program for Children with Special Needs.

Behl, D. D., Akers, A. L., & Roberts, R. N. (1997, Oct.). Addressing parent priorities through state-level policies. *Infants and Young Children, 10*(2), 36-45.

Center for the Study of Social Policy (1991). *Leveraging dollars, leveraging change: Refinancing and restructuring children's services in five sites*. Washington, DC: Center for the Study of Social Policy.

Gallimore, R., Weisner, T. S., Guthrie, D., Bernheimer, L. P., & Nihira, K. (1993). Family responses to young children with developmental delays: Accommodation activity in ecological and cultural contexts. *American Journal on Mental Retardation, 98*(2), 185-206.

Halpern, R. (1991). Supportive services for families in poverty: Dilemmas of reform. *Social Service Review*; *65*(3), 343-364.

Himmelman, A. T. (1992). *Communities working collaboratively for a change*. The Hubert Humphrey Institute of Public Affairs, University of Minnesota.

Individuals with Disabilities Education Act (IDEA) of 1990, PL 101-476, 20 U.S.C. § 1400 *et seq*.

Individuals with Disabilities Education Act Amendments of 1997, PL 105-17. 20 U.S.C. § 1400 *et seq*.

Kagan, S. L., Goffin, S. G., Golub, S. A., & Pritchard, E. (1995). *Toward systemic reform: Service integration for young children and their families*. Falls Church, VA: National Center for Service Integration.

Kahn, A. J., & Kamerman, S. B. (1992). *Integrating services integration: An overview of initiatives, issues, and possibilities*. New York: National Center for Children in Poverty.

Kysela, G. M., McDonald, L., Reddon, J., & Gobeil-Dwyer, F. (1988). Stress and supports to families with a handicapped child. In K. Marfo (Ed), *Parent-child interaction and developmental disabilities: Theory, research, and intervention* (pp. 273-289). New York: Praeger.

Mahoney, G., & Filer, J. (1996). Family service activities in early intervention: How responsive is early intervention to the priorities and needs of families? *Topics in Early Childhood Special Education, 16*(4), 437-457.

McPherson, M., & Roberts, R. N. (1997). *National Agenda for Children with Special Health Care Needs.* Technical paper, Maternal and Child Health Bureau, Division for Children with Special Health Care Needs, Rockville, MD.

McWilliam, R. A., Tocci, L., Harbin, G. (1995). *Services are child-oriented and families like it that way-but why?* Unpublished manuscript, Early Childhood Research Institute, University of North Carolina, Chapel Hill, NC.

Melaville, A. I., Blank, M. J., & Asayesh, G. (1993). *Together we can: A guide to crafting community-based family-centered strategies for integrating education and human services*. Washington, DC: U.S. Department of Education, Office of Educational Research and Improvement and U.S. Department of Health and Human Services.

National Early Childhood Technical Assistance System (NEC*TAS) (1995). *Helping our nation's infants and toddlers with disabilities and their families* (Office of Special Education Contract No. HS-91-01-1001). Chapel Hill, NC: Author.

New England SERVE (1997). *Assessing the quality of managed care for children with special health care needs: Summary of a regional survey of families, primary care providers & managed care organizations in New England*. Boston: Massachusetts Health Research Institute.

Ooms, T., & Owen, T. (1992). *Coordination, collaboration, integration: Strategies for serving families more effectively: Part two: State and local initiatives*. Washington, DC: AAMFT Research and Education Foundation, Family Impact Seminar (FIS).

Roberts, R. N., Akers, A. L., & Behl, D. D. (1996). Family-level service coordination within home visiting programs. *Topics in Early Childhood Special Education, 16*, 279-301.

Roberts, R. N., Akers, A. L., & Behl, D. D. (1997). *Best practices home visiting integration for early intervention* (Annual Report for Opening Doors, Grant #MCJ-495091). Logan, UT: Early Intervention Research Institute, Utah State University.

Roberts, R. N., Innocenti, M. S., & Goetze, L. D. (1999). Emerging issues from state level evaluations of early intervention programs. *Journal of Early Intervention, 22*(2), 152-163.

Roberts, R. N., Rule, S., & Innocenti, M. S. (1998). *Strengthening the family professional partnership in services for young children.* Baltimore, MD: Brookes.

Roberts, R. N., & Wasik, B. H. (1990). Home visiting programs for families with children birth to three: Results of a national survey. *Journal of Early Intervention, 14*, 274-284.

Trohanis, P. C. (1998). Changes through implementation of IDEA. In L. J. Johnson, R. J. Gallagher, M. J. LaMontagne, J B. Jordan, J. J. Gallagher, P. L. Hutinger, & M. B. Karnes (Eds.), *Meeting early intervention challenges: Issues from birth to three* (pp. 217-233). Baltimore: Brookes.

Wasik, B. H., & Roberts, R. N. (1994). Home visitor characteristics, training, and supervision: Results of a national survey. *Family Relations, 43*, 336-341.

Weisner, T. S. (1984). Ecocultural niches of middle childhood: A cross-cultural perspective. In W. A. Collins (Ed.), *Development during middle childhood: The years from six to twelve* (pp. 335-339). Washington, DC: National Academy Press.

White, K. R. (1990). *Final report for project period October 1, 1985 - December 31, 1990 of the Longitudinal Studies of the Effects and Costs of Early Intervention for Handicapped Children*. Logan, UT: Early Intervention Research Institute, Utah State University.

chapter 11

Community Efforts to Counter the Environmental Risks Children Face

Glenna C. Boyce
Diane D. Behl
Early Intervention Research Institute

Therese R. Johnson
Department of Human Services, Salt Lake City, Utah

The daily TV news as well as papers report that all is not well for many children in our society. One expert summarizes the concerns:

> More than one third of children in America do not enjoy good health, one fourth are raised in poverty, and an alarming number are inadequately educated and experience social and psychological distress. In the midst of plenty and progress, children in the United States are being robbed of childhood and its joys—the joy of learning, the joy of trust, and the joy of innocence....These statistics are documented in our scientific literature, with trends indicating that childhood problems, disorders, and maladjustments are increasing at an alarming rate. (Simeonsson, 1994, p. 4)

Yes, many of our children experience adverse environmental conditions in their homes or neighborhoods to the degree that they are at risk for poor health, developmental delay, psychological problems, and behavioral maladjustments. A number of risk factors that are associated with poor outcomes have been identified. Being poor is viewed as the primary risk. However, other family conditions, including chronic health and mental health problems, unemployment, illiteracy, drug and alcohol abuse, teenage child-bearing, single-parent households, limited proficiency in English, inadequate housing, and living in violent neighborhoods are also seen as "red flags." None of these circumstances necessarily result in developmental problems for children, but their presence, particularly in aggregation, is associated with subsequent developmental problems for children (Brooks-Gunn & Duncan, 1997; Masten & Coatsworth; 1998; Sameroff, Seifer, Baldwin, & Baldwin, 1993).

Who are the children who are "at risk" for developmental delay? Let us introduce several (names have been changed, to protect their anonymity).

> Barbara and her family including a father, mother and older brother moved to an urban area from a very rural area in a neighboring state. The family is living with relatives while they look for work. Barbara attends kindergarten sporadically. Her clothes are dirty and she is generally unkempt. She constantly has a runny nose and a cough. Her mother doesn't want to make her go to school when she cries. The older brother quit high school.

> Maria Rodriguez is a single mother raising two preschool-age daughters. She left an abusive marriage and she is faced with many stressors. She was not able to get child support for food and housing. Additionally, she feels frustrated in her efforts to get her daughters to mind her.

> Melanie and Jordan Truman are teenagers who lost their mother to cancer. Their father has a history of severe depression and struggles to maintain a job. Melanie and Jordan have been separated and shuffled from one relative's home to another. Both children have attempted suicide and have had psychotic episodes. With neither their father nor relatives equipped to deal with their needs, the children need full-time residential treatment.

> Jim, a second grader, is the fourth of seven children in the family. The family lives in a mobile home with rooms added on. The family's annual income is about $12,500. The stepfather works long hours to support the family. The mother tends other children in the home. Jim comes to school dirty and smelly. He gets very angry and aggressive at school. He wets and soils his pants when upset; his academic skills are very delayed.

> Emilia is a two-month-old infant. Her mother, Anna, is single and has recently moved from another state. Anna, Emilia, and Emilia's two brothers share an apartment with other relatives. Anna does not speak English and has had difficulty getting connected with needed services. Anna wants to get a job but cannot find affordable childcare. Her relatives see Anna and her family as a burden and would like to have her move out as soon as possible.

Children cannot counter the risk factors that may be present within the family or the larger neighborhood and community contexts by themselves. They need help. Likewise, the problems are often too great for families to solve on their own; they need assistance in understanding and accessing community resources and supports.

To this end multiple programs to help such children and families have been established by governments and groups at the federal, state, and community levels. Some programs have focused on certain risks (e.g., teenage mothers or drug users); others have focused on children who appear to be headed toward significant health, academic, or emotional-behavioral problems. The nay-sayers have been quick to point to "failures" and expense involved in many of these programs. In truth, all programs have not resulted in significant changes for children and families. However, such program efforts appear to be most successful when professionals across different agencies and interested citizens join with families to support the growth and development of children. One such success story was recently told to the first author by a university student who related her own family's experience of receiving coordinated services from such a team.

> This mother of five children had children attending school that was involved with a team of service providers, from the school and health, mental health, social work, work forces services agencies. Upon the recommendation of the school counselor, she and her family became involved. She reported that before she and her family were in the project, she felt she had no control over her children; she and her husband did not get along; her house was dirty; and she felt all was hopeless. She and her family received home visits, counseling, and other services over a period of two years. There were ups and downs with the services providers over that time, but through the experience she felt the program had "saved" her and her family—primarily in two ways. They helped her realize her own strengths and abilities—that she could effectively guide her children and maintain her household. Second, they taught her about the services available in the community and how to access them. Now she is enrolled in college; her marriage is succeeding and the children are doing better in school.

As was said prior to this example, programs are more likely to be successful when professionals across different agencies and interested citizens join with families to support the growth and development of children. How the personnel interact across agencies and with families, as well as how the state supports local efforts is crucial for positive outcomes for children and families.

Therefore, the purpose of this chapter is to highlight the community and state strategies necessary to integrate services for young children and their families who live in ecologically high risk environments. First, to set the stage for this discussion, the many types of risk factors that are associated with delays in children's development are reviewed to demonstrate the need for a continuum of services that include a wide variety of supports. Second, an historical overview of the efforts to integrate service systems is briefly outlined to delineate the strategies identified in the literature that appear crucial for success. Third, a case study, the community-statewide partnership initiative in the state of Utah, know as Families, Agencies, Communities Together (FACT), is presented. The strategies that have evolved at the state and community levels over the last ten years are discussed in order to assist others in their collaboration efforts. This discussion will include examples of a community site-based project and a local interagency council. Finally, a discussion of the issues that are still being faced and the direction the state's collaborative efforts are taking in the future, as well as a summary of the strategies necessary for success are presented. The authors of the chapter have been involved in the state FACT initiative over a number of years, either as evaluators or state level personnel.

RISK FACTORS

All children have certain basic developmental needs that include "sense of safety and structure, of belonging and membership, of self-worth, of independence and control over one's life, of closeness and participation in relationships, and of competency" (Pittman, 1991, as cited in Chaskin & Richman, 1992, p. 109). These needs are very similar to those identified by Maslow that were discussed in Chapter 2. Typically, these needs are met as children grow and develop within their ecocultural niche consisting of their families, peers, and neighborhoods. But, as was stated earlier, there are certain environmental factors that can disrupt children's development, resulting in health, learning, and/or behavioral problems.

The primary risk factor facing large groups of children is poverty. Since 1981, one in five American children (12-14 million) live in families whose income failed to exceed official poverty thresholds ("America's Children," 1998; Children's Defense Fund, 1997). Research has demonstrated that family income has selective, but sometimes quite substantial, effects on child and adolescent well-being. Poor children and adolescents show higher incidences of such things as growth stunting, lead poisoning, learning disabilities, grade repetition, school dropout, out of wedlock births, reported cases of child abuse, and experiences of violent crime (Brooks-Gunn & Duncan, 1997). Other familial risk factors that have been identified include mentally ill parents (Rutter, 1985), negative family interactions (Garmezy, Masten, & Tellegen, 1984), alcoholic parents (Werner, 1986), and mothers prone to child abuse (Farber & Egeland, 1987).

Research has also demonstrated that children are at greater risk when environmental risk factors accumulate (Rutter, 1979). For example, Sameroff, Seifer, Baldwin, and Baldwin (1993) assessed the cumulative effect of ten risk factors including (a) mother's behavior, (b) developmental beliefs, (c) anxiety, (d) mental health, (e) educational attainment, (f) family social support, (g) size, (h) major stressful life events, (i) occupation of head of household, and (j) disadvantaged minority status, and found that the total amount of risk present explained much of the variance in IQ scores at ages 4 and 13 and predicted IQ longitudinally. The research demonstrates the need for communities to have a continuum of services to support children and their families who face multiple risks.

THE MOVEMENT TO INTEGRATE SERVICES

As children grow, they need a variety of human services, including (a) health, (b) education, and (c) a variety of social services (Morrill, 1992). The number and type of services needed depends on the type and severity of needs. Because families vary greatly in their unique combinations of strengths and needs, communities must be able to provide a continuum of services that range from prevention and support services to intensive interventions that address serious problems. Multiple services mandated and funded by different federal and state agencies are usually available within a community. Therefore, families often must deal with a number of service agencies to receive needed services.

The federal government initiated programs in the early 1960s to address the needs of children in low-income families as part of the "war on poverty." As programs multiplied at the local, state, and federal levels, the fragmentation of services for children and their families became increasingly apparent. As Kagan and associates put it, "It became clear that attempts to fix the puzzle simply by adding more disjointed pieces would only exacerbate service problems" (Kagan, Goffin, Golub, & Pritchard, 1995, p. 6). Therefore, the federal government encouraged the integration of services. As early as the in the 1960s, the federal government recognized the importance of coordinated planning and service delivery in human service programs (Melaville & Blank, 1991) and provided significant leadership since then for the service integration movement (Kagan et al., 1995). In the 1970s, federal initiatives set in motion a wave of community-based and state-wide service integration systems (Agranoff, 1991). The efforts to integrate services for young children and their families became increasingly prevalent in the 1990s. (For a more complete review of the federal leadership of service integration efforts, see Kagan et al., 1995.)

The movement to integrate service systems has been based primarily on the belief that fragmented systems are not able to respond in a timely, coordinated, and comprehensive manner to meet the multiple and interrelated needs of children and families (Melaville & Blank, 1991). Accordingly, the goal of service integration is to:

> increase the efficiency and effectiveness of systems providing human services, though infrastructural reform...and direct service reform,...[while] positively impacting human outcomes, enabling children and families to experience a higher quality of life. (Kagan et al., 1995, p. 12)

The acceptance of these beliefs has resulted in many efforts to integrate services through agency collaborations at the local, state and federal levels for children whose development appears to be at-risk. Certain strategies have been identified in the literature as being necessary for successful collaborative service delivery. The following strategies (adapted from Behrman, Larson, Gomby, Shiono, & Lewit, 1992) have been considered important by those who have guided the FACT collaborative efforts in the state of Utah: (a) The participating agencies have to change the way they deliver services to children and families and how they work with each other; (b) Services should be comprehensive and tailored to the diverse needs of individual children and families; (c) The planning and implementation of services should not be dominated by any one agency; (d) Each agency should redirect part of its current funding to support the new collaboration; (e) Parents and other family members should play a key role in the development and monitoring of the service efforts; (f) Data about services provided and costs should be collected; and (g) Continuation of community collaboration efforts needs support from the state.

The major portion of the chapter discusses how these strategies have evolved and have been implemented at the state and community levels over time. Also, the collaboration issues the communities are still facing, the directions the collaborative initiative is taking, as well as the lessons learned will be summarized. To begin this discussion, a brief historical overview of the state-wide initiative is given.

THE STATE OF UTAH COLLABORATIVE INITIATIVE

The Utah FACT (Families, Agencies, Communities Together) Initiative has focused efforts to integrate services at the state, communities, and family levels in Utah. FACT's mission statement evidences the commitment to the standards of coordinated, community-based, culturally competent, family-centered services. It reads:

> Families, agencies, and communities together will develop, promote and deliver child-focused, family-centered, community-based, and culturally competent services which improve the health, safety, education, and economic well-being of the children in Utah. (Utah Department of Health, 1995)

This initiative serves children from birth (in some instances prenatally) to age 18 and children with disabilities to age 21 who require appropriate and uniquely designed interventions to: (a) achieve literacy, (b) advance through the schools, (c) to achieve commensurate with their ability, and (d) participate in society in a meaningful way as competent, productive, caring, and responsive citizens (Utah House Bill 39, Utah Code Annotated 63-75-2, 1992). Services are focused on families, as well, in order to support their attempts to meet the needs of their children. The community-based FACT projects, including (a) site-based kindergarten through sixth grade projects based in elementary schools, (b) site-based projects focused on infants and young children, and (c) county-based local interagency councils (LICs) that serve children and youth with multiple and enduring needs, demonstrate a continuum of care ranging from prevention, to support, to intensive interventions. The three types of projects and the continuum of care provided across projects are illustrated in Figure 11.1. The FACT initiative started with a few site-based projects located in elementary schools in 1990 and has grown to 112 site-based projects that served 1,766 children (ages ranged from birth through elementary school age) and 25 LICs that served 737 children and youth in 1998 (Boyce & Behl, 1998).

Historical Perspective on FACT Interagency Collaboration and Evolution

In 1989, the Utah state legislature directed the CEO's of three departments, Health, Human Services and Education, to develop a plan that was, for that time period, radical and innovative. Each department director agreed to contribute $100,000 of state money toward a pilot project that would provide coordinated case management services to children at

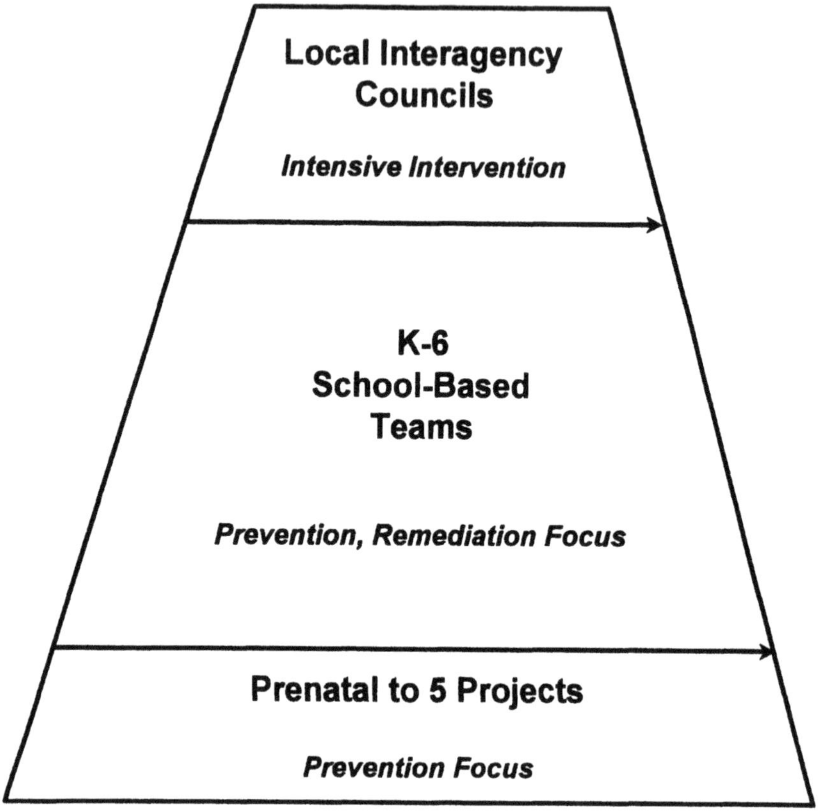

FIGURE 11.1. FACT service systems components.

risk. At that time, state governance structures were very categorical with each department (and even each agency within the department) providing services to clients using their own forms, assessment instruments, treatment models and protocols. Some of this was due to categorical and conflicting state and federal regulations; some was due to a business as usual attitude; and some was due to lack of creative leadership.

The 1989 agreement called for the identification of at-risk children who were receiving services from all three departments. Since this was a voluntary initiative, parents were asked to participate, and if they agreed, were enrolled in the program. Interdisciplinary teams of service providers were established at several elementary schools. Elementary schools were chosen because they were located within neighborhoods and were generally seen as being a neutral, non-threatening environment. The participating elementary schools were selected on the basis of having high populations of children who were low income and had low academic scores. The collaborative team consisted of personnel from the school; health, mental health, child, and family services; public assistance agencies; and a parent advocate. Upon referral, the teams conducted an assessment of the child and all family members. Assessing and serving all members of a family was a drastic change from the previous paradigm of providing services only to the family member who was referred. The family was viewed as an interdependent unit and the needs of all members had to be addressed in order to assist the child and help the family become self sufficient. A coordinated treatment plan was then developed. A single case manager was assigned to the family. The pilot project proved successful; the benefits reported by team and family members were a reduction in duplicated services (e.g., assessment and case managers), more holistic service plans, and a reduction in the amount of "red tape" for the family. The program came to be known as ACT, Agencies Coming Together, and provided prevention and remediation services to children from kindergarten to third grade.

With success came additional state funds allocated by the legislature and an opportunity to expand the program to more elementary schools. Predicated on the experiences reported from the pilot sites, it was determined that the program services must be delivered in a community-based, collaborative and family-centered manner. These components became the guiding principles of the initiative. This philosophy empowered local service delivery teams to provide services in new and innovative ways that would not have occurred under the traditional service system. As the initiative evolved, a stronger emphasis was made on family involvement in the identification of services. To publicly acknowledge the agencies' commitment to family involvement the word "families" was included in the name of the initiative (i.e., *Families*, Agencies, and Communities Together). A philosophy subcommittee was formed to formalize the mission and goals of the FACT initiative. The mission statement presented previously in the chapter was officially adopted in 1995. The components emphasized in the state's collaborative efforts included interagency composition of FACT teams, family involvement, private sector involvement, joint funding mechanisms, and the state-level organizations. These are discussed in the following paragraphs.

Interagency composition of FACT teams

Communities could participate in the FACT initiative by writing proposals for funding. Certain criteria had to be met in the proposals, but local communities were encouraged to write proposals that would meet the situations and needs of their community. First, the local community had to agree to support the FACT philosophy. Second, the five agencies (education, social services, public assistance, health, and mental health) had to be

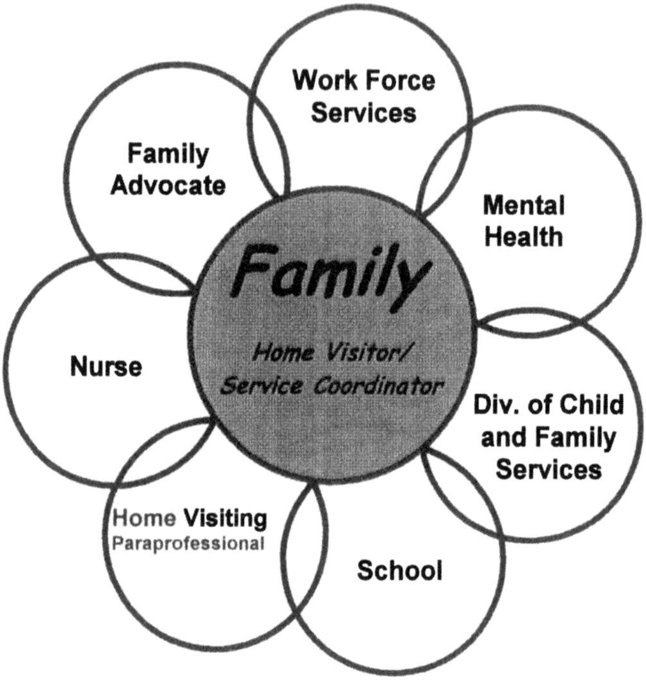

FIGURE 11.2. Site-based teams.

represented on the site-based team, but the team could be expanded to include other agencies or private organizations if that met the needs of the community. Services would be provided in the manner that best met the needs of the family. The composition of the FACT team with the focus on the family is illustrated in Figure 11.2. For instance, if a parent was ill, a case worker could go to the home for the interview and even assist the parent in locating needed documents, or a public assistance worker could take a client to the Social Security Office to obtain verification.

Family involvement

Requirements for FACT funding included involving parents in the development of the community's service plan and recruiting and training parent advocates to serve on the FACT team to help individual families through the assessment and service delivery process. Parents also played an integral role in the crafting and development of the initiative at the state and community levels. For example, when administrators began to fall back into a "business-as-usual" mode, parents effectively voiced their concerns. Parents also reminded staff, administrators, and legislators of the significant difference the program was making in their lives. Parents became the most effective advocates at the legislature and it was due largely to their efforts that additional funding was obtained. Parents and parent advocates involved in FACT acquired the courage to work with staff and identify the individual needs of their family members. This was sometimes a difficult transition for staff who were used to a system where professional staff "told" families what they needed. Under the traditional system, services had sometimes not been based on the needs of the family members, but upon the menu of services that the agency had available.

Private sector involvement in FACT

Concurrently, state representatives realized that the success of the initiative depended upon more than government entities. Government could not and would never be able to provide all of the resources that families needed to become self sufficient. Other partners were identified and requested to join in the initiative. Some of the key players included members of the business community, volunteers, and members of religious and civic organizations.

Funding mechanisms

At the state level, funding for the FACT initiative comes from an annual legislative appropriation of state general funds. These funds are then used in two ways. First, the funds are used to draw down federal funds for reimbursable case management services. Title IV-E and Title XIX funds are most frequently used. This increases the program budget and allows more families to be served. The program funds are also used to purchase goods and services for which federal funding cannot be used. Examples include car repair, noncovered medical bills, and housing deposits. These are labeled as "flexible funds" and each project area is allocated a set amount. The use of these funds is closely monitored to insure that they are spent on direct services rather than on administrative costs.

Each project area is given a yearly budget that breaks out the state funds, the federal funds and the flexible funds. A fiscal agent from each area is selected and her agency is then responsible for the disbursement of funds. A lesson learned early in the project is that the role of the fiscal agent must be clearly defined. The fiscal agent does not decide how the funds will be used, as this is the purview of the team; rather, the fiscal agent is the bill payer and contract monitor. The fiscal agent will also alert the team of potentially ineligible expenses.

At the local level, teams have been quite innovative in leveraging their funds in a manner that serves the greatest number of children. For instance, local communities work closely with businesses who regularly donate goods and cash for specific projects. They also work with religious and civic organizations, which provide untold numbers of volunteer hours. Often the collaborative efforts of the core service team leads to further collaboration with government and allied agencies that were not in the original FACT initiative. Many projects are realizing a greater degree of coordination with the inclusion of programs such as Head Start, community colleges, the 4H program and Extension services in their "teaming."

State-level organization and leadership

The FACT initiative is governed at the state level via a two tiered system. The enabling legislation mandated that a Council be established. The Council is comprised of the Executive Directors of the Department of Human Services, Health and Workforce Services,[1] the Superintendent of Public Education and the State Court Administrator. The statute further stipulates that the Council must meet at least quarterly and that all five of the individuals must be present for a quorum. The role of the Council is to take input from the State Steering Committee and the public and to provide direction and leadership to the initiative.

Also mandated in statute is a Steering Committee. This committee is comprised of state and local government officials, representatives of associations such as the PTA, Public Health Officers, parents and community representatives. The role of the Steering Committee is to assist the Council, monitor and solicit input for policy changes, provide technical assistance to the projects and make formal recommendations to the Council. The Steering Committee meets monthly and frequently establishes ad hoc committees to conduct research and make recommendations. Many local initiatives have chosen to model their local governance structures after the state system.

Professionals from the state agencies of education, human services, health, mental health, and welfare were chosen to serve as technical assistants for the community projects. Their role was to provide technical assistance and monitor the projects as to their compliance to the FACT philosophy and disbursement of funds. Statewide training meetings were held for project coordinators at which information such as the FACT philosophy, teaming concepts, and fiscal responsibilities were shared.

EXAMPLES OF FACT IN ACTION

In order for any service system effort to be successful, leaders must pay careful attention to the priorities of those they hope to serve. From

FACT families we learned which elements they considered the most important. They included (a) supportive relationship between provider and family, (b) easy access to help, (c) interventions that address family priorities rather than professional priorities, and (d) a continuum of services, offering various intensities of intervention, depending on need for support and remediation. An example of how these priorities are being addressed is featured in this description of how FACT operates in the west-central part of Salt Lake City. This community has a high Hispanic representation and a growing Vietnamese population; it is also one of the poorest sections of Salt Lake City. FACT is implemented via two primary infrastructures: the school-based project at Guadalupe School, and the Local Interagency Council (LIC). Together these projects demonstrate how FACT has been integrated into the existing infrastructure, expanding the continuum of services and support. The Guadalupe School will be highlighted first, followed by the LIC.

Site-Based Project: The Guadalupe School

The physical hub of an integrated service system must be one that is accepted in the community; the Guadalupe School represents such a site. A long-established and respected entity in the community, the Guadalupe School mission is to ensure that the children succeed in school. Originally established by the Catholic Church, the Center works as a public elementary school as well as a civic center for the community; 98 percent of children served are Hispanic. The school serves children from poor families (those eligible for free school lunch) and those who are at risk for educational delay. The center provides English as a Second Language (ESL) classes for adults, a home visiting program for infants and toddlers, a preschool program, and elementary school classes for grades kindergarten through three. Because of the supportive services it provides to the community, families do not feel the alienation that they might feel toward traditional schools as institutions. A FACT team was added to the preschool programs three years ago to improve services for those with more complex, multiple needs. This last year the FACT services were extended to the elementary grades.

Nurturing of healthy families via home visitors

Research suggests that the best interventions focus on nurturing general child development while also responding to specific problems/needs of individuals (Chaskin & Richman, 1992). This is the model followed by the Guadalupe home visitors (identified as parent educators) who serve families with children under 3 years of age. At Guadalupe home visiting, which has been documented as an effective way to reach families experiencing many challenges (Wasik & Roberts, 1994), serves multiple purposes, including child development, parenting training, parent support, and service coordination. Home visitors are most successful when they emphasize the strengths of the child and family, and truly listen to what the parent perceives as their needs (Bernstein, Hans, & Percansky, 1991). Focus group families described their parent educators (i.e, home visitors) as someone "who's easy to talk to," "who listens," "who cares about me as a person," "who makes me feel good about myself" (Boyce, Behl, & Price, 1998). This demonstrates that although a home visitor must be knowledgeable about the service system, the mechanism that brings about change is the personal trusting relationship program personnel establish with families (Larner, Halpern, & Harkavy, 1992). However, this can be a challenge for a home visitor who is working with families who have had negative experiences with agencies and are hesitant to trust someone new.

FACT team

The need to be able to procure additional resources for families was a major reason the Guadalupe pre-school program became one of the pilot site-based pre-school projects. The FACT team is comprised of a FACT preschool coordinator, public health nurse, a Division of Family Services worker, a mental health worker, a Work Force Services (welfare department) worker, and the Guadalupe Preschool Coordinator. A home visitor is included when the team is working with one of her assigned families. The FACT team augments the work of the home visitors by providing a broader continuum of services. For example, a family may have a child who demonstrates significant delays that are best addressed through the community Part C early intervention program (refer to Chapter 8 of this book for a description of Part C at the community level). Or, parents whose children are legal citizens but who do not have citizenship themselves may require additional support to access needed health care for their children. FACT teams are designed to meet such needs of families, providing enhanced communication, coordination and support from multiple agencies. The FACT team also provides a strong focus on well-childcare. The nurse from the health department can schedule childcare examinations, immunizations, and nutrition education; she also links families with affordable health services within the community.

The team obtains written parental permission for the home visitor to share referral information with needed agencies, particularly those on the FACT team. Usually the home visitor (who the family knows well) and the team member (who has been assigned to the family-based on the parent's report of needs) visit the family together. Often the FACT team member puts a service in place (e.g., discipline techniques) and the home visitor follows up weekly, with the FACT team member visiting less often.

Success can only be achieved if families want the services and view them as important. Home visitors are trained to address parental priorities first. Parents who were served through the Guadalupe project were interviewed, and they expressed their own personal growth and increased independence due to the continuum of care provided by the home visitor (Boyce, Behl, Akers, & Price, 1997; Boyce et al., 1998). Successful providers focus on empowering families, providing families with only as much help as they need (Wasik, Bryant, & Lyons, 1990). Families often have had negative experiences working with systems in the past or may not have the skills necessary to navigate the system on their own. For these families, a FACT team member may model a needed skill, such as calling for an appointment while the parent observes. The team member then works toward reversing this role, coaching the parent through the process and cheering her on as she learns to do for herself.

Understanding how to access services is a challenge for many families. Particular barriers preventing families from obtaining needed services typically include cultural/language barriers; distant location of services; mistrust of institutions; and citizenship status. Guadalupe home visitors or FACT team members help families overcome these barriers to services. Many personnel speak Spanish, or work closely with a translator. They also assist families with transportation to service agencies or bring the necessary application forms to families.

The Rodriguez story demonstrates how one FACT team worked. When Maria Rodriguez left her husband, she was struggling with raising two preschool-age daughters. As a young mother, she had little training in how to discipline appropriately or nurture growth and development. Also, Maria had added stressors associated with not having enough money for food and her apartment. Maria's home visitor recognized Maria's multiple needs, and she referred the Rodriguez family to the FACT team. Experience has demonstrated that when parents are invited to a FACT team meeting, they often feel outnumbered in a group of professionals. Therefore, the Guadalupe project has family advocates to support families during team meetings. A FACT team member was assigned to coordinate the interagency effort, and together the team connected Maria with needed financial support services and legal assistance for help in obtaining child support. The home visitor also worked closely with the social worker who provided parent training to Maria. As a result of this team effort, Maria felt more confident about her abilities as a parent and she suffered less stress as a result of the financial resources provided.

School-based program

The second tier of the triangle consists of the school-based projects. Located in elementary schools, FACT interagency teams work together to serve children and families identified as in need of resources and support. The focus of the school-based projects differs from the preschool projects in that it emphasizes school success, supporting children who are having academic, social, or health difficulties. Children involved in the school-based program are usually identified as candidates for FACT support by the classroom teacher, although parents may request participation. FACT teams meet with the child's teacher and family to discuss the child's needs in the context of the family. For example, Jim (described at the beginning of the chapter), was referred to the FACT team by his teacher who was frustrated with his poor attendance, acting out in class, and decreased interest in learning.

Although Jim was receiving resource room assistance for academics, his behavior was not being addressed. Based on conversations with Jim's mother, the team learned that Jim was acting out at home as well. Together, the team worked on helping Jim and his mother. The home visitor provided Jim's mother with some behavior management skills; Jim received social skills training in a small group at school to help him work on managing his own behavior; and the team used flexible funds to help Jim's mother obtain a washer so that Jim could come to school looking better.

One of the biggest challenges faced by the school-based FACT projects is overcoming multigenerational problems and attitudes. School-based teams have reported that it often takes several years for a family to solve their problems and be able to successfully support their children. For example, in the case of Barbara, the team first provided financial and material resources including shoes and clothes. Her father then found full-time work. Next the FACT team worked with her mother about Barbara's constant cough and nasal congestion, encouraging the parents to smoke outside. Barbara's health improved and she started coming to school in clean clothes with her hair curled. The home visitor also worked with the mother to counter her negative attitude and fear toward the school. At the time the mother was first interviewed, the family had been in the program almost two years and they had just attended their first family activity night at the school. Barbara's mother spoke of the activity in glowing terms, but it had taken a long time to get the family to one of the activities. A FACT team member tutored Barbara at school and her spelling papers and art work were displayed in the house. Later the FACT mental health team member convinced the mother that Barbara needed medication for ADHD. After that Barbara got along better with the other children and did better in her school work. Not all of the FACT team efforts were successful. Her mother and brother returned to school to get their general education degrees (GED), but they dropped out. When the mother was last interviewed, Barbara and her family had received FACT services for three years. Her mother was visiting with Barbara's teacher about Barbara's progress about once a week, instead of being afraid to speak to a teacher or principal. Barbara had just had friends over to a birthday party. Her father and brother were both employed full-time, and her mother had part-time employment.

Local Interagency Councils (LICs)

As mentioned earlier, the LICs represent the top of the FACT triangle, serving children and families with the most intensive needs that cannot be met through traditional service system or other FACT projects, such as the school-based efforts. The LIC team that services the central area of Salt Lake City is comprised of representatives from a broader range of agencies than the site-based FACT projects. Juvenile justice/truancy, mental health, residential treatment, and crisis intervention are strong participants in addition to the members found in the other FACT projects. Each LIC has a parent advocate to support families who are referred to the LIC. Typically, referrals are made to the LIC by one of the agency representatives after they have exhausted all sources of assistance through their usual channels. The families served by the LIC often represent those with serious behavioral/mental health problems, requiring intensive supports that are often very costly. The story of the Trumans is characteristic of a family served by an LIC.

Mr. Truman was a recently widowed father with a teenage son and daughter. Mr. Truman had a history of mental health disorders and had been receiving therapy for manic depression. His wife had been the sole financial support for the family. Following her death, Mr. Truman placed both children with relatives, which turned out to be emotionally abusive situations. After two years, both children had been returned to him; his son had committed serious acts of delinquency and violence and his daughter had attempted suicide. The Trumans were referred to the LIC by Mr. Truman's mental health provider to work toward achieving a coordinated, family-centered service plan. The LIC provided financial support for residential mental health care for the children paired with family therapy with Mr. Truman and his children. Additionally, the LIC connected Mr. Truman with Rehabilitation Services, which resulted in financial support for him to obtain a college degree in hopes of gaining employment. Given the volatile relationship between Mr. Truman and his children, a family preservation and support home visitor also worked with the family. LIC intervention with the Trumans was intensive and lengthy, which characterizes the majority of families served through this FACT component.

Although the LICs come together to address the needs of individual families and provide family-level service coordination, they also represent a movement toward systems-level service integration. These strategies involving the infrastructure reform are discussed in the next section.

COUNTY AND STATE SUPPORT FOR THE COMMUNITY'S EFFORTS

As described earlier in this chapter, the FACT initiative was created and initiated at the state level, and state-level policies were developed to support community efforts. When communities are given the authority to implement community-based solutions, creativity, energy and ownership are generated in a way that is typically not seen with the implementation of traditional state and local programs. This is not to say that state and federal entities do not retain a degree of stewardship and responsibility for the expenditure of state funds. But when programs become community driven, a state, federal and local partnership is formed. Communication becomes both bottom/up and top/down, which is needed to facilitate effective collaboration. These vertical integration supports, referring to integration among community, county, state, and federal levels, are depicted in the Central City example.

Community Autonomy

The first step in providing autonomy to communities within the FACT initiative was the state's invitation to school districts and other community-based programs such as the Guadalupe Center to participate in FACT by writing a proposal for the monies available. Certain requirements had to be met, such as having an interagency team to provide services, but they were encouraged to consider the needs and strengths of their families and community and devise projects that would work for them. For example, Central City has more cultural diversity than other areas of Utah. Accordingly, their proposed program took advantage of the available diversity by including a variety of cultures at the FACT table.

In addition, communities have been given autonomy to develop the infrastructure needed to ensure collaboration with key players. In the case of Central City, there is an additional support available via a county level FACT entity. Due to the size of the population and large number of key agency players, it was evident that collaboration at the county level would support the individual community efforts and avoid duplication of services in some instances. Therefore, they created a Salt Lake County FACT Policy Council that was parallel in function to the state FACT Council. This group consists of four school superintendents, parent representation in the form of a Parent Advocate and a PTA representative, and a representative from the United Way of Greater Salt Lake, the regional directors of participating agencies (including Division of Child and Family Services [DCFS], Valley Mental Health, Division of Services for Persons with Disabilities [DSPD], Health, Juvenile Justice, Division of Substance Abuse, and Work Force Services). Along with this Policy Council exists a Salt Lake County Steering Committee, which is similar to the State Steering Committee. This group is comprised of the middle managers of the agencies mentioned above, the Housing Authority, the four school district site-based coordinators and special education coordinators, and the county LIC coordinator. Both of these groups meet monthly to find ways to encourage community efforts to increase their service coordination and integration.

Blended Funding

Funds to support the FACT teams and family interventions are provided through state-designated interdepartmental funds from the Departments of Education, Health, and Human Services. These funds supplement the county and school district funds rather than draw upon the funds already in the community. These blended funds are a permanent line item in the state's budget and thus help ensure that this collaborative effort is institutionalized.

Public-Private Partnerships

The state FACT model has provided a structure for coordinating volunteers, business, religious groups, and private/nonprofit entities to come together. This prevents duplication of efforts from various subgroups and allows better leveraging of the community's resources. In Central City there are numerous agencies that work together. The Guadalupe School and the LIC are supported by the Children's Center, a private mental health provider in Utah. The FACT teams concentrate on ensuring that families are connected with other services that may be needed. For example, there is an agency serving teenage mothers specifically, which may be a better fit for some mothers than the Guadalupe project. The Guadalupe Center holds an annual auction, which is supported by contributions from the business community; thousands of dollars are raised annually thanks to this community support. In addition, United Way funds provide approximately 3 percent of the budget for Guadalupe.

Coordinated Application for Services

To expedite the receipt of services for families, FACT has facilitated exchange of information by accepting a multi-agency release of information form when helping connect families with state-funded programs, such as WIC. Additionally, all state-wide FACT forms are developed collaboratively among on-line workers (FACT team members), community administrators, and state-level staff. This has been critical to ensure that any forms developed are meaningful, functional and appropriate. These universal forms have provided a state-wide perspective on the number of types of families served, the needs of families, and the ability of the FACT communities to meet these needs.

CHALLENGES FACED BY FACT

As with all efforts to change the status quo, there were many lessons learned in regard to what works and what does not work in striving to integrate services to meet the needs of children and families facing multiple challenges. These challenges are discussed to demonstrate barriers that can arise and to share strategies for addressing these barriers. Many of these lessons learned were identified through the evaluation of FACT outcomes based on case study and focus group methodologies (Boyce et al., 1997, 1998).

Importance of Continuous Training

As demonstrated in the literature (Larner, Halpern, & Harkavy, 1992), training of providers and team members is a prerequisite to implementing a "new way of doing business," such as the FACT model. When FACT was initiated, there was a great deal of inservice training provided to policy makers as well as to direct service workers. Unfortunately, turnover in participants at the FACT table has made it difficult to ensure that all staff have the training needed to understand FACT's mission and its strategies. As with many projects, direct service providers and parents have been the ones who are left out of the loop, particularly in regard to the development of policies to support service integration. Collaboration among the direct service providers, families, and policy makers is needed to guide FACT as it evolves. In the case of FACT members at the Guadalupe School, the state level FACT technical assistants (TAs) played a key role in remediating the need for all staff to understand the common mission and approach of FACT. The TA's provided training for the FACT administrators as well as team members, emphasizing the importance of everyone's investment in the FACT philosophy and in ways to coordinate services. There was a need to train new FACT members in emphasizing coordination, shifting some time away from the traditional direct service mode.

Importance of Leadership

FACT's conception was due to a few key leaders from state-level departments who had a vision for a new way of doing business. However, it was sometimes difficult for other administrators, legislators, staff and allied agencies who were used to delivering categorical programs to understand the value of systems change and how it could be accomplished. State and federal administrators must rise to the challenge of letting go of some control for programs and be willing to let communities take the lead in establishing a system of service delivery that best meets the needs of their individual citizens. The top/down paradigm has been in effect for so long that it is incumbent upon state administrators to take a lead in this new endeavor. They must approach communities in an open and honest manner and must clearly articulate the overall goals, objectives and outcomes. They must be willing to assist communities in removing regulatory barriers that stand in the way of innovation. Fiscal barriers appear to be the most challenging to address. Although policy makers may be willing to share information and coordinate service delivery, they often remain territorial when it comes to coordinating funds. To continue the evolution toward service integration, leaders with vision must remain in place. FACT, like many other similar efforts, has been vulnerable to ebbs and flows in leadership, which has influenced the success of continued systems change. Yet the continued involvement of a few committed people maintains its presence.

Agency Professionals Who Can "Think Outside the Box"

Successful systems change is also dependent on the characteristics of the persons coming to the table. The director of the FACT project at the Guadalupe School described an important quality of a successful FACT team member as the ability to "think outside the box," meaning the ability to view her role beyond the limited agency job description and traditional bureaucracy. Successful team members base their efforts and policy making on the priorities of consumers rather than the priorities of the agency. According to the director of the Guadalupe School, the team members who have stayed with the project and enjoyed their jobs are the ones that are "self-starters," meaning that they are confident in their problem solving ability and initiate the action that needs to be taken rather than waiting to be told by the agency what to do next. This does not mean that good providers work "outside the system," disregarding regulations; rather, it means that those providers that are most successful are creative in meeting the needs of families within the confines of the system's regulations. These characteristics are equally as important for policy makers as they are for those who work directly with families.

Families as Key Players

The inclusion of families in the FACT system has been a gradual one. Because FACT family advocates serve on a voluntary basis, their active involvement often fluctuates. FACT state-level leaders are recognizing the need to have family advocates paid for their work, adding recognition to the value of their contribution. The consistent involvement of families and parent advocates is critical to ensure that the FACT model does not become provider driven. When family advocates have been included, they have typically been greatly under-represented. As emphasized by Roberts, Rule, and Innocenti (1998), true consumer involvement requires that consumers are confident in their representation. This requires that the ratio of professionals to consumers be balanced. This is particularly true for communities with under-represented populations. For example, the statewide evaluation revealed that those communities with relatively large Hispanic and Latino populations were not accessing the LICs (Boyce et al., 1997). Exploration of reasons for this and the identification of new outreach methods then became a focus of the FACT team.

FUTURE DIRECTIONS FOR FACT

Recognizing the success of the FACT method of service delivery versus the traditional system, state administrators are pursuing a policy change that would result in all services being provided in a "FACT-based" manner. The FACT philosophy would not be limited to communities proposing site-specific FACT programs for children and families. Rather, it would infuse the FACT philosophy and implementation strategies throughout the entire service delivery system. This is a paradigm shift from FACT as model programs to FACT as an applied, universal philosophy under which all services are delivered. The goal is to deliver services in a collaborative, family friendly manner. Communities will have responsibility for the development and administration of services that best highlight their strengths and address their individual needs. The state and the community will be partners in establishing and monitoring goals and outcomes. The intent of this legislation is to broaden the circle of those who are receiving the benefits of blended services. Thus, this change will have ramifications throughout the entire service delivery system.

SUMMARY

As stated in the introduction of this chapter, Utah's FACT initiative reflects the criteria necessary for a successful collaborative effort. These six criteria will be summarized below, emphasizing FACT's strengths and challenges.

1. *Participating agencies must change the way they do business.* As described in the history of FACT, there were leaders from key state departments that had the vision of "a new way of doing business." Thanks to the consistency in leadership over many years, FACT has been successfully implemented throughout the state. Transition and buy-in from the state to the communities was facilitated via training and technical assistance from the state-level leaders, yet it was not always clear sailing. Based on the FACT experience, it sometimes seems that everyone is in favor of collaboration until it infringes on their individual program. It is difficult to give up turf, and many conflicts have arisen with the implementation of this philosophy, particularly at the community level. Yet successes have been realized. Many local government officials and community leaders viewed the challenge of developing a new community-based service delivery system as positive. Since communities can be defined as geographical, ethnic and/or political units, by definition, each community has its own unique needs, organizations, and resources. Approaches and funding cannot come in a one-size-fits-all manner. It has taken many years, but the process has come full circle in Utah. State and federal authorities are recognizing what communities have known all along—problems must be defined and solved at the community level. Communities initially may be skeptical of a state-level effort to develop an integrated service system. This is after all a new way of doing business and few, if any, have had experience in developing local initiatives. To be ready to enter into this new partnership, the community must have local leaders with vision and a willingness to

take on the challenges of a new way of doing business. Even with this local leadership and enthusiasm, communities need assistance in developing systems of care to meet their needs. Success can be more readily achieved if communities have the support of the state-level policy makers not only in terms of technical assistance, but by modeling collaboration via changes in state policies and practices. Success can only be achieved with full involvement of families and other community members.

2. *Services should be comprehensive and tailored to the diverse needs of individual children and families.* FACT's success in improving child and family well-being has been linked to its ability to individualize services to meet the unique needs of families (Boyce et al., 1997, 1998). Although some FACT projects had some components that were offered to all children and families, such as home visiting, social skills groups, or parenting classes, the key component was individualized service plans. These service plans served as the method for ensuring the provision of comprehensive, coordinated services based on the needs of the individual children and families.
3. *The planning and implementation of services should not be dominated by any one agency.* At the state level, FACT has not been dominated by one agency; rather, there has been an equal partnership among the key agency leaders. This partnership is reflected at the community level as well. Although the FACT projects may be housed with one primary agency, such as the school, the school holds the same degree of authority as the other agency representatives at the table. However, there have been times when one agency has been viewed as the dominant leader. For example, many of the first local interagency councils (LICs) were organized by the mental health agencies in the communities. As a result, most of the children and families served by the LICs were referred by mental health, which resulted in the community's perception that the LICs existed to serve children with serious emotional disturbances, rather than a more heterogenous array of needs. This serves as an example of the importance of ensuring that one agency does not play so strong a role that those with other needs are not served.
4. *Each agency should redirect part of its current funding to support the new collaboration.* Ultimately, funding represents a strong infrastructural commitment to developing a sustainable service system. From its inception, FACT was based on blended funds contributed from the main state agencies. This resulted in strong agency buy-in from the start to develop a new way of doing business, and it quickly got communities on board who otherwise may not have participated without the additional financial support.

5. *Parents and other family members should play a key role in the development and monitoring of the collaborative effort.* As mentioned earlier, families are key players in the development of services to meet their own needs. The FACT initiative also reflects the importance of the role of families in the development of policies that drive the overall system. Parents, both independent and those representing organized parent groups, are members of the state-level steering committee. Community projects are required to have a family advocate on the FACT team. Unfortunately, family advocates do not have strong representation for two main reasons. First, they are not paid for their involvement as are their professional counterparts. Secondly, if one family advocate is overwhelmingly outnumbered by the professionals at the table, it can impact the family advocate's comfort level in taking a position on an issue, particularly if the position is different than that of the professionals. As has been learned through other efforts that have strived to be family-centered in their policymaking, it is important to have strong family representation at the table (Roberts et al., 1998) if the policy makers truly want family input to drive their efforts. It has been suggested that this should translate to one parent for each professional at the table. This also requires that family members be paid for their time, and that meetings are held at times that are convenient for families, and that childcare and transportation is supported if necessary.
6. *Collaborative efforts should collect data about services provided and costs.* FACT has required the collection of universal forms, which provides data on the types of services provided by each project. The costs of services is now being collected via expenditures of FACT-flexible funds. This has provided the FACT leaders and the community members with a basic overview of how their funds are being spent, which can help guide future budget decision-making. Yet true costs of services is much more difficult to capture. For example, some services or actual materials (e.g., wheelchairs, eyeglasses, therapeutic recreational activities) are donated by charitable organizations, and these funds expended are not recorded. Such cost studies are very time consuming and usually are only conducted by economists.

In sum, FACT is a realistic example of how state policies can support the development of community-based systems of care. Success can be more readily achieved if communities have the support of the state-level policy makers not only in terms of technical assistance, but by modeling collaboration via changes in state policies and practices. And this success can only be achieved by the establishment of partnerships with families and other community members. The lessons learned demonstrate that such efforts take a unified vision, perseverance, and continuous striving to improve the system to better serve the community.

NOTE

[1]The Department of Workforce Services began operation in January 1998. It combines public assistance programs, job training programs, and employment services.

REFERENCES

Agranoff, R. (1991). Human services integration: Past and present challenges in public administration. *Public Administration Review, 51*, 533-542.

America's children: Key national indicators of child well-being [Online]. (1998). Available: http://www.childstats.gov:80/ac1998/ac98.htm

Behrman, R. E., Larson, C. S., Gomby, D. S., Shiono, P. H., & Lewit, E. M. (1992). Analysis. *The Future Of Children, 2*, 6-18.

Bernstein, V. J., Hans, S. L., & Percansky, C. (1991). Advocating for the young child in need through strengthening the parent-child relationship. *Journal of Clinical Child Psychology, 20*, 28-41.

Boyce, G., & Behl, D. (1998). *Descriptive report of the general population of children and families served by the FACT initiative during fiscal year 1997*. Logan, UT: Early Intervention Research Institute, Utah State University.

Boyce, G. C., Behl, D. D., Akers, J. F., & Price, C. L. (1997). *Short-term evaluation of the impact of Utah's FACT projects*. Logan, UT: Early Intervention Research Institute, Utah State University.

Boyce, G. C., Behl, D. D., & Price, C. (1998). *Follow-up evaluation of the impact of Utah's FACT initiative*. Logan, UT: Early Intervention Research Institute, Utah State University.

Brooks-Gunn, J., & Duncan, G. J. (1997). The effects of poverty on children. *The Future of Children, 7*, 55-71.

Chaskin, R. J., & Richman, H. A. (1992). Concerns about school-linked services: Institution-based versus community-based models. *The Future of Children, 2*, 107-117.

Children's Defense Fund. (1997). *Big economic gains lift very few children out of poverty* [Online]. Available: http:///www.childrensdefense.org/release092997.html

Farber, E. A., & Egeland, B. (1987). Invulnerability among abused and neglected children. In E. J. Anthony & B. J. Cohler (Eds.), *The invulnerable child* (pp. 253-288). New York: The Guilford Press.

Garmezy, N., Masten, A. S., & Tellegen, A. (1984). The study of stress and competence in children: A building block for developmental psychopathology. *Child Development, 55*, 97-111.

Kagan, S. L., Goffin, S. G., Golub, S. A., & Pritchard, E. (1995). *Toward systemic reform: Service integration for young children and their families.* Falls Church, VA: National Center for Service Integration.

Larner, M., Halpern, R., & Harkavy, O. (1992). The fair start story: An overview. In M. Larner, R. Halpern, & O. Harkavy (Eds.), *Fair start for children: Lessons learned from seven demonstration projects* (pp. 3-19). Binghamton, NY: Vail-Ballou.

Masten, A., & Coatsworth, J. D. (1998). The development of competence in favorable and unfavorable environments. *American Psychologist, 53,* 205-220.

Melaville, A., & Blank, M. J. (1991). *What it takes: Structuring interagency partnerships to connect children and families with comprehensive services*. Washington, DC: Education and Human Services Consortium.

Morrill, W. A. (1992). Overview of service delivery to children. *The Future of Children, 2,* 32-43.

Roberts, R. N., Rule, S., & Innocenti, M. S. (1998). *Strengthening the family-professional partnership in services for young children*. Baltimore, MD: Brookes.

Rutter, M. (1979). Protective factors in children's responses to stress and disadvantage. In M. W. Kent & J. E. Rolf (Eds.), *Primary prevention of psychopathology, Vol. III - Social competence in children* (pp. 49-74). Hanover, NH: University Press of New England.

Rutter, M. (1985). Resilience in the face of adversity: Protective factors and resistance to psychiatric disorder. *British Journal of Psychiatry, 147*, 598-611.

Sameroff, A. J., Seifer, R., Baldwin, A., & Baldwin, C. (1993). Stability of intelligence from preschool to adolescence: The influence of social and family risk factors. *Child Development, 64,* 80-97.

Simeonsson, R. J. (1994). Promoting children's health, education, and well-being. In R. J. Simeonsson (Ed.), *Risk, resilience, and prevention: promoting the well-being of all children* (pp. 3-12). Baltimore, MD: Brookes.

Utah Department of Health, Utah Department of Human Services, Utah State Office of Education, & Utah Administrative Office of the Courts. (1995). *FACT: Families, agencies, & communities together.* (Mission statement, available from the FACT Steering Committee, 120 North 200 West, Room 319, Salt Lake City, UT 84145)

Utah House Bill 39, Utah Code Annotated 63-75-2, Coordinated Services for Children At Risk (1992).

Wasik, B. H., Bryant, D., & Lyons, C. (1990). *Home visiting: Procedures for helping families*. Newbury Park, CA: Sage.

Wasik, B. H., & Roberts, R. N. (1994). Home visitor characteristics, training, and supervision: Results of a national survey. *Family Relations, 43,* 336-342.

Werner, E. (1986). Resilient offspring of alcoholics: A longitudinal study from birth to age 18. *Journal of Studies on Alcohol, 44,* 34-40.

chapter 12

A Community-Based Approach to Preventing Child Maltreatment

Sharon Carnahan
Rollins College

Carnot E. Nelson
Thomas R. Gordon
University of South Florida

INTRODUCTION

Children have the fundamental right to grow and develop in a family where they are nurtured, rather than neglected, and affirmed, rather than abused. Community-level programs aimed at the primary prevention of child maltreatment seek to secure this right for every child. Though these issues are not new, and our efforts at helping families deal with the issues of abuse and neglect are as old as social services programs themselves, the renewed interest in prevention rather than rehabilitation has been rapidly growing throughout the country. As one response to this concern, in 1991 the U.S. National Advisory Board on Child Abuse and Neglect recommended the implementation of a national system of neonatal home visiting and support to prevent physical child abuse and neglect (Guterman, 1997). In 1992, the National Committee to Prevent Child Abuse (NCPCA), in partnership with the Ronald McDonald House Charities, began a major effort to encourage the prevention of child maltreatment before it occurs, rather than to restrict intervention efforts to the prevention of recurrence. This emphasis on primary prevention was based on the success of the Hawaii Healthy Start system of home visitation and support for new parents who were judged to be at risk for child abuse and neglect (Center on Child Prevention Research, 1996; Mitchel & Cohn Donnelly, 1993). The Healthy Families America initiative now has more than 250 sites in all states and the District of Columbia. This chapter concerns the rationale for a community-based approach to the prevention of child maltreatment, implementation of this model in two communities in Florida, the results these sites have obtained, and the lessons learned in the process. A special emphasis is placed on the history of the community integration of services within these programs.

DEFINING CHILD MALTREATMENT

Although the definitions of child maltreatment remain controversial, child neglect is generally defined as an act of omission committed by parents or caregivers that results in harm or endangerment of children or the failure to meet a child's most fundamental physical needs, whether physical, emotional, educational, or medical. Child abuse is defined as an act of commission that results in physical harm to children; depending on the definition, this harm may have been intentional or unintentional (Knutson, 1995). Research indicates that neglect and abuse may have different precursors. For example, the incidence of neglect is strongly associated with family poverty and neighborhood risk factors, while child abuse is more strongly associated with parental factors, such as a lifetime history of affective disorders (Egami, Ford, Greenfield, & Crum, 1996). In addition, sexual abuse is generally viewed to be etiologically distinct from other forms of abuse, and harder to predict and prevent. One form of abuse is often accompanied by another (Ney, Fung, & Wickett, 1994). Most prevention programs are aimed at both abuse and neglect; this mixed approach leads successful interventions to simultaneously target factors within the parent, within the family and child, and within the community.

Effects of Maltreatment on Children

The effects of child maltreatment on development vary widely. Sequelae depend on the transactional nature of the abuse: its frequency, severity and duration; the timing, especially the developmental level of the child at the time of the abuse and at the time when effects are measured; whether the abuse event was perceived as traumatic by the child; and the prior and subsequent life events surrounding the abuse, including the influence of protective or buffering factors. These protective factors may include the presence of naturally occurring social supports such as a community, school, or church, which aids children in their recovery from trauma; more often, the ecological context is bleak, and includes neighborhoods plagued by violence and poverty. Thus, to paraphrase psychiatrist D.W. Winnicott, there is no such thing as just a child: there is always a child with a parent and a family, existing in a community, surrounded by a culture (Winnicott, 1996).

We do know that maltreatment affects a child's future in multiple domains. These can include developmental regression and delay, especially communication disorders (Katz, 1992); disturbances in the attachment relationship, including disorders of attachment; disturbances in personality development, including a poorly developed self concept or lowered self-esteem; and deteriorating school performance (Blount, 1992). Maltreated children are also at increased risk for the extremes of risk-seeking or risk-avoiding behaviors, and long-term damage to their mechanisms of self-regulation and arousal modulation have been hypothesized (Cicchetti, Barnett, Rabideau & Toth, 1991).

Who Is at Risk?

The community-based approach to prevention posits that families at increased risk for child maltreatment can be identified before the fact by a combination of demographic, community, and family history predictors, and that this approach is more effective than one that relies on identifying potential abusers through personality characteristics or personal history alone. The transgenerational assumption of child abuse, very popular in the public forum, has been that the experience of abuse predisposes one to abuse one's own children. This assumption is widely questioned. It is clear that most abused children do not grow up to be abusers, but that an abuse history in parents, as well as a history of alcoholism, anxiety disorders, or other psychiatric problems, increases the likelihood that the parent will be a perpetrator of future abuse (Egami et al., 1996; Knutson, 1995). Severe neglect remains the most common form of maltreatment, and all nonsexual forms of abuse are statistically linked more closely to poverty than to any other single factor (Besharov & Dembosky, 1997).

Based on reports such as the Third National Incidence Study of Child Abuse and Neglect (NIS-3) (Sedlak & Broadhurst, 1996), it is possible to identify factors that increase the likelihood that child maltreatment will occur. First, the NIS-3 found *no significant race differences* in the incidence of child abuse and neglect. The findings suggest that the disproportionate number of minority children in child protective and welfare services is the result of "differential attention somewhere during the process of referral, investigation and service allocation ... (not) inherent differences in the rates at which they are abused and neglected..." (p. 7).

Next, there are *age differences* in the incidence of abuse. A greater proportion of neglect victims were less than eight years old, while a greater proportion of physical, sexual and emotional neglect victims were older. This may reflect differential surveillance; children less than five do not come into contact with professionals as frequently as older children, and NIS-3 reports that nearly two-thirds of the substantiated reports in this study came from professionals (Sedlak & Broadhurst, 1996).

Child maltreatment is also predicted by *family status*. Family *income* is the strongest single predictor of an incidence in nearly all categories of child maltreatment. Children from the lowest income strata in the NIS-3 study were more than 22 times more likely to experience maltreatment, and 40 times more likely to experience neglect. *Children of single parents* had a 77 percent greater risk of physical abuse, an 87 percent greater risk of neglect, and an 80 percent greater risk of suffering serious harm, than did children in two parent homes, independent of income status. Maternal drug use, while not systematically studied, was frequently noted in maltreatment cases. Sedlak and Broadhurst (1996) contend that these results cannot be explained on the basis of the higher visibility of low income families in the welfare system; to equalize these numbers across income levels, nearly four million cases of substantiated maltreatment would have to exist in middle and upper income groups, and go completely undetected (p.11).

Certain *community factors* are common in areas of the country where increased maltreatment is seen. In one study, factors that explained nearly half the variance in rates of child maltreatment, violent crime, and juvenile delinquency included impoverishment, geographic and economic isolation, population instability (frequency of moves), and "childcare burden," the ratio of children to adults in a community (Korbin & Coulton, 1996). These factors, taken together, may result in a cumulative risk (Sameroff & Fiese, 1990) leading to a breakdown of the family, which can no longer provide a minimally adequate environment for a child's safety and development.

The influence of community risk factors has strong implications for interpreting the results of Healthy Families and other interventions. Suppose, for example, that we worked with mothers in a high-risk community, characterized by geographic and economic isolation, poor public transportation, and therefore poor access to health care. As part of the Healthy Families America intervention, transportation to the health clinic would be provided and the program, therefore, would lead to improved rates of immunization, utilization of a medical home, access to contraceptives, and prevention of repeat pregnancies. However, community risk factors such as levels of unemployment, housing shortages, crowding, and drug abuse could not be directly affected by the home visiting program and could be so high in the community that the program was unable to have any effect on rates of child maltreatment. As this example illustrates, evaluations of the success of child maltreatment prevention programs must also consider ecological, community-based factors, as well as changes in individual family functioning (Rauh & Brown, 1996). Thus, as this chapter will discuss, isolated child abuse prevention programs may be doomed by the enormity of challenges facing high-risk families. Approaches that integrate multifaceted solutions in a coordinated way may be more likely to achieve the desired outcomes.

THEORETICAL RATIONALE FOR A PREVENTION APPROACH TO MALTREATMENT

The identification of families at risk for child maltreatment has followed a framework based on an integration of psychoanalytic, learning, and environmental theories, and ecological models of human development (Daro, 1993). Screening to identify families at risk has sought to find parents who came from high risk communities, and were themselves abused, lacked social support, or were otherwise isolated. Learning theory approaches suggest that parents would not abuse their children if they knew how better to care for them. Environmental and ecological approaches focus on making resources available to parents to compensate for shortcomings in areas such as financial support or job training (Daro, 1983).

The theoretical rationale for the prevention approach to child maltreatment within the Healthy Families America model is straightforward and simple (Daro & McCurdy, 1994). Child abuse is seen as the result of a predictable series of events, and early intervention can prevent these events from occurring in at least some cases. Child maltreatment is the result of increased family stress, leading to problems in the family's ability to cope, and the parents' attachment relationship to their children. The program philosophy or theory of change is eclectic, and includes efforts to promote improved attachment relationships (reparent the parent—a psychodynamic approach), model supportive relationships and encourage parents to generalize these behaviors to interactions with their children (drawing upon social learning theory and in support of the parent's sense of self-efficacy), and improve knowledge of child development, especially the realistic understanding of appropriate maturity demands (in an effort to change the parent's schema of the child, a cognitive/developmental approach). The program also seeks to support mothers as they improve their maternal life course, through encouraging continued education, training and employment, and prevention or wider spacing of subsequent pregnancies. Finally, the programs seek to reduce overall family stress by helping families to build on their own strengths, and to access community resources, both economic and interpersonal, through the use of case management services provided by the agency (an ecological approach). Some Healthy Families sites are active in promoting community change, often by providing officials with an assessment of the needs of families in areas such as domestic violence intervention, public transportation, and accessible health care.

IMPLEMENTING THE HEALTHY FAMILIES AMERICA APPROACH

In order to prevent child maltreatment, a system of care must either provide universal service delivery, or provide services to those families who are most at risk. Deciding who will be served is the first and most crucial program step. Universal screening and service delivery is favored by the NCPCA and others, but is often not tenable due to fiscal constraints. In addition, the incidence of child maltreatment in the general population may not warrant a universal approach.

Next, this chapter presents a summary of the HFA model, followed by details of the implementation of two Florida Healthy Families sites, in Orange County (Orlando) and Pinellas County (St. Petersburg and Clearwater). Both programs begin by targeting communities whose social ecology (demographics and status on key variables of risk) is associated with an increase in child maltreatment. Within each state, a few communities have a disproportionate share of cases of maltreatment, especially child neglect. Next, within these areas, they screen all new births for family-based psychosocial risk factors, previously associated with increased risk for child maltreatment. Third, programs provide families with social support, case management services, and parenting training, timing the onset of these interventions to a hypothesized "window" of opportunity for establishing a therapeutic relationship with a new mother, prenatally or at the birth of a child. Finally, these programs seek to strengthen communities as well as families through systems of interagency and community collaboration and coordination.

The Healthy Families America Model

The HFA model has been described elsewhere (see, for example, Daro & McCurdy, 1994), and will be briefly summarized here. The overall approach of HFA is to offer all new parents some supportive and referral services, and to offer intensive home visitation services to those most at risk of child abuse, neglect, and other poor health outcomes for children. Services must include certain critical elements. Technical assistance is available from the NCPCA in implementation of these standards, and includes on-site training of home visitors, supervisors, and other staff. A system of voluntary credentialing is in place, with external evaluators provided in cooperation with the Council on Accreditation of Services for Children and Families.

Critical Elements of the Healthy Families America Model

This section summarizes the critical elements of the Healthy Families America model (Table 12.1).

TABLE 12.1.
Critical Elements of the Healthy Families America Model

1. Services are initiated prenatally or at birth
2. Services are voluntary, and positive, persistent outreach efforts are used to engage families initially
3. If universal service delivery is not possible due to fiscal constraints, systematically identify those families most in need of services due to the presence of factors associated with increased risk of child maltreatment
4. Offer services intensively (at least once a week) and for the long term (i.e., 3 to 5 years)
5. Services should be culturally competent, and materials should reflect the diversity of the population to be served
6. Services should focus on supporting the parent as well as positive parent-child interactions and child development outcomes
7. Families should be linked to a medical home. Depending on the family's needs, they may also be linked to other community services
8. Services should be provided by staff with limited caseloads (recommended: no more than 15 of the most stressed families; no more than 25 overall)
9. Service providers should be selected because of their personal characteristics (nonjudgmental, compassionate, ability to establish rapport), their willingness to work with culturally diverse populations, and their skills to do the job
10. All service providers should receive basic training before beginning their contact with families
11. All service providers must receive intensive, didactic training specific to their role in understanding the critical elements of successful early identification and home visitation
12. Program staff should receive ongoing, frequent, effective supervision

Services are initiated prenatally or at birth

Programs identify families in the target population for services either prenatally or at the birth of the baby. Programs identify characteristics of the target population, and where the mothers can be found (hospitals, clinics, community centers, high schools, and so on). Organizational agreements with community entities, such as prenatal clinics and hospitals, must be comprehensive and efficient, as the goal is universal screening of all members of the target population. Once families are screened, they are further assessed for program eligibility; if eligible, they are offered voluntary services. Programs track the rate of program acceptance. For those who accept home visitor services, the first visit occurs either prenatally or within three months after the birth of the baby.

Programs use a standardized assessment tool to systematically identify families most in need of services

This assessment tool identifies the presence of various factors associated with increased risk for child maltreatment or other poor child outcomes (e.g., social isolation, substance abuse, and parental history of abuse in childhood). The screening tool is used uniformly with the target population to determine eligibility for services. Training in the assessment process is standardized, as is determining interrater reliability. Until recently, our programs used the Kempe Family Stress Checklist (FCS) (Orkow, 1985), an interview-based measure conducted prenatally, during, or soon after, the mother's hospital stay for the birth of the target infant. We now use a similar instrument, developed by Healthy Families Florida, specifically for our target populations. This phase of the program is called *family assessment.* Families scoring sufficiently high on the FSC are offered services, typically about 25 percent of families originally screened. Others are given appropriate referrals to services within the community. Risk assessment is an inexact science, under constant examination and revision.

Services are offered voluntarily, using positive, persistent outreach to build family trust

Participants sign a voluntary agreement for services. The programs have guidelines specifying a variety of positive outreach methods to build family trust, engage new families, and maintain family participation in the program (such as telephone calls, visits, mailings, and parenting groups). Outreach is continued for three months until the family is either reengaged or moved from the area. Families frequently take up to six months to fully engage in the program and establish a regular pattern of home visits.

Intensive services are offered at the beginning, with well-defined criteria for increasing or decreasing intensity of service over the long term

Participants receive the number of home visits commensurate with the level of family stress and coping they demonstrate. Services are typically weekly or more for the first six months after birth. Criteria for moving participants from one level to the next are clearly defined and linked to family progress and the intensity of services required. For those families who wish to continue participating, the program ensures that it offers home visiting services to participant families for three to five years (depending on the program).

Services are culturally competent

Staff understands and respects cultural differences among participants. Moreover, staff and materials used reflect the cultural, linguistic, geographic, racial and ethnic diversity of the population served. The programs maintain a description of the cultural, racial/ethnic, and linguistic characteristics of all groups in the service population. The program promotes culturally competent practice among program staff through agreements with appropriate community entities for client-centered services, in-service training and staff assignment, and annually evaluates (and reports to higher authorities) the extent to which services accommodate cultural differences and use cultural and family strengths/ resources, based on established criteria.

Services focus on both supporting parents and supporting parent-child interaction and child development

In Florida, delivery of services to families is guided by the Individual Family Support Plan (IFSP). The process of developing the IFSP uses family support practices in which the home visitor and the family collaborate to identify family strengths and competencies, family needs, problem areas, and the services necessary to address them. Of particular importance is the development of family goals, which are integrated into the IFSP. Review of the plan by the family, the home visitor and, when appropriate, the supervisor, occurs on a regular, scheduled basis (in most cases, at least semi-annually). The program promotes positive parenting skills, knowledge of child development, and parent-child attachment relationships, using established curricula. Developmental surveillance is completed at specified intervals through use of established, validated instruments, and staff training is provided in their use. When developmental delays are discovered, appropriate referrals are made and follow-up instituted.

All families accepting services are linked to community resources according to their needs, as documented in the individual family support plan

As a minimum, linkages include a medical provider to ensure optimal child development and to address health issues (such as timely immunizations and well-baby care). The linkages act as collaborations among families, home visitors and the service providers.

Home visitors have limited caseloads, ensuring that they have adequate time to spend with each family

In general, no full-time home visitor has more than 15 families on the most intense service level (requiring weekly visits) and no more than 25 families total. The program carefully manages its caseload size per home visitor to ensure that maximums are not exceeded.

Home visitors and program management staff are selected on the basis of a combination of personal characteristics, as well as experiential, training and educational qualifications

Screening and selection of home visitors includes consideration of such personal characteristics as acceptance of individual differences, ability to establish trusting relationships, and willingness to work with the culturally diverse populations present among the program's population. Typically, home visitors are paraprofessionals who meet educational and other requirements established by the program. All Family Support Workers (FSWs) in our Florida programs are high school graduates, and about half have some additional coursework in child development or human services related fields. Managers and field supervisors are professional social workers with experience in managing and administering human service programs that embrace the concepts of family-centered, strength-based service. A Master's degree in human services is the preferred educational level for field supervisors and managers. In those instances where volunteers and interns perform program functions, the same selection criteria apply.

Intensive training is provided to those who assess families and visit families in their homes

All service providers receive basic training in such areas as cultural competency, substance abuse, reporting child maltreatment, domestic violence, drug-exposed infants, program evaluation, and services available in the community. They also receive training specific to their roles on the essential components of family assessment and home visitation. For the most part, staff receive necessary initial training within six weeks of hire, and before assuming caseload or management responsibilities.

Training consists of one week of core subjects, prescribed by HFA and taught by HFA trainers, and four weeks of program-specific training conducted by local trainers. Four hours of monthly in-service training are also provided on a routine basis.

Direct service staff receive regular, ongoing, effective supervision

Weekly supervisory time is provided to all direct service staff. The ratio of supervisors to direct service staff is sufficient to permit effective supervision to occur (normally 1:5 or 1:6). In our programs, supervisory relationships are supportive, and often focus on the FSW's personal development as well as on their relationships with families.

The program is governed and administered according to principles of effective management and ethical practice

Our programs have a board, which oversees their work and provides feedback on program effectiveness. The content of the board and the method of supervision of the program varies from site to site; this is an important way for communities to take ownership of an HFA program and stay involved in its implementation.

Our Florida programs also have independent evaluators (the authors of this chapter), who have an ongoing relationship with the agencies, and provide feedback on a monthly basis. Staff at all levels, as well as community leaders, participate in the evaluation process. This participatory evaluation style has resulted in mid-course corrections and a high level of accountability for completion of program goals on the part of both agency staff and community leaders.

HEALTHY FAMILIES AMERICA IN CONTEXT: IMPLEMENTATION IN TWO COMMUNITIES

A Community-Based Approach

The two HFA sites described here are in urban central Florida. Table 12.2 describes the programs, their participants, and selected outcomes. In the high-risk neighborhoods served by our programs, if 100 percent of births are screened, about 25 percent will ultimately enroll in the program. In order to succeed, the HFA approach must be embedded in a supportive network of community connections. Cooperative arrangements with community groups for recruitment of family support workers and client families, with hospitals for early identification and assessment of families, with resources for ongoing training and referral, with funding sources for long term support, and with the academic community

TABLE 12.2.
Program Characteristics of Healthy Families in Florida

Program characteristic	Healthy Families Pinellas	Healthy Families Orange
Target area served	Twenty-eight census tracts in Pinellas County	One urban ZIP code in downtown Orlando
% of births whose medical records are screened annually	100%	100%
Limits on target population	No current CPS cases or drug involved families; periodic cap on Spanish-speaking families if workers not available.	No current CPS cases, drug involved families, medically fragile newborns, or children with disabilities. Periodic cap on Haitian families if workers not available.
# of families served	801 families	253 families
Mean age of mothers	22 years, 8 months	25 years
% less than 18 years of age at program entry	15% adolescents at entry	39% adolescents at entry
Marital status	92% unmarried, 8% married	93% unmarried, 7% married
Ethnicity		
African American	77%	85%
White, Hispanic	16%	1%
Haitian	7%	3%
Asian, Other	0%	11%
Selected results		
Immunization rates	97% immunized at 24 months	100% immunized at 24 months
Reports of abuse or neglect	<1.50% of children served by the program; county-wide rate is 5.5%	< 2.05% of children served by the program; county-wide rate is 2.60%, but our best comparison ZIP code rate is 5.88%.
Repeat pregnancies	no data	86% of program participants (90% of adolescents) did not have a repeat pregnancy within two years of program entry.

(continued)

TABLE 12.2.
Continued

Program characteristic	Healthy Families Pinellas	Healthy Families Orange
Community partnerships & primary funders	Juvenile Welfare Board of Pinellas County	Heart of Florida United Way/ Success By Six, Ounce of Prevention Fund of FL, Department of Children, Youth & Families Family Preservation and Support Services, Orange County Healthy Start Coalition, Arnold Palmer Hospital for Children & Women.
Administrative structure	Program manager reports to the Director, Community Health division, Pinellas County Health Department; governing body is a management team of collaborating agencies, funders, and program management.	Program manager reports to the Director of the Center for Children & Families at APH; governing body is a Steering Committee of funders and the project evaluator.

for evaluation of client progress and community impact, are essential for the HFA approach.

Both counties described here are models of a community-based, collaborative approach to the prevention of child maltreatment and the improvement of child health outcomes for high-risk communities and families. Although both programs adhere to the Critical Elements of the HFA model, their unique community contexts have led to an adaptation process, and two quite different programs have emerged. For example, Healthy Families Pinellas, the older of the two, has steady, county-level funding and a broad community base of support. The newer program, Healthy Families Orange, occasionally finds its community collaboration strained by the competition for scarce intervention resources.

Each of these programs measures similar outcomes for children and families: improvements in parent and child functioning, family stress, and family health. Each uses a quasi-experimental approach, in which outcomes for Healthy Families participants are compared with available comparative data on key variables, or a pre/post-test design is used to measure progress in parenting skills. However, each is also charged with evaluating the service integration effort itself. "Human services integration is a process by which two or more entities establish linkages for the purpose of improving outcomes for needy people" (Konrad, 1996, p. 6).

If this linkage is successful, then services should be less fragmented, duplicative, and more responsive and efficient.

Konrad (1996) defined a matrix of services integration dimensions and levels of integration of services. We describe each Healthy Families Florida project in terms of its place on this matrix. In the intensity of integration continuum, at the simplest level, services may share Information and Communication. Next, they may move to Cooperation and Coordination, followed by Collaboration, Consolidation, and finally true Integration of Services. Some aspects of a multiagency activity may be well integrated, while other components are struggling to share information. For example, several community agencies may have fully integrated goals shared among themselves, but have separate and competing lines of governance and authority or they may compete with one another for adolescent clients. We will describe each Healthy Families program, and place it on this continuum of integration.

Healthy Families Pinellas

History of the collaboration

Healthy Families Pinellas (HFP) is an HFA program in Pinellas County, an urban area on the West Coast of Florida. It is a cooperative effort among the Pinellas County Health Department, Family Service Centers, Inc., and the YWCA of Tampa Bay, as well as Bayfront Medical Center, Morton Plant Mease Health Care, and other hospitals and clinics for family assessment (Nelson & Gordon, 1996). All workers in the program are employees of one of the cooperating agencies. HFP is funded by the Juvenile Welfare Board (JWB) of Pinellas County, an independent taxing authority. HFP is available to families of newborns, as well as prenatally, in designated census tracts in north and south Pinellas County. Families are referred by the appropriate medical facility based on risk factors indicating potential for child maltreatment, using the Healthy Families Florida assessment instrument. In comparison with other areas in the county, the service area has a maternal population that is younger, more likely to be unmarried, less educated, and has a higher percentage of teenage mothers and minorities. Service areas also have a high incidence of domestic violence and substance abuse.

Although prior to the Healthy Families Pinellas project, Family Service Centers, Inc. and the YWCA had worked with the Health Department, they did not have the degree of collaboration necessary for HFP. The funding agency, the Juvenile Welfare Board (JWB) of Pinellas County, made it a requirement in the request for proposal that this project be a true collaboration. JWB staff believed strongly that no single agency could successfully undertake this program on its own.

The impetus for HFP came from the JWB. Statistics had shown a high rate of child maltreatment in the county. A rise in the *ad valorem* taxes provided JWB with resources, which could be directed toward new initiatives; JWB staff had become aware of and had carefully evaluated the Hawaii Healthy Start Program. Because of results from Hawaii, the program was implemented in south Pinellas County on a trial basis, with later expansion to other high-risk areas in the county.

Project description

HFP began in October 1992, as a cooperative among the Pinellas County Health Department, Family Service Centers, Inc., and the YWCA of Tampa Bay, funded by the Juvenile Welfare Board (JWB). The Robert Wood Johnson Foundation provided some additional funding. HFP began with one team in St. Petersburg, covering seven designated census tracts. Additional teams have been added over time, with a concurrent increase in the number of census tracts. There are now 10 teams operating throughout Pinellas County.

The governing body of HFP is the Management Team, which consists of selected staff representatives from the Juvenile Welfare Board and the collaborating agencies, the program manager, three assistants, representatives from the participating hospitals, and a representative of the program field supervisors. Major program policy issues are considered, discussed and approved by the Management Team.

Dimensions of service integration

In terms of Konrad's (1996) intensity of integration continuum, HFP has consolidated separate agency activities into a cohesive, integrated program on nearly all dimensions. For example, members of the collaboration (Pinellas County Health Department, Family Service Centers, Inc., and the YWCA of Tampa Bay) are full partners in the operation of the program. There is complete agreement on the target population, program goals and policies, the operation and authority of the management team, implementation of the HFA model, accountability, and desired program outcomes. Budgeting is a function performed by the Juvenile Welfare Board, with other members of the collaboration providing resources in kind. Integration is achieved by a combination of formal agreements and less formal cooperation, coordination, and communication. In almost all instances, HFP family support workers are the primary case managers for client families, even if these families are receiving services from other agencies. Moreover, regardless of whether family support workers are employed by the Pinellas County Health Department, YWCA, or Family Service Centers, Inc., the program is the same. The Management Team, in its role as the policymaking body for

HFP, tries to maintain the salary structure and benefits for family support workers equitably across agencies, so that there will be no substantial differences based on the agency of assignment. Our research has shown that the family support workers clearly identify with Healthy Families Pinellas rather than their parent agencies. Moreover, the collaborative acting in concert makes hiring decisions, again regardless of the agency that will carry the new employee on its books. All project personnel use the same data system; all reports to JWB are generated by HFP without reference to the collaborating agencies. Thus, HFP has consolidated many of each individual agency's administrative functions.

An independent evaluation of the program is provided under a contract between the University of South Florida and the Juvenile Welfare Board of Pinellas County. Evaluators attend all management team meetings, as well as selected team meetings, and have provided training in goal setting, a key part of the program. The evaluators are *ex officio* members of the management team, consistent with maintaining objectivity for the independent evaluation. Program objectives (both goals and activities) include:

1. Low rates of maltreatment in families;
2. Families appropriately referred by the medical facilities agree to accept services;
3. Families will be referred to community based resources, will follow through on referrals, and will increase their knowledge of community resources;
4. Families will care for their medical needs, including immunizations;
5. Where a need for improvement is initially indicated, parent-child attachment will be enhanced;
6. Child development will be assessed at specified intervals;
7. Actively enrolled families will be referred for family planning;
8. Subsequent pregnancies will receive pre-natal care in first trimester; and
9. Parents will participate in support groups and/or other parent education activities.

Other people in family households benefit from services provided by HFP. A recent review indicates there were an average of 4.4 other people living in each household, including siblings, parents, relatives, and others. Thus over 2,000 people are directly or indirectly benefiting from and otherwise being influenced by the program.

Individual family support plans

One of the major cornerstones of Healthy Families Pinellas is the development and implementation of sound individual family support plans (IFSP). Considerable effort has been put towards these plans. An effective family support plan should be a living document that represents the goals of family members and has utility in tracking family empowerment over time (Dunst, Trivette, & Deal, 1994). The distinction between long-term goals and the steps needed to achieve them is an important one. This is an area in which the family support worker is vital. The family support plan is a joint effort between the family support worker and the family; as goals are achieved, additional goals are set. The principle at work with family support plans is to encourage the family to focus on their individual and collective goal accomplishment rather than become frustrated as goals seemingly become more distant and difficult to achieve (Cassidy, 1996; Locke & Latham, 1990; Paulson, 1977). On balance, family support workers, as well as families, have accepted goal setting as a worthwhile endeavor, as shown in the following example.

> **Mary Beth** is a 28-year-old, single African American mother with three children. Prior to enrolling in Healthy Families Pinellas, she had a confirmed report of child abuse, with two children removed from the home and placed in state custody. Healthy Families became involved with the birth of her third child in March 1993. Mary Beth was ready to set new goals for herself, and very much wanted to keep this new baby. Her family support worker referred Mary Beth for counseling and to parenting classes, modeled appropriate parenting skills during home visits, encouraged Mary Beth through difficult times, referred her for training at a local vocational school, helped her get her children back, and helped her reach her goals. Mary Beth now has custody of her children, has completed vocational training as a legal and medical secretary, has a full-time job, has purchased a home, and is a successful graduate of Healthy Families Pinellas.

As Table 12.2 indicates, the programs emphasize strong rates of immunizations. In addition, attachment between mother (and father when present) and infant is an issue of considerable importance to family support workers and field supervisors. At least 90 percent of those who initially showed attachment problems have demonstrated improvement.

Attrition

The drop out rate is about 20 percent annually. On average, about 75 percent of the families leaving the program are no longer eligible because they have moved from the designated census tracts. Almost without exception, these families are moving to better housing in more secure areas, which is a positive reflection on the program.

Child maltreatment

Since program inception, confirmed reports of verified maltreatment by program participants represent fewer than 1.50 percent of target children enrolled in the program and their siblings. This is a significantly better record than that of Pinellas County as a whole, where the verified abuse rate is approximately 5.60 percent for children under the age of seventeen. This is an excellent record, notwithstanding the absence of experimental, causal data that would show conclusively that these results are due solely to HFP interventions. The facts are that these mothers live in extremely high-risk communities, that some of the mothers were themselves past victims of abuse and some had been perpetrators prior to enrolling in the program. At present, they are not now maltreating their children. It is reasonable to conclude that HFP is at least partially responsible.

Summary

Healthy Families Pinellas is made up of a consortium of three different agencies. Family support workers are employees of the various agencies, although they operate under the direction of the program manager. The administrative procedures frequently differ among the agencies, but concerted efforts on the part of all members of the program have minimized problems. Of particular note is the loyalty demonstrated by family support workers to Healthy Families, as opposed to their parent agencies. By all measures, they identify with the program, and deal with their home agencies only when necessary on administrative matters. This unique feature of Healthy Families Pinellas makes a strong program even stronger.

All process and outcome measures examined to date show very positive indications that the Healthy Families Pinellas Program is succeeding in its stated objectives and is reflective of all that is best in home visiting programs (Powell, 1993). Families are coalescing, infants are thriving, inappropriate parenting behaviors have generally been reduced, and JWB approved objectives are substantially being met.

Healthy Families Orange

The Healthy Families Orange (HFO) early intervention project, which began in 1995, is implemented by screening the medical records of every mother who has a baby while living in zip code 32805. This area, known as the Parramore/Washington Shores neighborhood, has demographics that indicate a high percentage of poor birth outcomes, births to adolescents, and reports of child maltreatment to the state registry (see Table 12.2). It is located near the heart of Orlando, an urban area in central Florida. Housing in the area consists predominantly of single family housing and duplexes, with a few large, rent-subsidized, three-story apartment complexes. HFO is housed at the Orange Center Elementary School Service Center, on the school campus, and shares space with WIC, immunization clinics, Head Start, and other community-based programs. As such, it is identified in the community as a part of the school, rather than as a part of the child protective services agencies.

The goals of HFO are to prevent child maltreatment and improve child and family health outcomes in zip code 32805 through a program of selective, systematic, intensive home visiting and case management services that are part of a comprehensive, coordinated, community-wide effort. Program objectives (both goals and activities) include:

1. Reduction in levels of family stress;
2. Improvements in parent-child interactions;
3. Reduced child maltreatment reports to the state registry;
4. Conformity with standards for EPSDT Checkups and Immunizations;
5. Reduction in repeat births and births to teens;
6. Improved access to prenatal care; and
7. Improved collaboration and effectiveness of referrals between agencies.

Early identification procedures are completed in five local community-based hospitals by two family assessment workers, who review medical records and interview mothers and fathers. Teams of paraprofessional home visitors, themselves from the neighborhood to be served, visit no more than 15 of the most stressed families (or no more than 25 families total) per week. The paraprofessionals are supervised closely by a master's level clinician (usually a social worker) who meets with each worker individually each week. The team includes a child development specialist, who trains workers in administering the Denver II Developmental Screening Test and supervises assessments using the NCAST measures.

An independent evaluation team from Rollins College, funded by the Heart of Florida United Way, conducts a quarterly review of data on all goals and objectives, and provides feedback to funders and the agency through annual reports and presentations (Carnahan, 1998a, 1998b). The senior evaluator has at least weekly contact with the agency, and serves as a member of the multiagency steering committee that governs HFO efforts.

Child maltreatment

In the first three years of operation, HFO reports a child maltreatment rate of 2.04 percent. This is less than the 5.88 percent reported for the 32805 zip code, and lower than the 2.60 percent reported for Orange County as a whole. This is a good record. HFO families are themselves at higher risk for child maltreatment than the population as a whole, even within zip code 32805. Although the NIS-3 notes the probability of reduced surveillance of children less than five (Sedlak & Broadhurst, 1996), this is certainly not true for families enrolled in intensive home visiting programs. HFO families are subject to intense scrutiny, and have an FSW, supervisor, and Child Development Specialist present in their home on a regular basis; they are more likely than their neighbors to be reported for abuse or neglect, should it occur. In fact, the one removal of a child from the home this year was initiated by HFO. Further, we note that 37 percent of the mothers were in the state mandated reporting system prior to the birth of their target (program entry) child. They were victims either of abuse while a child, a family member where abuse was alleged, or as a perpetrator or alleged perpetrator in the distant past.

Family activities

As Table 12.2 indicates, HFO has been successful in immunizing 100 percent of participating 2-year-olds, and 86 percent of mothers (90 percent of adolescents) have not had repeat pregnancies. In addition, 89 percent of mothers who did have a second pregnancy, and disclosed it to their FSW, received prenatal care in the first trimester. In cases where repeat administrations of parent-child interaction measures are available, 74 percent of mothers improved their NCAST scores, indicating an improvement in infant feeding or teaching skills, and an improvement in mother-infant interaction. These gains are made despite the difficulty in initial engagement of these high-risk families in therapeutic relationships. Following is a case story that describes the year long process of engagement between one mother and HFO; it is not unlike a dysfunctional but ultimately successful "dance" of attachment.

Case Story: The Dance of Engagement

Patricia, 24 years old, entered the HFO program at the birth of her fourth child, Tyran, January 22, 1996. Patricia scored a 60 on the Kempe Family Stress Index with highest scores in the areas of substance abuse, multiple stresses, potential for violence, harsh punishment, and child unwanted/at risk for bonding/attachment. Her response to the birth of her son was, "No man's going to want me now." Patricia was known to local Child Protective Services personnel from previous child abuse/neglect reports. She had already failed to respond to the services of Family Builders and Homemakers, as well as protective counseling/supervision.

Engagement was a difficult process. Patricia refused to sign an IFSP, fearing its possible use in any future interaction with child protective services. She had no knowledge of child development or the importance of parent-child interaction, and she was resistant to any avenues of discipline other than yelling and spanking. Her finances were in jeopardy due to her lack of budgeting and planning. Immunizations for all children were spotty or non-existent. She refused to take her children out of the apartment area because they were so "bad." She refused services and ordered her FSW out of her home approximately every other week. Nevertheless, her FSW kept returning. The supervisor made home visits with the FSW, counseling her not to take this "rejection" of the program personally, but as a symptom of the mother's feelings of rejection by others. The worker focused on establishing pleasant, noncoercive visits, playing with the children and modeling parent-child interactions for this mother. Gradually, a relationship was established, building on this mother's will to keep her children and her powerful opinions.

By August 1996, the FSW had established a supportive, working relationship with this mother. Patricia was no longer under supervision by Child and Family Services. Her C&F worker had witnessed Patricia's active resistance to other programs, her negative interaction with her children, and her precarious economic situations. He could not believe this was the same mother. "I don't know what we're paying you for your program," he said, "but whatever it is, you're worth it!" The C&F worker had witnessed Patricia's substantial improvement with parent-child interaction, her expanded knowledge of child development, her use of positive reinforcement versus physical punishment, and her use of budgeting to use her financial resources wisely.

When Patricia's oldest child, Jayna, entered kindergarten that fall without benefit of prior experience with day care or Head Start, she had substantial problems with attention span and behavior. The principal sent Jayna home in the back of a police car when she could not control the child. HFO staff accompanied Patricia to subsequent conferences with the principal to advocate for Jayna. HFO's offices are physically on the grounds of the public elementary school, facilitating interagency work in this setting.

With great strength, Patricia calmly and competently, despite her underlying anger, explained the positive reinforcement program she used in the home, Jayna's need for recognition as a leader and a caregiver as her preferred role in the home, and the need for the school to use the methods Patricia found successful in molding Jayna's behavior. A behavior program was developed with positive reinforcement measures to be given in both the home and the school, counseling services were implemented, and Patricia volunteered her services to the school. By January 1997, Jayna was doing well in school in all domains.

By March 1997, Patricia had obtained her first job in her life, takes great pride in her children, takes her children for outings on the bus, and believes in herself and her children. She is still resistant to the IFSP process, once again "firing" her FSW when her worker pressed her to complete an updated IFSP that was two months late. But, once again, her FSW refuses to be "fired," knowing that Patricia has ultimate confidence in her worker and is simply flexing her newly found empowerment. This mother now keeps in constant touch with HFO, using a pay phone to call about changes in her life.

HFO recently became accredited by Healthy Families America and the Council on Accreditation as an HFA site. External evaluation indicates that its implementation of the model is sound, with hospital screening, home visiting, supervision, child and family assessment, interagency coordination and referrals implemented as designed. Outcome measures indicate improvements in parent child interactions relative to a parent's own earlier performance, and in immunizations, child maltreatment rates, and repeat pregnancies relative to county or zip code data from the same area.

HFO in its community: history and implementation

The HFO program began three years before the first staff was hired, a product of sustained community-wide planning and cooperation. A group of agency staff and academics became interested in implementing the HFA model. Considerable time was spent in reviewing the demographics of three high risk zip codes, as well as identifying the level of services available in each community. The area with the worst demographics and the least available services was chosen for intervention.

The group wrote and submitted a Community Integrated Services Systems (CISS) grant proposal in 1994. The key innovation of the proposal was a unique system of shared accountability for the intervention program. Each member agency would contribute an employee, space, or materials directly to the shared project. After the proposal failed, representatives of the hospital and the Healthy Start Coalition convened a meeting of interested parties to discuss the future of the plan.

At the same time, the Heart of Florida United Way and local businesses were initiating the Success by Six Campaign, a national United Way project that organizes work in local communities to assure that all children reach six years old ready to be successful in school. Success by Six includes service projects and a media campaign to raise awareness of children's issues. Representatives of the community group held several meetings with the Success by Six Steering Committee, which agreed to take on the HFO Project as its first venture in central Florida.

The community group members joined Success by Six as *ex officio* members of several implementation committees, which met for the following year. Letters of agreement were written to detail the contributions and responsibilities of each member agency. These letters were important cornerstones of the developing collaboration. To maintain the collaborative nature of the project, several features were included.

1. Program funding came from multiple sources (see Table 12.2).
2. Initial staff were hired by a multiagency committee.
3. Program oversight and supervision were provided by a multiagency steering committee.
4. Program staff were "members" of several different agencies.
5. The program was housed in the Community Services Center of Orange Center Elementary School, in the heart of the neighborhood to be served.

A multiagency Evaluation Committee chose program goals and objectives, and United Way agreed to fund an independent evaluation component. Initial funding was available for one high-risk zip code, rather than countywide implementation.

Collaborative progress

During the first year, each of the funding agencies, in addition to HFA and the NCPCA, asked HFO for data on a quarterly basis. Some agencies also conducted site visits on a quarterly or annual basis. Some agencies who participated by funding a "position" wanted HFO records to meet the standards of their own host agency's accrediting boards. Some funders ended the year in December, while others ended in July. At the end of Year I, the evaluators noted that HFO had experienced audit visits from six different entities, and recommended that the entities meet to discuss areas of common concern and calendar.

The Department of Children and Family Services/Family Preservation & Support Services took the lead in this effort, establishing a *Monitoring Committee* composed of members of each funding source, plus the evaluator of HFO. As a result of six months of effort, the agencies established a *joint monitoring tool* for review of records, and all but one agreed to a joint site visit every six months. All agreed to accept the quarterly reports of the external evaluator on outcome related data. This innovative, collaborative approach has resulted in a significant saving of time to HFO staff, and an increase in cooperation between agencies.

Community-based services must be embedded—not just located—in the community. The placement of HFO in the public school proved to be very important. Perceived of as a part of educating the family, not as a "social service" or child abuse program, HFO has avoided much of the resistance to such programs often exhibited by local residents. Cooperative ventures, such as "Play Shops" parenting groups, expedited Head Start referrals, and immunization clinics for HFO families have evolved naturally from the agency's placement within the family services center. Staff of HFO frequently eats lunch in the school cafeteria, mingling with students and teachers. The school has designated one employee as an official ambassador to the program, and she participates in many programs. The Project hopes to involve community leaders (such as ministers and PTA officials) in further planning for HFO.

Dimensions of service integration

In Konrad's (1996) terms, HFO's most integrated services are at the administrative level of operation. HFO shares fully integrated goals for improvement in the lives and health of children and families with all of its partners. These written goals are part of letters of agreement and cooperation with each partner agency. At the level of funding, HFO is consolidated as well; partner agencies contribute funds or in-kind contributions to a central pool, do not require a separate accounting for the funds, and see the services of HFO as meeting their own goals. For example, the Orange County Healthy Start Coalition contributes its enhanced services dollars to HFO, which does home visits with many Healthy Start clients in the zip code.

Other services remain more fragmented; formal collaborations with partner agencies result in agreements for specific services, but these must be ironed out one problem at a time. For example, HFO is currently at work on a transition plan for children as they reach age 3 (Head Start and public school ESE program age). Despite close relationships with the local elementary school, this transition plan must be worked out with ESE and childcare officials locally.

Lessons Learned in Implementation

Healthy Families America in Florida (Pinellas and Orlando) has gone to scale very rapidly, from a dream to two fully accredited programs serving nearly 900 clients in less than five years. Although the programs are different, they share common successes. Among the more important factors we believe necessary to success are adherence to a national model, leadership, administrative structure, choice of the target population, and the nature of the collaboration.

A national model

The Healthy Families America model is empirically and theoretically sound. Adherence to the 12 core principles of the model, the process of accreditation, and the presence of external evaluation has made our programs accountable to outside forces. For example, in the face of fiscal pressures, it is difficult to maintain the low worker to family and supervisor to worker ratios we believe are essential to success. The national model has made it easier to convince funders of the importance of such standards.

Leadership

Strong leaders with vision began both programs. Continued advocacy for program support and expansion is important. In addition, it is critical to have the leadership of the collaborating agencies engaged. Perhaps the most difficult part of the process is for the leadership to relinquish control to a trusted representative who works with the collaboration, and to empower that person to make decisions in the name of the agency. Likewise, a strong program manager who is seen as "in charge" by all associated with the program allows the program a measure of autonomy. A management team, such as that of Healthy Families Pinellas, is also a useful tool for generating ideas, discussing program issues, and providing support to the program.

Administrative structure

Administration should be consolidated and simplified—not an easy task in a collaborative venture—so as to avoid interfering with the operation of the program. Every attempt should be made to retain administrative functions at the collaborating agencies to permit the program leadership to concentrate efforts on delivering services to client families. Issues of "turf" should be worked out in advance, and aggressively reworked as needed, again to avoid distractions to program operation.

Choosing the target population

In cooperation with families, programs must decide who they can help—and who is best served by other agencies. Target populations are selected from areas where the demographic characteristics suggest a high probability for child maltreatment, but mothers who are perpetrators in an open CPS case at the time of their child's birth are generally not invited to participate. Healthy Families is a strength-based program. The model is designed to build on the strengths families bring to the program; it is generally *not* designed for rehabilitation. Healthy Families Orange and Pinellas also do not normally accept families with current Child Protective Services involvement nor who are drug-involved; there are other programs better suited for families with these particular challenges.

HFO also refers families of infants with disabilities, newborns less than 1500 grams, or mothers with a diagnosed psychiatric illness, to other programs. This decision is problematic, as a lifetime history of alcoholic, affective, or anxiety disorders has been associated with increased risk for maltreatment (Egami et al., 1996). HFO has judged that the paraprofessional home visitor is not equipped to intervene in these cases, and is actively seeking funds to add a mental health component to service delivery.

The nature of the collaboration

Interagency collaborative agreements, painstakingly written and reviewed annually, are important; they help to define the nature of the collaboration. However, they are supplemented by the informal agreements and supports worked out between program level staff on a daily basis. The informal collaborations take place after the community trusts workers in a program to do a good job and keep their word. Both administrative and program level collaboration are essential for success.

Gordon (1998) suggests that these issues are important to collaborations: How does the collaboration develop its missions, goals, and objectives? Are they internally or externally directed? What does each member of the collaboration bring to the table? How permeable are the boundaries between agencies? How willing are the members of the collaboration to subordinate the interests of their agencies to the interests of the collaboration? Where applicable, how does the collaboration deal with power imbalances among agencies? How trusting are the members of the collaboration? The way the members deal with these and other questions define the nature of the collaboration. In our experience, trust and good will among the members is the most important determinant of successful collaboration.

HEALTHY FAMILIES FLORIDA: STEPS TOWARD A STATEWIDE PROGRAM

The 1998 Florida Legislature enacted legislation and appropriated $10 million to the Department of Children and Families to implement the Healthy Families Florida program. Funds are insufficient for a statewide program, but a significant expansion will be supported. The legislation requires the Department to contract with a private, nonprofit corporation to develop, implement, and administer the program. The Ounce of Prevention Fund of Florida is the organization selected to work with communities to implement Healthy Families Florida (HFF). Both existing and new sites have received HFF funding. HFF encouraged applications from collaborative partners and limited applications to one per county.

The HFF expansion legislation passed with bipartisan support. The campaign to implement HFF has involved Florida Sources, the state affiliate of the National Conference to Prevent Child Abuse, and local Healthy Families programs who have worked closely with both the legislative and executive branches of the government. In addition, the Secretaries of Health and of Children and Families each provided both personal and staff support for HFF. The bill came under opposition in the House by the Christian Coalition; a ramification of this opposition was the elimination of the Kempe Family Stress Checklist as the assessment tool on the basis that it was perceived as too intrusive.

HFF is a program whose time has come. The former governor was a prime mover in bringing great visibility to Healthy Start, also a home visiting program, designed to reduce the incidence of low birthweight and infant mortality; child maltreatment was receiving extensive media coverage throughout the state; Healthy Families is voluntary on the part of participants, essentially eliminating any appearance of coercion; the program has been successfully implemented in several areas of the state with positive results; and a strong economy makes funding less of a problem than in leaner times. Taken together, these facts suggest that there may never again be a more propitious time than now to implement a wide-ranging, proven program to reduce child maltreatment.

CONCLUSIONS, CHALLENGES, AND RECOMMENDATIONS

There is substantial opportunity for further research into the efficacy of intensive home visiting programs provided by the HFA model, some of which is being undertaken by the HFA Research Network, a loosely organized consortium of program evaluators from throughout the United States. We could be on the threshold of a major breakthrough in abuse prevention programs, but we need to verify that this model is as effective as it appears to date. Additional research issues include the need for selected randomized trials of the model; improvements in risk assessment at all levels of income; description of the subpopulations for whom the model is most successful; issues in the engagement and retention of high risk populations in intervention programs; and reduction of community level risks for child maltreatment by political or economic means.

Schorr (1988) identified the following characteristics of successful programs, which we believe hold true for the Healthy Families Florida model. Successful programs are *comprehensive*, providing a broad spectrum of services through interagency collaboration. Each Florida program is embedded in a functioning network of interagency collaboration and coordination. Next, HFA programs *focus on relationships,* both among staff (through intensive supervision) and with families, maintaining low ratios throughout. Through the use of the IFSP and the adjustment of service delivery intensity according to the level of stress and empowerment in the home, services are individualized for clients and families. Services are *intensive*—averaging once a week in the beginning. Primary prevention of maltreatment is the program's aim. *Funding is stable* (in the Pinellas County program) and broad based (in the Orange County program). Finally, there is an *evaluation component* built into each program, providing accountability and feedback.

As Florida supports a statewide expansion of this community based approach to child maltreatment, we offer these lessons learned in implementation, and wish for an improvement in the lives of Florida's children and families at risk for child maltreatment.

REFERENCES

Besharov, D., & Dembosky, J. (1997). The politics of child abuse in America: A review. *The American Political Science Review, 91,* 184.

Blount, K. (1992). Chronic psychological manifestations. In S. Ludwig & A. E. Kornberg (Eds.), *Child abuse: A medical reference.* New York: Churchill Livingstone.

Carnahan, S. (1998a, August). *A community-based approach to preventing child maltreatment.* Paper presented at the annual meeting of the American Psychological Association, San Francisco.

Carnahan, S. (1998b). *Third annual report of the Healthy Families Orange Evaluation Project.* Orlando, FL: Heart of Florida United Way.

Cassidy, K. D. (1996, April). *The application of goal setting theory to a framework for home visiting.* Unpublished honors thesis, University of South Florida, Tampa.

Center on Child Prevention Research. (1996). *Intensive home visitation: A randomized trial, follow-up and risk assessment study of Hawaii's healthy start program* (NCCAN Grant No. 90-CA-1511). Chicago: National Committee to Prevent Child Abuse.

Cicchetti, D., Barnett, D., Rabideau, G. J., & Toth, S. (1991). Toward the development of a transactional model of risk taking and self regulation: Illustration through the study of maltreated children. In L. P. Lipsett & L. L. Mitnick (Eds.), *Self regulatory behavior and risk taking: Causes and consequences.* Norwood, NJ: Ablex.

Daro, D. (1993). Child maltreatment research: Implications for program design. In D. Cicchetti & S. Toth (Eds.), *Child abuse, child development, and social policy.* Norwood, NJ: Ablex.

Daro, D., & McCurdy, K. (1994). Preventing child abuse and neglect: Programmatic interventions. *Child Welfare, 73*, 405-430.

Dunst, C. J., Trivette, C. M., & Deal, A. G. (1994). *Supporting and strengthening families, volume I: Methods, strategies and practices.* Cambridge, MA: Brookline.

Egami, Y., Ford, D., Greenfield, S., & Crum, R. (1996). Psychiatric profile and sociodemographic characteristics of adults who report physically abusing or neglecting children. *The American Journal of Psychiatry, 153*, 921-928.

Gordon, T. R. (1998). *Anatomy of collaborations: Theory and practice.* Unpublished manuscript.

Guterman, N. B. (1977). Early prevention of physical child abuse and neglect: Existing evidence and future directions. *Child Maltreatment, 2*(1), 12-27.

Juvenile Welfare Board of Pinellas County. (1994). *Goals report for fiscal year 1992-1993.* St. Petersburg, FL: Author.

Katz, K. B. (1992). Communication problems in maltreated children: A tutorial. *Journal of Childhood Communication Disorders, 14*, 147-163.

Knutson, J. F. (1995). Psychological characteristics of maltreated children: Putative risk factors and consequences. *Annual Review of Psychology, 46*, 401-420.

Konrad, E. J. (1996). A multidimensional framework for conceptualizing human services integration initiatives. *New Directions for Evaluation, 69*, 5-19.

Korbin, J. E., & Coulton, C. (1996). Understanding the neighborhood context for children and families: Combining epidemiological and ethnographic approaches. In J. Brooks-Gunn, G. J. Duncan, & J. L. Aber (Eds.), *Neighborhood poverty: Context and consequences for young children*. New York: Sage.

Locke, E. A., & Latham, G. P. (1990). *A theory of goal setting and task performance.* Englewood Cliffs, NJ: Prentice-Hall.

Mitchel, L., & Cohn Donnelly, A. (1993). Healthy Families America: Building a national system. *AMAC Advisor, 6*, 9-10.

National Committee to Prevent Child Abuse. (1997). *Healthy Families America Credentialing Self-Assessment Tool.* Chicago: NCPCA.

Nelson, C. E., & Gordon, T. R. (1996, April). *Healthy Families Pinellas: A program to reduce child abuse and neglect.* Paper presented at the meeting of the International Society for Prevention of Child Abuse and Neglect, Dublin, Ireland.

Ney, P. G., Fung, T., & Wickett, A. R. (1994). The worst combinations of child abuse and neglect. *Child Abuse and Neglect, 18*, 705-714.

Orkow, B. (1985). Implementation of a family stress checklist. *Child Abuse and Neglect, 9*, 405-410.

Paulson, R. I. (1977). *A behavioral view of goal displacement in a social welfare agency.* Unpublished doctoral dissertation, University of California, Berkeley.

Powell, D. R. (1993). Inside home visiting programs. *The Future of Children, 3*, 23-38.

Rauh, V., & Brown, E. (1996). *Community level factors: A discussion document for the HFA Research Network*. Unpublished manuscript.

Sameroff, A. J., & Fiese, B. H. (1990). Transactional regulation and early intervention. In S. Meisels & J. P. Shonkoff (Eds)., *Handbook of early childhood intervention* (pp. 119-149). Cambridge, England: Cambridge University Press.

Schorr, L. B. (1988). *Within our reach: Breaking the cycle of disadvantage*. New York: Anchor.

Sedlak, A. J., & Broadhurst, D. D. (1996). *The Third National Incidence Study of Child Abuse and Neglect*. Washington: U.S. Department of Health and Human Services.s

Winnicott, D. W. (1996). *Thinking about children* (R. Shepherd, J. Johns, & H. T. Robinson, Eds.). Reading, MA: Addison-Wesley.

Author Index

Subject Index

www.ingramcontent.com/pod-product-compliance
Ingram Content Group UK Ltd.
Pitfield, Milton Keynes, MK11 3LW, UK
UKHW020233290926
15470UKWH00002B/514

9 781567 504408